NEW LIVES FOR OLD
HOW TO CURE THE INCURABLE

NEW LIVES FOR OLD
HOW TO CURE THE INCURABLE

By J. ELLIS BARKER

Editor of " Heal Thyself (*The Homœopathic World*) "
Author of " Good Health and Happiness," " Cancer: How it is
Caused, How it can be Prevented," " Miracles of Healing and
how they are Done," " My Testament of Healing," etc., etc.

With an Introduction
by Sir HERBERT BARKER

SECOND EDITION

B. JAIN PUBLISHERS (P) LTD.
An ISO 9001 : 2000 Certified Company
USA — EUROPE — INDIA

NEW LIVES FOR OLD

Reprint Edition: 1999, 2003, 2007

Published by Kuldeep Jain for
B. Jain Publishers (P) Ltd.
1921, Street No. 10, Chuna Mandi,
Paharganj, New Delhi 110 055 (INDIA)
Phones: 2358 0800, 2358 1100, 2358 1300, 2358 3100, 5169 8991
Fax: 011-2358 0471, 5169 8993; *Email:* bjain@vsnl.com
Website: **www.bjainbooks.com**

Printed in India by
J.J. Offset Printers
522, FIE, Patpar Ganj, Delhi - 110 092
Phones: 22169633, 22156128

BOOK CODE / ISBN: 978-81-319-0225-7

DEDICATED TO

THE MEMORY OF

TWO GREAT PHYSICIANS:

MY FATHER,

AND

DR. JOHN H. CLARKE,
MY FRIEND AND TEACHER

CONTENTS

CONTENTS

INTRODUCTION

I HAVE much pleasure in introducing Mr. Ellis Barker's work *New Lives For Old—How To Cure The Incurable.* I owe much to homœopathic treatment at Mr. Barker's hands and at the hands of others. Besides, and chiefly, I firmly believe that the methods of treatment discovered by that great medical genius Hahnemann are destined before long to be universally recognized and practised by the medical profession, to the great advantage of suffering humanity.

Of late years orthodox medicine has drifted farther and farther away from Nature. The medical profession seems to be ruled by the surgeon and the laboratory man to a far too great extent. Operations have increased incredibly and, according to some surgeons, many of these are unnecessary and therefore merely mutilations.

I believe that the art of healing has lost its way and that the future belongs to less risky and more natural measures. The curative powers of a wisely chosen natural diet, of air, sunlight, exercise, baths, massage and manipulative surgery are great, especially if, where necessary, these natural methods of treatment are reinforced by wisely chosen homœopathic medicines which can do much good, as I can testify from long personal experience, and which cannot possibly do harm. To these forces, I think, belongs the future of healing.

The evidence which Mr. Ellis Barker adduces in order to show that very few diseases are incurable, that even the apparently most intractable maladies can be treated and cured, is so overwhelming that one is irresistibly imbued with the enthusiasm and conviction which carry the author through chapter after chapter of his amazing work, and I can only say, as Sir Arbuthnot Lane said of his former book on cancer, that the present volume is "a very remarkable production indeed."

Just such a work as Mr. Ellis Barker has written was never more clamantly called for and more urgently needed than at the present time, when cancer, heart disease and many other maladies are destroying ever-increasing numbers. The oft-times unsatisfactory methods employed by medicine and surgery should be replaced by saner, safer and far more efficacious therapeutic measures. Mr. Ellis Barker has such truly encyclopædic knowledge of his subject, such a catholicity of understanding and so high a degree of analytical and selective acumen as to render him superlatively fitted to write the book I have the honour to present to the world.

Humanity already owes the author a very heavy debt of gratitude for other literary efforts. His latest work will only increase the public's obligation to this most able and most worthy disciple of the famous founder of homœopathy.

HERBERT BARKER.

THE GROVE,
  ST. LAWRENCE,
    JERSEY,
      CHANNEL ISLANDS.

FOREWORD

MEDICINE is an art. Physicians and other artists are born, not made. The greatest healers of all times from Hippocrates and Celsus to Hahnemann, Mesmer, Priessnitz, Kneipp, Kellgren, Coué and Sir Herbert Barker were self-taught, and many of them were laymen, keenly interested in the art of healing. In all the arts and sciences outsiders have been pioneers. The schools produce chiefly mediocrities, Cromwell, England's greatest soldier, was a farmer, and Ulysses Grant, America's greatest soldier, was a shopman. Leeuwenhoek, who discovered the micro-organisms of disease, was a draper; and Pasteur, who created modern medicine, was a chemist. England's greatest medical men, Harvey, Sydenham and John Hunter, were treated as quacks by their orthodox contemporaries.

This book may enable thousands of thinking men and women to improve their health and that of their families, and to cure disorders and diseases declared incurable by the medical profession. Its teaching will increase very greatly the power to heal of those doctors and surgeons who are willing to learn much that is new to them—and to unlearn still more. Laymen and doctors who desire to study the new art and science of healing should read the companion volume to this book, *Miracles of Healing and How They are Done,* published by John Murray, which contains details of a large number of wonderful cures of diseases, usually considered incurable, which were effected by about a hundred highly qualified physicians in accordance with the teaching of Dr. Samuel Hahnemann.

This volume owes its origin to the inspiration of my friend, the late Dr. John H. Clarke, a great physician, a great thinker and a great character, who introduced me to the new healing art. I am under the highest obligation to my friend, Sir Arbuthnot Lane, whose teaching is of the utmost value to mankind. His teaching, applied to thousands of my patients, has mightily helped in their recovery. He has inspired my activities. I am grateful to Mr. Alfred Kohnstamm for suggesting to me the title of this book and to the proprietors of *Heal Thyself* for allowing me to reprint those pages which were previously published in their journal.

Open-minded doctors and surgeons who wish to study the new art and science of healing may find this difficult. I shall gladly help them all I can, as far as my limited time allows. They should not disdain to learn from a layman. Hippocrates, the Father of Medicine, wrote 2,300 years ago in his *Precepts*: " In medical matters experience and commonsense are far more valuable than scientific theories, however plausible. Do not hesitate to enquire of laymen if their opinion is likely to advance medical science and the treatment of the sick." It may interest them to learn that I have been able to help a considerable number of doctors and surgeons who had considered themselves incurable.

                                        J. ELLIS BARKER.

ALBION LODGE,
   FORTIS GREEN,
      EAST FINCHLEY, LONDON, N.2.

CHAPTER I

There are no Incurable Diseases—Why
Medicine Fails to Cure

NEARLY fifty years ago my father was dying of
an aneurysm of the aorta, a grave and protracted
disease, which had been declared incurable by the leading specialists of his time. I know now that this
malady, though still considered incurable by orthodox
medicine, has frequently been cured by homœopathy,
which might have saved his life. I was at the time a
youth of 14 or 15, and I vividly remember the tragic
months during which my father, who possessed Hercu-
lean strength and a wonderful constitution, struggled
bravely with his insidious enemy. Although he suffered
physical agonies, his brain remained clear and active
to the end. During the last few months of his life, he
often expressed deep regret that he could not hand on
to a successor, or to the medical profession as a whole,
the rich experience which he had acquired in the course
of decades. He had been an excellent doctor, beloved
by his patients, and he had worked without a holiday
during more than twenty consecutive years up to the
time of his final breakdown. Many other able doctors
have expressed similar sentiments when they had
become incapacitated or were dying.

There is a gigantic medical literature which is added
to from month to month. Unfortunately, practically
all the books published are dry and tedious and they are
as uninteresting as is the railway time-table. In the
textbooks diseases are classified under general headings, such as bacterial diseases, poisonings, diseases of

1

the digestive tract, the respiratory system, the liver, the kidneys, the heart, skin diseases, etc. This classification is purely fictitious. There is no such thing as a skin disease, seated only in the skin, or a heart disease which affects only the heart, etc. Most diseases are general and constitutional. For instance, faulty nutrition may produce a so-called skin disease, a disease of the liver, of the kidneys, of the heart, asthma and so forth. It would obviously be a mistake to treat in such cases the skin with an ointment or to give the textbook treatment for stomach, liver or heart.

The medical student is taught to mistake the local manifestations of a constitutional disorder for the whole of the malady and to treat his patients faultily. The usual physical examination of patients is concentrated upon the important organs, such as the heart, lungs, liver, etc., and if the doctor cannot find any obvious fault, he considers that there is no serious disease. Distinguished specialists habitually cover their lack of knowledge of the art of diagnosis and of the art of healing by telling the suffering individual, who is obviously ill, that he is " organically sound " and that his sufferings are " merely functional."

Under general headings, such as Diseases of the Digestive Tract, Diseases of the Stomach, Diseases of the Bowel, etc., the textbooks enumerate individual diseases, and the student is not warned that these specific diseases have no existence in fact, that the names and the classification of the so-called diseases continually change and that what is called a disease is merely a more or less arbitrary collection of symptoms.

The recognised textbooks are filled with scientific padding and are very useless for practical purposes. Under the heading of every disorder pages and pages are given to the definition of the disease, its history, its distribution, and particularly to its " morbid anatomy," which means the appearance of the diseased body and of its organs after death, information which interests chiefly anatomists and pathologists. This information is followed by a lengthy description of all the changes which, in the course of the disease, take place in the composition of the blood, of the spinal fluid, and of all the secretions and excretions, etc., which is of interest chiefly to laboratory workers.

After having waded through a mass of useless information, the busy doctor discovers at last the heading Treatment. While the theoretical part of the so-called local disease is discussed at wearisome length, the information under the heading Treatment is only too often scrappy and more or less valueless. We frequently read " The disease is incurable," or " There is no medical treatment," or " The case should immediately be handed over to the surgeon." It would be dangerous to give in the textbooks full details regarding treatment, because treatment varies from year to year and there is no unanimity in the profession regarding treatments.

The majority of the textbook writers are sceptics with regard to the efficacy of treatment. They half-heartedly recommend, or merely enumerate, the latest drugs or serums which may be untried, unsafe, or dangerous.

One of the leading textbooks is the late Sir William Osler's *Principles and Practice of Medicine*. After having glanced through numerous pages devoted to the purely theoretical side of the various diseases, we read with wearisome iteration in the few lines devoted to treatment that such-and-such medicines " may be tried."

Medical students are forced to acquire the useless information contained in the textbooks in order to pass their examination and to obtain their degree. When they begin to practise, they jettison very promptly the whole of this scientific ballast and rely for guidance in treatment on booklets of the size of a pocket diary.

The busy general practitioner is inadequately paid. He can make a living only by seeing every day a much larger number of patients than he can properly handle.

He works all the time at high pressure, giving to each patient the minimum of time. He has no leisure for study and usually has few, or no, books. He learns in course of time that a perfunctory and purely formal examination will serve because it will satisfy the patient, and that he can carry on his rushwork with little knowledge and few prescriptions. Often the sum and substance of his knowledge of the healing art may be summarized in sentences such as " For fever give Quinine, for heart disease give Digitalis, for epilepsy give Bromide and Luminal, for rheumatism give Salicylates, for pain give Aspirin or Morphia, for sleeplessness give Veronal," etc.

Apart from the exceedingly unsatisfactory official and more or less standardized art of healing with treatments based on the delusive name of the disease, not on the condition of the patient, there is an extremely valuable unwritten art of healing which the able and successful practitioner acquires by decades of experience and observation. Unfortunately this wonderful and invaluable knowledge is only too often lost to mankind, as it was in the case of my father. Every successful doctor is besieged by those in search of health. He has scarcely enough time for meals, sleep and the most necessary relaxation. He has, therefore, no opportunity to write down his experiences. Besides, such publication might lead to severe criticism on the part of his colleagues. For years I have urged in vain friends of mine, eminent physicians and surgeons, to write down, or dictate, their practical experiences for the benefit of all. Books of this kind are infinitely more important than the bulky, but largely useless, textbooks.

This volume bears the sub-title, " How to Cure The Incurable." The writers of medical textbooks, who usually have little, or no, practical knowledge of the healing art, are far too ready to declare that certain diseases are " incurable," or are " incurable, except by surgery." Every day we are informed that " Cancer is incurable, except by surgery." Nevertheless, all cancer specialists and almost every busy doctor has seen spontaneous cures of undoubted cancer cases. In the special literature devoted to cancer, hundreds of spontaneous and of art cures of undoubted cancer may be found, as I have shown in my two cancer books. The surgeons have monopolized cancer treatment to the great injury of those who suffer from that horrible malady.

Some of the most distinguished surgeons, such as Sir Alfred Pearce Gould, Sir Arbuthnot Lane, and Erwin Liek, have little faith in operation for fighting cancer. They rightly rely on prevention as the safer remedy. It is worth pointing out that cancer is almost unknown among primitive races, leading primitive lives, that the cancer mortality is approximately twice as great in the towns as in the country districts, and that it is about three times as great among butchers, merchant seamen and men occupied in the alcoholic drink traffic as among clergymen and agricultural labourers. This significant difference is far more important than all the so-called discoveries made by cancer researchers in the course of the last fifty years.

Surgery has failed disastrously to stem the flowing cancer tide. Drowning men clutch at a straw. The floundering medical profession, feeling helpless in the face of cancer, has grasped at X-rays and radium for the treatment of that disease. Unfortunately, leading surgeons have told me that they have not seen a single cure of undoubted cancer effected by radium or X-rays, but that they have seen innumerable cases in which the disease had been terribly aggravated by their use. After all, cancer is not a local disease, but a constitutional malady, whatever the surgeons may say, and a constitutional disease cannot be cured by cutting or burning away its local manifestation.

Many diseases apart from cancer are declared to be incurable in the textbooks. The printed assertion of incurability is readily believed by medical students and doctors of insufficient experience. A long life and the

B

careful observation of actualities have taught me that
there are no incurable diseases. If, as happens not infrequently, a disease disappears which the doctors had
declared to be incurable, the patient is shown mislead-
ing textbooks containing this statement and he is told
that in his case a miracle has happened. Such miracles
occur every day—especially to competent doctors.
The incompetent never see such miracles among their
patients.

Orthodox medicine considers as incurable not only
cancer and numerous other grave maladies, but every
long-established disease. Sir Arbuthnot Lane wrote:
" By no known means can we *cure* any chronic disease.
Therefore prevention is infinitely more important than
cure."

The new science and art of healing, called homœopathy, which was founded more than a century ago
by Dr. Samuel Hahnemann and which has been practised ever since by thousands of highly qualified doctors,
knows no incurable diseases. It specializes in the cure
of chronic diseases. Hundreds of undoubted cancer
cases have been cured by homœopathy. My friend,
the late Dr. John H. Clarke, has performed numerous
cures of cancer after the diagnosis of cancer had been
established by the microscopic examination of excised
tissue. He likewise cured a number of cases of
aneurysm of the aorta, from which my father died,
and numerous other diseases proclaimed incurable by
orthodox medicine. I had urged him for years to put
on paper the sum and substance of his experience.
Unfortunately he died prematurely and with him were
buried fifty years of unusual success in the true art of
healing.

In 1931 I published a book in which I described
several hundreds of cures of diseases which are incurable by orthodox medicine and which were performed
by more than a hundred homœopathic doctors.   I
gave the volume the title *Miracles of Healing and How
They Are Done.* The book created much interest and
it was widely reviewed in the professional journals.

Some of the representatives of orthodox medicine sneeringly stated that my book was "a mere compilation," that the cures described could not have taken place in reality, that only a layman, unacquainted with practical medicine, could have written such a book.

It is true, I am a layman, but I am not devoid of clinical experience. Being interested in health—I was an invalid for years—I had written some books devoted to the prevention and cure of disease by diet and common-sense measures. They were successful, I was visited by sick people who had read them, and who told me that their diseases had been declared incurable by high authorities and they implored me to help them. My hesitation was overcome by their entreaties. My first case was a man with pernicious anæmia. He came to me before the liver treatment was known. He told me: "You must treat me. I have been given up by all the doctors. You are my last hope." My second case was a man who had been sent home from a hospital with the diagnosis that he suffered from inoperable cancer of the bowel and bladder and that he had only a week to live. I had not the heart to refuse these unfortunate people. Success in both cases led to my becoming known to the friends of the sufferers and to others.

Careful study of the medical literature and personal experience and observation of an unusually large number of desperate cases have convinced me that there are incurable individual patients, but *there are no incurable diseases*. Cancer, disseminated sclerosis and all the chronic diseases are difficult to treat, but not infrequently they can be cured.

As I had failed in my attempts to cause some of the ablest doctors to give their experiences to mankind, I reluctantly resolved to describe myself the methods whereby the most intractable diseases may be cured, drawing upon my experience. I have described the cures contained in this work in simple and untechnical language and have withheld no information. There is no mystery about them. I have put all my cards on the table. Therefore the readers of my book, both professional and lay, if they have any aptitude, may be as successful as I have been, or more successful. Moreover, I have described all cures, as far as possible, in the language of the patients themselves, quoting their actual letters. The whole of this book is based on documentary evidence which may be scrutinized and which, with the permission of the patients, I shall gladly place at the disposal of any duly accredited and impartial medical body interested in the subject-matter of this book, provided professional discretion can be guaranteed.

CHAPTER II

How to Cure Heart Disease

PEOPLE in general have a great dread of heart disease. Their instinctive fear is perfectly justified. When the great pumping apparatus of the body is injured, the position is indeed serious. However, one must not exaggerate the significance of the disorders of the heart. Looked upon from one point of view, the heart is a most delicate piece of machinery. Looked at from another point of view it is a tough muscular structure which readily adjusts itself to changes, abnormalities, etc., which are comprised under the general heading " heart disease."

Very frequently one finds that people who complain about their heart have a perfectly sound heart. Abnormalities, such as palpitations, feeling of faintness about the heart, fluttering, clutching pain, irregularity of the heart's action, etc., may be due to some extraneous factor, such as chronic indigestion, which causes the inflated stomach to press upon the heart, constipation and accumulation of gas in the bowel, which have a similar effect, nervousness, which causes the heart to act in a nervy, irregular way, abuse of tobacco, or of drugs which temporarily upset the heart, anæmia, which weakens the heart by failing to supply it with adequate food, obesity, which puts an additional and severe strain upon the heart, etc. On the other hand, we find that people who actually suffer from heart disease have frequently not the slightest notion that anything is wrong with that wonderful organ, and they may die suddenly of heart failure.

9

The orthodox treatment of heart disease is rather pitiful. The general practitioner and many consultants test the heart's action in the usual way, and then inform the unfortunate patient that he suffers from fatty degeneration of the heart, or from an injury to one of the valves, etc. That information has naturally a most serious result upon the patient's spirit. A man who boldly goes into the doctor's study, complaining about pains in the left arm, breathlessness or something of the kind, and who is informed that his heart is " diseased " often comes out utterly crushed. He has received a deadly injury by the information rashly given to him. Furthermore, the treatment of heart disease is incredibly faulty. The motto of the medical profession seems to be " For Heart Disease give Digitalis." With unbelievable recklessness Digitalis is prescribed to all and sundry, to heart cases where it may suit and to those where it is utterly unsuitable. It is an exceedingly dangerous drug, the cumulative action of which often kills the patient. Eminent medical men whom I could quote have stated that more people die of Digitalis than of heart disease, and very possibly that assertion is true. If Digitalis fails to relieve, the patient may be given Strophanthus, Nitrate of amyl, or any of the other so-called "specifics" habitually used for heart disease, which are enumerated in the books on treatment. Hardly ever one finds that a heart patient has been treated constitutionally. A perfunctory prescription of Digitalis and perhaps another dope or two for the patient's nerves, sleep, or bowels is all that is given. The all-important carefully individualized regulation of the patient's life in general is left out. Possibly it is considered as unimportant by the average practitioner and specialist. At any rate I have found in scores of cases the shoddiest of shoddy treatment for heart disease which is in most cases quite easily curable, even if declared absolutely incurable by the leading specialists.

Those who wish to treat heart cases successfully must not fill their patients with despair, but buoy

them up with hope. Despair and worry are the most
powerful depressants, while hope and confidence are
the most wonderful tonics. If a man comes to me
declared absolutely incurable by the highest authorities
in Harley Street, I am apt to challenge their gloomy
prognosis with indignation, and if I am told that such-
and-such a heart valve is " incompetent," which means
that it is gravely injured or diseased, I may tell the
patient: " That information is of no interest to me
and is quite useless, and the man who gave it to you
is 'incompetent.' It would be of great use if one
could take out your heart and send it to the plumber
to have another valve fitted to it. The heart is not
an ordinary piece of machinery, like a clock or a motor-
car, but it is a piece of machinery which happily
is self-adjusting and self-repairing. I myself have
suffered from heart disease many years ago, and the
doctors wanted to send me to Nauheim for treatment.
I met a sporting doctor who told me that an enlargement of the heart, from which I suffered, was nothing
serious, that most athletes who went in for vigorous
exertion have enlarged hearts and that these hearts
become normal again through automatic self-adjust-
ment if Nature is given a chance. There was a time
when I could not walk up a short flight of stairs without
sitting down every few steps. I can now walk up the
highest staircase of any tower or spire and eat a meal
while doing so. There is plenty of good stuff in you.
Your heart will probably adjust itself if reasonably
treated. Has your pessimistic specialist asked you
anything about your diet, your way of living, your
exercise, your occupation, etc.? " As a rule one
gets the reply: " The specialist has forbidden me to
smoke, I must not eat potatoes, abstain from exercise,
live on a white diet, composed of white fish, breast of
chicken, milk pudding and milk, and that is all."

White is the colour of innocence, but milk and rice
pudding, given in abundance, though nominally very
digestible and therefore helpful to the heart, fatten
up patients, and this is particularly dangerous if heart

patients are stout.   Furthermore, most heart cases
are constipated, and their trouble is largely due to
constipation and vitamin starvation. Now the milky
diet is constipating and devoid of vitamins and of the
indispensable mineral elements which the heart needs.
Putting people with heart disease into bed has, of
course, some justification, at least in theory.   The
pumping function of the heart is greatly eased if the
pumping has to be done along the level of the resting
body instead of up and down, the standing or moving
body.   In extreme heart cases it may be justified to
put the patient on his back for some length of time. In
other cases it produces obesity, staleness of the body as
a whole, constipation and auto-intoxication and, before
all, deep depression which harms the patient greatly.

As soon as a man is told: " You must lie in bed
without a pillow, you must not move at all, you must
not even wipe your nose, or scratch your back," he
believes that his life hangs by a thread and that haunting thought may prove worse than the disease itself.
As a rule it is far better to keep the patient out of bed,
keep him busy, keep him interested, and before all,
keep him hopeful. Besides, the unforunate bed case
is apt to be drugged to death. He is given Digitalis
in large doses because it is recommended in the textbooks. When he gets depressed he is given a tonic.
When he gets constipated he is given Cascara sagrada
or Castor Oil, two of the most dangerous bowel irritants,· or salts, which are weakening.   If he cannot
sleep, he is given some dope which benumbs the nerves
of the body as a whole and therefore gravely impedes
the healing process.

The fact that a man has heart disease can easily
be ascertained by means of the stethoscope and various
other instruments and appliances. However, the fact
that a man has heart disease or some heart anomaly
is of relatively little importance. If the body is given
an adequate chance, it will patch up the heart and
it may go more or less irregularly, but quite satisfactorily, until the patient is 90 or 100. Such cases

are known to every medical man. The all-important question is not whether a patient suffers from this or that nameable disorder of the heart, but *why* he suffers from endocarditis, myocarditis, or whatever may be the outlandish official name of the trouble.

Some years ago I was travelling by railway. There were a man and a lady in my compartment, and they noticed that I was reading a medical book. The lady started a conversation and told me that she and her husband had just returned from a six month's holiday on the Continent, recommended by a specialist, and that her husband had not received any benefit for his heart. I immediately asked who was treating Mr. B. and I was informed that he was under an excellent practitioner, and that he had consulted three leading specialists in Harley Street. I asked: "Were you given any advice about diet or were you asked any questions about diet?" The reply was "No, but I was told not to eat any potatoes because they were too starchy." I glanced attentively at the man. He looked more like a kidney case than like a heart case, and I concluded that his so-called heart disease was due to abuse of alcohol, condiments, tobacco, or some other irritant. On my inquiry, the wife informed me to my horror that her husband took mustard by the tablespoonful. "He puts it on chicken, fish, bread and butter and eats it neat. I told the heart specialists about it, but they thought it of no importance." I told Mr. B. to his face that he suffered not from heart disease, but from too much mustard. He exclaimed: "You can give me what diet you like, but you must leave me my mustard." A few earnest words caused him to change his mind. There and then I administered to him a solemn oath that he would not touch mustard for a month, and would write to me when the month was up. In a month's time I had a most gratifying letter telling me of vast improvement. My advice had done him more good than six months' leisure, combined with treatment, on the Continent.

On the 1st April, 1928, a Mr. T. W. B. wrote to me

from Carbis Bay that he was dying of heart disease, that the doctors had given him only a few weeks to live, that he was lying in bed, that his wife had to turn him in bed, because he was not allowed to do so himself, that he had read some of my books, whether I could help him. I asked him to let me know in full detail what he ate and drank at every meal and when, what medicines he was taking, what was the cóndition of his bowels, age, height, weight, and, most important of all, he was to send me his prescriptions, and his photograph. After a few days I received all the details. Mr. B. was a well-to-do man who had been engaged in the grain trade. He had led a sedentary life. He had fed and feasted unwisely and had become flabby and very obese. He weighed 17 stone 4 lbs., was constipated, lived on a most unsuitable fattening diet, was given the usual Digitalis for the heart, medicine to help him digest the food for which his body had no need and which it refused to elaborate, medicine to empty his bowels, dope for the nerves, dope for sleep. His so-called heart disease was obviously not a primary disease but a consequence of faulty living and of faulty treatment. At a distance of several hundred miles I diagnosed his case more correctly than the doctors and specialists who had used all the scientific appliances of their calling. I wrote to him on the 2nd April:—

" I am sure that you will agree with me that your great trouble is overweight. Your heart has to work against resistance and it got enlarged through trying to overcome that resistance, and it probably became flabby through infiltration of the heart muscle with fat. Flabbiness of the muscles in general and flabby heart muscles often go together. That flabbiness is caused largely by auto-intoxication following upon chronic constipation, which in turn is responsible for acidity of the stomach which cannot be properly combated by neutralizing medicaments. The health of the heart depends on the quality of its food, of the blood with which it is nourished."

A few days later I received the details which I

required and I sent him on the 10th April my directions. They began with the words:—

"As I wish to bring down your weight by about 2 lbs. per week, I want you to weigh yourself regularly. For the time being I wish to cut out flesh, fish, fowl and their products, and I want you to subsist on a somewhat meagre, lacto-vegetarian diet. You will get milk, which is liquid meat, eggs and cheese, which are meat in another form, and your body will be encouraged to live on your surplus fat to the extent of a quarter of a lb. per day."

I gave him liquid paraffin for bowel regulation and Kaylene for absorbing the toxins in his bowel. Moreover, I told him to take regular exercise, one or two walks on the level during five minutes by the watch on the first day, a minute to be added every day so that he would do one or two walks of 35 minutes after a month and one or two walks of 65 minutes after two months. Digitalis and all other drugs were immediately taken away. The only tonics which he was to receive were my letters of encouragement.

So far all his doctors and consultants had depressed Mr. B. by frightening technicalities of the heart condition and by depressing forecasts made to him and to his wife. As soon as his dopes and the over-heating and totally unsuitable diet had been taken away, Mr. B. began to flourish and he devoted himself with the greatest enthusiasm to the progress of slimming and of building up his strength. In six months his weight had gone down by more than four stone. I explained to him that this was equivalent to the weight of two buckets filled with water. He became lithe, young and bright once more. He extended his walks from day to day and from month to month. Gentle homœopathic medicines were sent to him in accordance with his needs.

By Autumn he had so much improved that he could travel to Scotland, and he, who in the past had taken no exercise, who had habitually overfed on rich food, was able to go for non-stop walks of from 10 to 12 miles in the Scotch hills. He became a young man once more.

In February, 1929, an article of mine was published in the *Sunday Graphic*, in which I referred incidentally to the danger of using Digitalis for heart disease and to the possibility of curing heart disease mainly by dietetic measures. A few days later I received a letter from a well-known city man, Mr. L. H. Q., addressed to the *Sunday Graphic*, worded as follows:

" A week or so ago I am told you had an article in the *Sunday Graphic* referring to the cure of heart trouble by dieting. I am 61 years old, and have a none too good heart for which I am taking Digitalis." He came to my house on the 5th March, 1929. He arrived in his car, and he got out with difficulty and walked slowly along the front garden, leaning heavily on his wife, fighting for breath all the time. He was tall and well made, had been a great athlete, had been in the habit of going for 40-mile walks, and now he could scarcely stagger along my front garden. He had been to the best Harley Street specialists, and he had been told that nothing would keep him alive except Digitalis, that he must not spend the winter in England, that he should immediately go to the Riviera and take gentle exercise on the level, either walking or being pushed along in a bath chair. When I touched the question of diet I was told, exactly as in the case of Mr. B., that he could eat and drink what he liked, but that he was not to touch potatoes, which were " too starchy." I remarked thereupon: " Potatoes are your best friends." He lived in his opinion "very simply." However, he lived on the same kind of food which had nourished him at the time when he had been tremendously active with games, sports and pedestrianism. When he had finshed his story and I had ended my interrogation he asked me with surprise: " Are you not going to examine my heart? " " No," I said, " that has been done sufficiently in Harley Street and with very indifferent results." " Are you not going to feel my pulse either? " " No," I replied, " I am not much interested in your pulse, but I am immensely interested in your breath, which is pestilential." He turned to his wife: "Is that true?" "Yes." "Why did you not tell me?" There was no reply. I explained to him that in my opinion he did not suffer from heart disease but from the pressure of a foul, gas-inflated stomach upon the heart, and I sent him my directions, which were introduced by a sketch of his condition, worded as follows:

"You are 61 years old, tall, well-proportioned, have good hair, a rather florid complexion, have no natural teeth, the whites of your eyes are yellow, the tongue is white, and you have a very unpleasant bitter breath. Your hands and feet are apt to get cold and numbed in bed, you are much troubled with flatulence of stomach and bowel, you take no laxatives or purgatives, you take Digitalis twice a day by doctor's orders, and you go once a day to stool, stools being dark. In my opinion you do not suffer from heart disease or heart weakness, but from protein poisoning, from a totally unsuitable concentrated diet, with plenty of alcohol and strong coffee, although you take no exercise whatever."

Before sending the man away I "tested" his heart by asking him to walk up and down a small flight of stairs. He did it with the greatest difficulty and told me that for three and a half years he had not been able to put on or take off his socks.

In addition to a carefully selected vegetarian diet, I gave him Carbo vegetabilis and Nux vomica combined in very small doses to regulate his gastric digestion, pig bile tablets to activate his liver, gall bladder and bowel, and Crataegus to strengthen the heart. When he was at my house, his stomach felt like a balloon, and he was in acute misery day and night with flatulence. In two or three days his stomach had gone down to a normal size and the tumultuous beating of the heart had disappeared.

A few weeks later, Mr. L. H. Q. visited me again, radiantly happy. He told me: "I can race you up any staircase," and informed me that, when going to his office in the city, he did not wait for the lift but walked upstairs like a youngster. He, like Mr. T. W. B., had been put upon very short walks to be increased by a minute every day.

On the 5th May, two months after the beginning of the treatment, an anonymous doctor attacked me in the *Sunday Graphic*, pouring contempt upon my assertion that many diseases incurable to orthodox medicine could easily be cured by a common-sense diet, aided by mild homœopathic drugs. This attack aroused the anger of Mr. L. H. Q. He sent a letter to the Editor, worded as follows:—

" I am (or was) a ' heart ' case, complicated with ' chronic bronchitis.' For over three years I was under a leading heart specialist and my own doctor. By January of this year I could no longer dress or undress myself, or put on or take off my boots, or get into bed and lie down (with five pillows) or walk upstairs without resting continually, and this, although assisted. The least exertion prostrated me.

" My doctor told me early this year he could not do any more for me. I was as well as I should be. He advised me to keep on taking Digitalis, to give up business altogether, to have a bed made up on the ground floor and, when well enough to do so, to go abroad and live there permanently. I should not go out except in warm weather. A fog would, he said, ' kill me.' I was to reconcile myself to the inevitable.

" With this sentence I went to my office on Monday to clear up things. By one of those queer accidents which do happen in real life, I heard that day by chance that a Mr. Barker had written an article in your paper, which, my informant said, referred to a case which seemed similar to mine. I had never heard of Mr. Barker, but as I stood to lose nothing by having a try in another direction, I wrote to him, caie of your paper. He made an appointment with me, and I am still under treatment by him.

" For some weeks now I have dressed and undressed unaided and stairs have almost ceased to trouble me. I get into bed as easily as when I was 50 years younger, and I sleep eight hours on end. My breathing is normal. I have even been out in fog without bad effect. I hardly know that I have a heart. My daily Digitalis doses ceased the first day of my treatment, and I have religiously obeyed instructions as to diet, which are almost exactly contrary to all previous instructions. I put in seven and a half hours' work at the office daily."

Mr. Q. used to take for breakfast 2 eggs, or 3 rashers of bacon and 1 egg, white bread and butter and strong coffee. For luncheon he took some sandwiches. In the afternoon he took two glasses of sherry and at the evening meal he took a kind of alderman's dinner, not disdaining the most indigestible food, such as salmon, mince pies, pork pies, washed down with half a bottle of sherry. None of these foods had been forbidden by his doctors. This was another case in which the patient did not suffer from heart disease but from faulty feeding. The original disease had, of course, been aggravated by supplying the heart with dope instead of dealing with the causation of the trouble.

On the 26th February, 1930, I received a letter from a poor widow, a Mrs. J. L. B. of Southampton:—

"I am a sufferer from heart disease. The doctors here say that the muscles of my heart are affected and they give me medicines to keep me going to a certain extent, for I can't work much, only light duties, resting on my couch in the kitchen most of the time. I am a heavy woman, 49 years old, and have been troubled with simple palpitation since I was 21 years of age. Every time I was examined by doctors they said there was nothing much wrong with my heart, until about 8 years ago, when one doctor told me I had heart block. Well, I did not take much notice and still went on, palpitations getting a little worse, until last August, when I got very severe palpitation and the doctor ordered me to rest. I have been resting ever since but feel no better. I am now writing to ask if you think there is any cure for me or if I can be so far improved as to be able to work in my home for my children."

I told Mrs. J. L. B. to send me the fullest details, asking: "What do you eat and drink at every meal and in between, what medicines do you take, condition of bowels, sex organs, motions, urine, sexual discharges, what improves and aggravates your condition?" After receiving all the details I sent her my directions, in which I described her case as follows:—

"You are 49 years old, and, although you stand only 5 feet 2, you weight 11 stone 2 lbs. 14 ozs., carrying at least 30 lbs. of overweight, to the great injury of your weakened heart, which has to work against the resistance of surrounding fat. No wonder that the doctor told you that the heart muscle was affected. If it becomes fatty, it loses its strength. In addition you are somewhat constipated, live on concentrated food, suitable for people who take plenty of exercise, although you take no exercise at all. You were vaccinated three or four times in India, and only the first vaccination took. It is most essential to get your weight down; otherwise there will be disaster."

I gave Mrs. J. L. B. a reducing diet of a vegetarian kind, and told her that she was to lose 2 to 3 lbs. a week. As in nearly all my heart cases, I told her to disregard the orders of her doctor forbidding exercise, and gave her the usual five minutes' walk or walks, a minute to be added every day. I helped her digestion and excretion with Nux vomica and Carbo vegetabilis and liquid paraffin.

For some reason or other the people who come to me as a rule willingly adopt the régime which I give them, even if it involves abstention from their favourite foods. Mrs. B., like most of my heart cases, enthusiastically cut down her food and threw away the doctor's medicine. She had been in the habit of hobbling about with a stick. On the 28th March, a fortnight after she had begun, she wrote to me: "I am going on nicely and have discarded the stick as I find I can walk without it now, thank God. I still go along very slowly, especially up a steep incline." On the 16th April she wrote: "I find I have lost 2 lbs. 2 ozs. during the last week. It seems to be making a world of difference to me, and I am now able to come downstairs at 7.30 a.m. and get the breakfast ready for my two daughters." On the 29th April she was well enough to travel to London and to call upon me. On the 17th June she wrote: "I have reduced still more and am now 9 stone 5 lbs. 2 ozs., having lost 25¾ lbs. since I started, and I feel worlds better for it."

I have not mentioned the medicines which I gave to the three heart cases described so far. I have not done so because the experienced homœopath has no specifics for diseases. He is not taught parrot-like: "For heart disease give Digitalis." He gives those medicines which are indicated by the momentary pressing needs or symptoms of the patient, and every change of symptoms must be countered by a corresponding change in medication. Mrs. B. suffered from vaccinial poisoning, having been vaccinated in India three times, vaccination not taking. I had to treat her for this and for many other things as well and it would only confuse non-expert readers if I gave the full list of medicines which Mrs. B., or the previous two patients, were given in the course of their treatment. Incidentally the cases of Mr. T. W. B. and Mrs. J. L. B. show that it is not indispensable for a prescriber to see his patients. These two cases were grossly mismanaged by the doctors who frequently saw and treated them and whose whole knowledge of the treatment of heart cases seemed to consist in the formula: "For heart disease give Digitalis."

Dr. Thomas Sydenham, the English Hippocrates, one of the greatest medical geniuses which Britain has produced, wrote bluntly 250 years ago: "The sick man dies of his doctor" and help up to scorn the incompetence of the medical profession. Naturally his colleagues denied his charge. Every modern doctor realises that it was justified. In Sydenham's time bleeding, purging and salivating by huge doses of mercury were generally accepted methods of treatment, exactly as the abuse of Digitalis, of serum treatment, unnecessary surgery, etc., are now generally accepted. The Registrar-General publishes every year detailed statistics from which we learn that the people die only

c

from the various diseases known to medical science. According to the official statistics they never die from over-eating, self-drugging, medical incompetence, etc. "The doctor buries his mistakes"—and he writes the death certificates.

On the 22nd June, 1931 a Mrs. M., of Oldham, Lancashire, wrote to me:—

"I am a working man's wife, and I am suffering from heart trouble. I am a woman of 56 years of age, with one daughter. I went to the doctor some years ago and he said my heart was very bad.

"I did not want to think he was right. Anyhow, I find there is something wrong somewhere. Last year I was in bed five months, but I have done no good since. I am in bed at the present time and have been eight weeks, and the doctor does not want me to get up as he says there is nothing but rest for it. The doctor says it is the muscles of my heart that are sagged, and that I shall never be able to do a hard day's work again. The other doctor I saw told me that they would have to keep their eye on me as long as I lived. So I take it they are never going to be able to cure me. I have no pleasure in walking about as I cannot get my breath. I do not seem to stand anything. If I talk it is an effort to me and I am getting tired of it."

In immediate reply I wrote:—

"I very much hope to improve the condition of your heart and your general health, fetch you out of bed and get you to walk, etc., provided you are willing to carry out my directions. However, I am afraid I cannot help you unless I have full details of your condition. Tell me what brought about the heart trouble. Was it through overstrain, rheumatism, or is it inherited? What illnesses have you had? What is your height and approximate weight? Tell me in full detail what you eat and drink at every meal and what medicines you are taking and have been taking. Are your bowels in good order or not? Have you any difficulty with your urine or sex organs, has your trouble come on after the change of life, do you suffer with violent flushes, do you perspire much, little or not at all, have you taken much sugar, salt, pepper, mustard, pickles, vinegar, alcohol, strong tea, strong coffee? Send me your photo."

Her doctors had examined her heart with a stethoscope, but had not asked a single question about her diet and way of living. Her reply disclosed clearly to me the causation of her trouble. In my directions, sent to her on the 29th June, I summed up her case as follows:—

" You are 56 years old, a working man's wife, and have come to me complaining of heart trouble which has been diagnosed by the doctor as *angina pectoris*. You find it difficult to walk about because you cannot get your breath, find it difficult to talk, and seem altogether in a very unsatisfactory condition. You stand 5 feet 4, weigh 10 stone 9, and seem to me much too heavy. You eat very faultily, taking much salt and pepper, lots of butter, sugar and cakes, take brandy first thing in the morning and Port wine, have a poor circulation, are chronically constipated. It seems that the heart trouble was intensified by the change of life. Four years ago you had apparently vomiting and diarrhœa which compelled you to be in bed for three weeks. Ten months afterwards your heart trouble became very noticeable and the doctor told you that your heart muscles had sagged much. Very likely your abdominal organs have sagged as well and I want some information on that important point. Ten years ago you had a severe itching eruption which was treated with a lotion."

I gave Mrs. M. a reducing diet, told her " Avoid flesh, fish, fowl and everything made of them, condiments and spices, take the absolute minimum of salt, apparently you are salt-poisoned, the absolute minimum of milk and butter and abstain from sugar, cake, jam, marmalade, sweets of every kind, strong tea, coffee, alcohol in every form." She was to lose 2 lbs. per week.

I have two photographs of her, one taken at the beginning of the treatment, and the other a year after. On the first Mrs. M. looks flabby, heavy, shapeless, with big bags under her eyes. On the second photo she looks distinguished, with an excellent figure, clear-cut features, scarcely recognizable as the same woman.

My first letter had given hope to Mrs. M. She proved a woman of sterling character and she made magnificent progress. On the 7th July, one week after the beginning of the treatment, Mrs. M. wrote to me:—

" The doctor has been coming to see me ever since I began to be ill. He visits me once a week to examine my heart. After all this time I am not able to go upstairs to bed, or up the least incline. Now I have come in touch with you, I am sure before long I shall be able to get about better. I have been up to-day since 12 o'clock and I have walked about the house nicely. I have had my evening meal which I enjoyed, and I am going to tell you all about myself and then I am going to bed, thanking God I am so much better. I feel better than I have been for some time. I feel so much lighter in my body. As for my talking, if you heard the difference, you would be surprised. I can talk and take my breath without any difficulty. My medicine is suiting me fine and my diet also. I feel so comfortable after I have had a meal and I am enjoying my meals and am liking them well. I hope this letter will be satisfactory to you for I am so satisfied myself."

In a week a few doses of Sulphur 6X night and morning and a little Nux vomica and Carbo vegetabilis combined, together with a reducing diet and bowel activation with liquid paraffin, had produced a wonderful improvement in her heart condition and general health. Where the doctors, who had mechanically examined her heart with a stethoscope, had failed, I, a layman, who had never seen or examined her, had succeeded. A week after, on the 15th July, Mrs. M. reported:—

" I am much better, I am walking about a little, and am just going outside the door. I can take my breath better when I am talking and walking, my motions are wonderful. I am fine in my body, I feel so different, my friends are seeing a change in me already—I do not look so haggard. I have had a big load taken off me when I got in touch with you, who is going to cure me. I had almost given up."

On the 29th July, a month after the beginning of the treatment, she wrote:—

" My doctor came to examine my heart yesterday, and he told my husband I was better than I had been for some time. The doctor asked my husband if he had noticed the difference in the colour of my lips."

On the 7th October she wrote:—

" I am much better. I went out yesterday morning for a short walk in the sun and I felt fine. What do you think my doctor said to me when he saw me? I was sewing when he came bounding in. He looked at me and said, ' My word, Mrs. M., you look as if you were almost ready to give me the sack. Anyhow,' he said, ' we will see what that heart of yours has to say for itself.' When he had examined my heart he said: ' My word, your heart is a lot stronger than it was.' "

On the 28th October she wrote:—

" I am so much better, I wonder sometimes if I am the same woman that could not stir and be able to get a mite of breath. Do you know I can walk at my own speed, and it is not a bad one, and never be short of breath, and I can tell you it feels grand. I wonder where I should have been if I had not got in touch with you. I feel this morning I could do almost anything."

The letters of Mrs. M. became more and more joyful. With the greatest enthusiasm she carried out everything I advised, practising self-denial in many ways, and she was richly rewarded. On the 16th December she told me:—

" My heart is more steady than it was. My doctor has been to see me and he was surprised. He said: ' Mrs. M., you are wonderful. How long is it since you had any medicine?' I told him I had had none since last June. He asked how I slept and if I could eat, and I told him I could do both. He sat and talked with me a long time and at the finish I think he was puzzled. You know when doctors tell you that you will never do this and never do that and in so short a time they see a different woman, like me, they are bound to be wondering what has caused it, and you know I have been examined by more than one doctor and they will all be wrong. I wonder what he would say if he knew who it was that made such a difference in me. I would just like to tell him but I guess he would never forgive me. I was talking to a person last week and she said you are a different woman. We thought you were never going to be right again. She heard the doctor tell me I should never cook a dinner again. I felt this morning I could do all the work there was to do."

Later on she wrote:—

" My doctor has been. I am going to be a young woman again. My eyes are doing grand. I can see to pick a pin off the table without glasses and that is something for me. I can tell you if I had put my glasses down anywhere in the past, I could not see enough to pick them up without my husband telling me where they were. I am glad to be able to say that I am better than I have been for years. My doctor knows it. He has not been in to see me for six weeks."

I had given her eye exercises which had helped her. She was very poor, her husband was out of work, but I was well rewarded for the trouble I took by the joy I gave her and myself.

I have described a few of my successful heart cases, but, of course, I have had failures. Unfortunately many of my failures were caused by my patients. Nothing is more dangerous for a patient than too rapid a recovery.

I had a very similar case to Mrs. M. The woman in question was doing wonderfully well and I had told her very strictly not to rush, and to avoid excitement. Her daughter-in-law was to have a baby. She went around at the critical moment. Labour pains began as soon as she arrived. There was no nurse and the doctor had not come. She got excited, rushed about, trying to fetch help, collapsed and died.

There was in the West End of London a most devoted couple, a Mr. and a Mrs. A. F. D. They were childless. They lived for one another. Mr. D. was fond of social life, and he had a weak heart and a high blood pressure, which frequently go together. One day he went to a Harley Street consultant and he was horrified to be told that he had a blood pressure of 300 and that his heart had gone to pieces. He went immediately to two other consultants, who confirmed the verdict, sought his wife and told her that all was over. With tears in her eyes she knelt down and prayed that God should send her a saviour.

At that very moment a friend of mine, Sir R. P., was near by and it occurred to him that he might call on Mrs. D. He found her in tears and suggested: "Send for Mr. Ellis Barker." I saw the pair on the next day and I noticed that the husband's face was jaundiced, drawn, greasy looking, and that his eyes were very watery. These are indications of salt-poisoning. He told me about his blood pressure and his symptoms and showed me his prescriptions. "Did your doctor or did the consultants tell you anything about your diet?" "Not a word." The man took large quantities of meat, strong coffee, strong tea, alcohol, and smoked numerous cigarettes, a deadly combination in a heart case. He took in the course of the day a tablespoonful of salt and other condiments as well in huge quantities. In view of the very clearly marked symptoms of salt-poisoning, I gave him a diet from which all heating and irritating things were eliminated, forbade salt in cooking and at the table, and gave him Natrum muriaticum 30, a dose of 3 pilules to be taken three times a day.

Natrum muriaticum is table salt, and I gave it to him in the 30th potency, which means by the decillionth of a grain. A decillion is 1 with 60 noughts behind it. In this high potency salt is a very powerful remedy. It is my favourite prescription in cases of salt poisoning. Mr. D. started improving at once and the homœopathic medicine caused him to sweat salt from every pore. A few days after our first meeting he told me laughingly: "You can't deprive me of my beloved salt. If I want to have a taste of it, I need only lick my lips or my hands. They taste like concentrated salt." In a few weeks he had improved greatly. His blood pressure rapidly went down from 300 to 180.

A little while after this he went to his club in the West End, where he met some of his friends. They celebrated his recovery with cocktails and wines with which salmon, beef and game pie were washed down. There were Stilton, ices and strong black coffee and brandy to wind up with, and then they smoked. Mr. D. took all these things which I had strictly forbidden. When the meal was over he stepped into his car to drive home. Suddenly he felt like dying. He pulled up and sat helpless for more than two hours, gasping for breath. That meal was the turning point. He went down steadily. The utmost skill of doctors, both allopathic and homœopathic, proved unavailing. He had improved too quickly.

Frequently people with high blood pressure report that they have been told by their doctors that nothing can be done for high blood pressure, that the hardened pipes through which the blood is running with difficulty cannot be widened by any possible means. I habitually explain to patients that far more pressure is required to drive a thick liquid through a system of pipes than a thin liquid. Usually people with high
? blood pressure have thick blood. In the olden times such people were bled profusely. The loss of blood was immediately made good by water from the tissues and the thick blood was promptly made thin.

The thinning of the blood can be effected by dietetic regulation which is apt to reduce blood pressure gradually in practically all cases, especially if it is accompanied by bowel regulation. People with high blood pressure usually suffer from constipation and auto-intoxication and live on a concentrated, stimulating and heating diet, which is supposed to give them strength, but which weakens them, keeping the blood thick and the blood pressure high. In nearly all cases which have come under my care I have been able to reduce blood pressure considerably by dietetic means. If the blood pressure is brought down by drugs, the improvement will not last. As soon as the drug is withdrawn, blood pressure shoots up again.

On the 4th February, 1929, Mrs. B. A. B. wrote to me from Birmingham:—

"My mother-in-law, who is 70, has had two very severe heart attacks, and other minor ones. Up to this age she has enjoyed fairly good health, and had no attack whatever. These attacks come on at night and the specialist says she will always be subject to them and that to the end of her days, which will be short if she has any severe ones. She must consider herself an invalid. The trouble is high blood pressure which causes the walls of the heart to collapse. It is really tragic for her to realize what all this means."

With the usual brutal crudeness, a specialist, considering only the mechanical action of the heart and the deteriorated state of the arteries, had made a statement which gave the invalid no hope, aggravating her condition. I asked the usual questions, which the specialist had not asked, as to her way of living, diet, etc. Her daughter informed me that Mrs. B. lived on white meat and fish, milky foods, etc., by doctor's orders. A white diet may be very artistic. It harmonizes with the white walls of hospitals, the white dresses of nurses, and it may suggest purity or cleanliness to the brainless. But white meat and fish become as putrid in a stagnant bowel as "butcher's meat" which was not allowed by Mrs. B.'s advisers. She was very constipated, and had been given tonics for her heart. She did not perspire at all. On the basis of the information given by her daughter and of a photograph, I sent on the 2nd March directions to the old lady whom I had never seen, worded as follows:—

"You are 70 years old, not a very great age, you look somewhat flabby, and you are troubled with your heart and nerves. The health of the heart and of the nerves depends on their nutrition. I hope to strengthen both vastly by purifying and strengthening your blood and body, and I hope you will help me and become rejuvenated. I have handled successfully far more serious heart cases than yours.

"Go to stool three times a day, whether you feel the need or not, but do not strain.

" Take three times a day, three-quarters of an hour before meals, about a tablespoonful of liquid paraffin, you regulating quantity by results. Stools should be as loose as cow dung and as yellow as mustard. Having swallowed the paraffin, sip half a tumblerful of cold water.

" Breakfast. Thick barley gruel with plenty of milk in it, a lightly boiled, poached or a raw egg stirred in milk, stale wholemeal bread and thin butter, grated mild meagre cheese, 2 cups of very weak China tea, slightly sweetened.

" Mid-day meal. Vegetables boiled without salt or soda in the minimum of water, vegetable water to be reduced by cooking separately, and to be drunk at some convenient time, mashed potatoes done with plenty of milk—the potatoes used for this purpose should be boiled in their jackets—a lightly boiled, poached, or a raw egg stirred in milk, milk pudding or macaroni cheese.

" Afternoon tea. 2 cups of very weak China tea, slightly sweetened, with a little stale wholemeal bread, thinly buttered, and honey if liked.

" Evening meal. More or less like mid-day meal.

" After evening meal. Sip vegetable water.

" Before going to bed, take hot footbath, strengthened with mustard to improve circulation, and to draw blood away from heart and head. Have the headposts of your bed gradually raised with the same object in view, have some extra pillows under your head, and have two hot-water bottles to your feet. Get up very slowly and gradually, particularly if you have to make water or empty your bowel.

" Report progress once a week and act with wise discrimination, not with mechanical obedience to these directions, for no one understands the working of your body better than you do yourself. If you are in difficulties, write at once."

She was given a small dose of Sulphur 3X night and morning to clear the blood and re-establish perspiration, and she was to take between meals a dose of Crataegus 1X. The diet was rich in mineral elements and vitamins, was not heating and was likely to strengthen her body. In the introductory paragraph and in an accompanying letter I had given the patient every possible encouragement. She felt hopeful and confident and gradually forgot the gloomy forecasts of her doctor and the heart specialist. Medicines were frequently changed. She was given Ceanothus 1X because her spleen was enlarged, etc. On the 18th April, six weeks after the beginning of the treatment, her daughter-in-law wrote: "My mother-in-law is doing remarkably well and has gone out to tea, looking quite well and walking with quite strong steps and upright. Various people have seen her lately and remarked how very much better she is doing and looking." She improved steadily and became a totally different woman. Her daughter-in-law wrote to me on the 21st June: —

"I know that my mother-in-law is ever so much better. The doctors and the specialist said she would be a confirmed invalid. When she started your treatment, she spent all her hours lying down. Now she rests in all about two hours each day."

On the 10th October I was told: —

"My mother-in-law has had a most wonderful summer, walking a good deal and everybody remarking how well she looked. It is a twelvemonth now since she had her first attack."

A few months later the daughter-in-law considered Mrs. B. cured.

The cases described so far were cured, or vastly improved, after many months of treatment. Occasionally one is able to produce a cure in a few weeks or days by means of a clearly indicated homœopathic medicine.

On April 27th, 1933, Mr. B., a major in the Army, came to me complaining about his heart. He was a man of magnificent physique, 41 years old, had never been ill, was made prisoner during the Great War, and was ill-fed and maltreated for two years in Germany, and then sent to Switzerland, a wreck. He was to come before a medical board for examination. Previously he took an enormous quantity of the strongest black coffee and smoked a huge number of cigarettes in order to upset his heart and to be repatriated on account of permanent and incurable invalidism. When seen by the doctors, his heart was indeed in a terrible condition. He was considered to be a permanent invalid and was sent home to England. His general health improved rapidly, but his heart never got well.

At odd times and for no obvious reason he had frequent attacks which forced him to stand still and to fight for breath. There was severe constriction of the chest. He went to doctors and specialists. Their treatments were unsuccessful and he came to me, after fifteen years of suffering, believing his heart to be incurable. I discovered that there was a definite feeling of constriction which suggested Cactus grandiflorus. I gave him that medicine in the 1X strength, three pilules to be taken three times a day. He rapidly improved. After a few weeks I gave him Cactus in the 30th potency, a dose of three pilules to be taken after every attack. I saw my patient again on September 6th. He told me that he had not had an attack for months and he declared that he was completely cured.

Mr. J. B., a business man of Belfast, wished to consult me and arrived at my house on the 17th June, 1931. He looked a very sick man, was fat and flabby, he had a poor complexion, yellowish whites to the eyes, which lacked sparkle, he had hard, tortuous arteries on the temples, looked aged, exhausted, had headaches at the back of the head, a very bad sign, pain in the kidney region, radiating toward the bladder, sore feet, legs, arms and hands, he was, and always had been, constipated, had much catarrh. He was 51 years old and looked 70. Big bags under his eyes suggested kidney trouble. His doctor had recently told him that he suffered from valvular heart disease, a dilated heart and high blood pressure. Two and a half years previously he had been informed that he suffered from chronic Bright's disease. Naturally his physical condition and the cruel information given to him had deeply depressed him. He looked stricken and desperate.

I told him that there was an unlimited reserve in most people, that his troubles were largely due to an unsuitable diet, and that he was likely to mend if he mended his ways. Not one of his doctors and consultants had made any enquiries about his nutrition. He took enormous quantities of salt with his food and large quantities of Epsom salts every morning, huge quantities of butter and cream, masses of mustard, plenty of alcohol, was fond of meat. Salt, mustard and alcohol were fearfully injurious to his kidneys and liver, and the malfunctioning of these organs was bound to upset the body and particularly the heart. He had been given large doses of Digitalis for his heart and much Quinine and Iron as a tonic, although bowel regulation would have been by far the best tonic.

I prescribed a mild, non-irritating and weight-reducing diet, forbade Epsom salts and the medicines he was taking, particularly Digitalis, and as he had to stick his over-hot feet out of bed—a leading Sulphur symptom—I gave him Sulphur 6X night and morning which would clear his blood, skin and complexion, a change which was bound to encourage him. I also gave him Natrum muriaticum 30 for his salt craving and the salt-poisoning from which he suffered. In such cases Natrum muriaticum, table salt, in a high potency, is helpful, and often curative. In view of his desperate condition, I had very little hope for him, but I have not the heart to say to a patient: " I am afraid I can do nothing for you."

He reacted splendidly. On the 26th June, after a week's treatment, he wrote: " I feel somewhat better, I sleep much better, my colour is somewhat better, my heart has a very steady beat, my tongue is cleaner, I feel brighter, but I still have the exhausted beat-up feeling in feet, legs and body if I walk any distance." I sent him Arnica 3X for his feeling of weakness, and he wrote on the 10th July: " When taking the new medicine I feel the effect almost immediately. It seems to stimulate me and give me a brighter feeling." On the 18th July he reported: " My face is not nearly so flabby, my eyes are much brighter and have some sparkle, the yellowness of the whites has greatly gone, the soreness at the back of the head still troubles me occasionally, not continually, I am sleeping better."

I then gave him for his heart Crataegus, mother tincture. When he complained about nervous fears, I gave him Ignatia. When he complained about wheezing, I sent him Bryonia and he improved steadily. When he came to me, he had been too ill to work. He was now able to go back to work. On the 28th August he wrote:—

"I am again carrying out my every-day work and feel no ill effects. My strength is well maintained. In fact, I am stronger. My heart is greatly improved, I have no jingling or unsteady beats, but occasionally I feel it beating or thumping, but there is no shortness of breath. I have been only a little over two months on your treatment and it has made a wonderful change. The soreness in the back of my head has partly disappeared."

On the 25th November he had an attack of sickness, pain in the head, giddiness, and his left arm and leg felt quite numb. Probably a small artery had burst in his head, producing a "stroke." A doctor was called in, and he was informed that he suffered from disseminated sclerosis, and was advised to eat half a pound of liver per day. He wrote:—

"I enquired from the doctor to-day how my heart was, and am delighted to tell you that he said there was *little the matter with the heart to worry about. When I questioned him about my blood pressure, he said it was 30 points over the normal, but this was probably due to my nervousness. After he had taken my urine and tested it, he said that there was practically nothing the matter with my kidneys. All this great improvement of heart, blood pressure and kidneys is due entirely to your treatment, and I cannot thank you enough for all you have done for me, and I have every faith in your making my left side all right again.*"

The italicized passages were underlined by Mr. J. B. I could not believe my eyes when I read what the doctor had said.

I helped him onward with Arnica 3X to absorb the clot on the brain. He recovered, but, later on, there were numerous ups and downs, and he sent complaints about this or that organ. He also was troubled with chills, attacks of influenza, had difficulties with the bladder, etc. The destroyed tissue of kidneys and liver cannot be re-created. I felt doubtful of the results of my treatment. Various relapses occurred, but I always succeeded in getting his condition back to something like normality and he frequently expressed to me his boundless faith in me which was, perhaps, not shared by his family. Occasionally his wife made complaints, writing to me directly. I frequently suggested that if he or his wife would like to have additional advice, they should call in any doctor and that I would welcome such action.

Towards Autumn, 1933, there was a distinct aggravation in Mr. J. B.'s condition, and his letters ceased. I thought that he had died suddenly and that his family had not informed me. To my great surprise I received on the 15th November a long letter from Mr. J. B. himself, written in bed in pencil, with a very shaky hand, so shaky as to be almost unreadable: —

" You will be surprised to hear from me again. My wife tells me that she wrote you twice, to which she had no reply (I never received the alleged letters). Well now when I wrote you last, you were treating me principally for the heart. Your attention was very great and I did appreciate it very much, but the fault of not being able to explain everything to you thoroughly was probably due to my mistake.

" I have been confined to bed since the 27th July—nearly three months—and as far as I can find out, one day, recently, I got about two days to live. The first doctor who examined me informed me I was suffering from heart valvulitis, low pressure, and kidney disease. The next doctor said the same. Then a professor was brought in. I think it was he who said I would live only a few days. That was about the 12th September. The fourth doctor was a Dr. G., a young man, who is said to be clever as well as being an able practitioner. He examined me and said if some certain thing responded, I would live for several months longer and if something else responded to his treatment I would live for years. He seems to be young and inexperienced and could say nothing for certain. Anyhow, Mr. Barker, I have got no satisfaction from any of them. They have ordered me tea, Hovis bread and butter and scrambled egg for breakfast, bowl of chicken soup, chicken, bread, etc., and a cup of tea for dinner, tea, toasted Hovis bread and butter, and scrambled egg for supper.

" I have been troubled terribly with insomnia and can sleep only on injections of Morphia. I do want natural sleep badly. Sometimes my urine is very thick, and I was wondering if drinking any amount of parsley, as well as taking it in other ways, would stop the progress of the kidney trouble. I have been taking pills, etc., from the doctor.

" Naturally I am very weak, but, until I went under their treatment, I was not nearly so bad. The doctor told my wife last night that it was now not so much the heart, although it is still bad, but the kidneys, the urine from which was poisoning my system.

" Mr. Barker, you are a man I have always had wonderful confidence in, and I certainly think if anyone can help me and prolong my life, it is you. I shall expect you to be prompt, as usual."

With a trembling hand and with his last ebbing strength poor Mr. J. B. wrote this letter. I immediately sent him by registered post my reply and some medicine, but I never heard from him again.

Before he came under my care, he had been depressed and injured by being told that he suffered from valvular heart disease, a dilated heart and Bright's disease. During my treatment he had had a slight stroke which ought to have been explained to him as a fainting fit or violent indigestion, but he was crudely told that he suffered from disseminated sclerosis. When, towards the end of his life, he was in a very low condition, three doctors and a consultant were called in who told him that he suffered from " heart valvulitis, low blood pressure and kidney disease " and that he could not live long. Thus they poisoned his mind and destroyed his vitality.

The treatment by the four doctors consisted in the usual doping with Morphia, etc., which, of course, aggravated his complaints. The treatment which he was given was unconscionable, both from the medicinal and from the psychological points of view. I had given the poor man more than two years of comfort, hope and happiness. I feel certain that if he had been given orthodox treatment at the time when he placed himself under my care, he would have died in a few months. The health foundation which I had laboriously created in that poor wreck in the course of two years was rapidly destroyed by daily injections of Morphia and other maltreatments.

CHAPTER III

Migraine and Neuralgic Headaches

MIGRAINE is a violent, long-lasting and one-sided headache. Frequently one meets cases where it has been in evidence 10, 20 or more years. Occasionally migraine is due to a cerebral tumour, or to chronic nephritis, but in the vast majority of cases the cause is a mystery. Like all chronic diseases, it is considered practically incurable by most doctors and medical writers. The information contained in the standard textbooks on treatment is discouraging. In Letheby Tidy's *Synopsis of Medicine* we read: " It often defies treatment. Among drugs best are Bromides, long course, as in epilepsy, Nitro-glycerine, etc." Continued use of Bromides produces Bromide poisoning and a Bromide skin eruption. Besides, it injures the brain. During attacks Aspirin, Phenacetin, and other drugs are recommended in the textbooks but they do not cure. Some doctors try to cure the disease by methods of violence. They have all the teeth extracted, frequently without benefit, and they suggest operations on the antrums, etc. Neuralgic headaches and face aches are treated with poisonous drugs, and if they fail, operation on the nerves is proposed which often results in partial paralysis, blindness, etc.

A considerable number of migraine cases have come my way, and I have been fortunate in the great majority. A vegetarian diet will frequently produce great relief and occasionally a cure. In some cases migraine is due to coffee which may agree well with the victim who has not the slightest suspicion that it produces these temporary prostrating attacks. In his paper *On the Effects of Coffee*, published by Hahnemann in 1803, we read: " If the quantity of coffee taken be immoderately great and the body very excitable and quite unused to coffee, there occurs a semi-lateral headache from the upper part of the parietal bone to the base of the brain. Very slight things cause in the coffee-drinking lady migraine, or a frequent, often intolerable, toothache on one side of the face. The migraine alluded to only appears after some exciting cause, such as vexation, over-loading of the stomach, chill, etc., and differs entirely from the so-called nervous hemicrania. The pain is almost intolerable. In very bad cases I have seen it last 36 hours."

Some years ago a young married wife, Mrs. L., living in the south of London, came to me. She was a woman of magnificent physique. She had never been ill in her life, but she suffered frequently from maddening migraines which the best doctors and consultants had failed to cure. A vegetarian diet and complete abstention from coffee, of which she was extremely fond, cured her rapidly.

There is not a single cause for migraine and neuralgic headaches. Not every case can be cured by a non-flesh diet and abstinence from coffee. The benumbing drugs employed by orthodox medicine have not cured a single case, while homœopathic medicines, indicated not by the name of the disease but by the individual symptoms of the sufferer, have cured numerous cases.

On the 19th April, 1932, I received a letter sent by Mrs. C. R. B., from Berners Street, London: —

" I have just arrived from South Africa, and, having read on the voyage, your book *Miracles of Healing and How They Are Done*, I am so desirous now of trying homœopathic methods to cure my migraine headaches."

She arrived at my house on the 26th April. I went thoroughly into her case and sent her directions, in which I summarized her condition as follows: —

" You are 48 years old, wife of a retired school inspector, have four healthy children, had three miscarriages, chiefly due to violent vomiting, and you have come to me complaining about violent headaches on the right side of the head above the eyes, from which you have suffered ever since you were 10 years old. Headaches start at the back of the skull at the top of the spine and radiate from there to the right temple. They last either 24 or 48 hours, they are accompanied by nausea and liverishness, they usually start early in the morning, are relieved by lying quiet and heat, you feel worst about 3 or 4 in the afternoon, get a pain which radiates from the liver to the face, are excessively fond of bread and butter, take much salt, drink numerous cups of coffee, greatly over-sweetened, have cold feet in bed. You had eclampsia after the first baby, your mother died of pneumonia at 68, and she suffered from petit mal after the change of life."

The lady looked ill, worn and anxious, had swollen toe joints, had lost all her teeth through abscesses, and was altogether in a very poor condition. Bowels were in excellent order. I took the view that her right-sided headache might be due to large quantities of coffee or to auto-intoxication. I forbade flesh, fish, fowl and everything made of them, coffee, and told her to take the minimum of sugar and salt. As she suffered from sleeplessness, I gave her Coffea in the 30th potency, which would probably give her sleep and antidote at the same time the coffee. In addition I gave her Sanguinaria 1X, which is an excellent medicine for many right-sided headaches.

Mrs. B. thought it quite out of the question that she should lose a headache which had been with her for 38 years. I did my utmost to raise her hopes and she started treatment immediately and enthusiastically.

On the 1st May she sent me her first report and, referring to the sketch of her troubles which I had given in my directions, she gave me a few supplementary facts which proved her salvation : —

" I think I ought to mention a sympton which may be trivial or may be helpful and that is that when my headache is bad, I am always conscious of a mass of phlegm, which seems to have gathered at the back of my nose. It is peculiarly noticeable when I am lying down and I keep wanting to swallow it away. And there is also a slight neuralgic pain down the ridge of the nose coming from the eyebrows more or less."

An orthodox physician would immediately have thought of the cavities which stand in connection with the nasal passages and would have explored them for inflammation and the accumulation of pus, and would have proposed a draining operation. It occurred to me that the orthodox proceeding might be correct. At the same time I have so often seen pus-filled cavities become normal by the use of the indicated homœopathic remedy that I had no desire to send Mrs. B. to a surgeon. Besides, an operation might not have cured the migraine for which she had consulted me. Lastly, I thought that the numerous doctors and specialists whom she had previously consulted would in all probability have examined the cavities of the skull.

There are various remedies which are indicated if there is a sense of fullness at the root of the nose, such as Gelsemium, Kali bichromicum,^{200} Paris quadrifolia, Sticta pulmonaria and seven or eight others. Among the various remedies Sticta pulmonaria, the old-fashioned Lungwort, seemed to me most indicated. I wrote to her on the 3rd May:—

" I send you a new medicine Sticta pulmonaria 1X, marked ' Fullness back of nose, catarrh, headache.' I suspect that your headache is catarrhal and I would like you to give this medicine a good trial. Take 3 pilules three times a day between meals."

Her next letter was dated the 18th May. She complained about pain in her left foot, a headache on the top of the head, which she attributed to suppressed menstruation, and a gouty tendency which was in her family. Her right-sided migraine headache was not mentioned. I was surprised and sent her some medicine to regulate her period. Her next letter, dated 30th May, amazed me:—

"I should have written last week to thank you, but I was prostrated with an attack of lumbago and could not write. This is my leave-taking letter. You have cured miraculously the headaches from which I have suffered so much and I do thank you with all by heart. If I feel one coming on in the early morning, I take 3 of your Sticta pulmonaria pilules and to my great joy the headache fades away in a few hours. It is marvellous, for they used to continue for a day or two days."

She told me that she would write to me from Africa if she wanted more homœopathic medicine for her headache. I sent her a helping of Sticta pulmonaria, but as I never heard from her, I assume that the cure was permanent.

The most interesting point about this case is the fact that Sticta pulmonaria is not enumerated in the textbooks of homœopathy among the right-sided migraine remedies. Homœopaths have no specifics for the names of diseases. They are guided by the totality of symptoms, or by the most urgent symptoms, or the most telling symptoms, without regard to the name of the disease. That makes homœopathy so puzzling to the orthodox physician who has been taught to make an exact diagnosis and who then looks for the "specific" in his literature. If a good homœopath is asked: "What medicine do you give for right-sided migraine?" he will truthfully answer: "One can give Sanguinaria, Chelidonium, Iris,[30] and a few others, which produce and cure right-sided headaches, but any of the other thousand remedies may be indicated by the symptoms of the patient."

Mr. J. C., a busy dentist in Northumberland, told me on the 30th September, 1928:—

"I am 37 years of age and blessed with what has been diagnosed as a chronic appendix. I will not bother you with a recital of medical attention and chemists' nostrums of the last ten years, except to say that about July, 1927, while busy with the 50th bottle of medicine of that particular series, I had the good fortune to become acquainted with your book, *Good Health and Happiness*. Following its advice, I scrapped the medicine and gradually improved in health so much that this summer has been a real joy to me, for which many thanks.

"Unfortunately a month ago I had an attack of gastric influenza, and this looks like reducing me to the same state of chronic indigestion that existed prior to July, 1927. My doctor, an excellent fellow and a dear friend, merely scoffs at diet, as interpreted by yourself and others of like opinion. Can you tell me how to get back to the period of improvement that existed a month ago? The desire for work and exercise is going rapidly, and I find medical advice on diet just as useless as that which I received during my hospital training. One has to be careful not to give offence when working so closely with the medical profession, but I am sorry to say their knowledge of diet, as you know it, is practically nil."

Doctors must not treat a case which they have not seen, although the patient may not be able to travel to the doctor or the doctor to the patient. I never hesitate to treat by letter people far away if the case is clear. I asked Mr. J. C. for further details and a photograph of his face, addressing to him numerous questions relating to his medical history and inheritance, etc. On the 4th October he told me that he had had double pneumonia, had never been robust, had had migraine from childhood onward. The migraine was aggravated by lack of exercise, he being a very busy man: —

"The migraine attacks have also returned and my doctor says he thinks they are due to worrying about a tremendous amount of masonic work I have to do, in conjunction with the indigestion caused by the appendix. I have had indigestion more or less for the last ten years and have treated it by the usual method of chemists' dope. Since abandoning this method and trying to follow your diet, I have benefited much."

In a further letter of the 11th October he wrote:—

"The migraine starts with disordered vision, with partial blindness. I can only see part of a word or part of a person's face when looking at them. Then a most peculiar feeling, a sort of contracted stiffness, spreads down the left side of my face, tongue and arm. Speech is affected. A violent boring pain over the right eye follows, which finishes up with a general headache which sometimes lasts for days at a stretch. My indigestion is usually bad at the same time."

It was quite clear to me that this fearful migraine was due, at least in part, to indigestion, chronic constipation and auto-intoxication. I sent him a diet sheet and, notwithstanding the delicate state of his stomach, he was to take large dishes of bran porridge made of equal weights of coarse oatmeal and ordinary bran, boiled a few minutes. Flesh, fish, fowl and everything made of them were forbidden, he was put on a milky diet, large quantities of bran were to be added to his milk puddings, and, as a digestive help, I gave him some Carbo vegetabilis 3X and Nux vomica trit. 3. On the 18th October the dentist wrote:—

"Unfortunately I had an attack of migraine just a few hours before receiving your directions. When I received your letter, I was taking a Bismuth mixture for my stomach and a bottle for my headache, which I think was Luminal. These I dropped, as requested. I am pleased to say that I have felt a little better the last couple of days."

With extraordinary brainlessness people suffering with indigestion are given every day the Bismuth mixture, which is also called the white mixture. Hundreds of patients have come to me with indigestion and when I ask them, "Are you having the white mixture?" they usually answer "Yes." Occasionally I ask the second question, "For how long have you been taking it?" and I may be told, "Oh, I have been taking it for years." And if I ask, "Has it done you any good?" I may be told, "Not to my knowledge." Probably the majority of my readers have received at one time of their lives the useless and dangerous Bismuth mixture, which is just as worthless as Pepsin, which was handed to all stomach sufferers a few decades ago and which is no longer the fashion. Luminal, which that poor fellow was given for his headache, is a habit-creating poison which has never cured a headache, exactly as the Bismuth mixture has never cured faulty digestion, but both medicines may relieve for a time and both can be prescribed without examination of the patient and without giving any thought.

Mr. C. immediately abandoned his dopes, took his horse fodder cheerfully and hopefully, and did well. On the 1st November, after three or four weeks' treatment, he wrote:—

"I am very pleased to say I have not had an attack of migraine since commencing your treatment. My bowels are working well and my appetite is very much improved."

On the 16th January, 1929, he reported:—

"I am very much better indeed. I feel better, look better and eat better and with relish, of course. in accordance with your instructions. I have never had a real attack of migraine since commencing your treatment. I think this proves the migraine was due to faulty diet and not to any nerve complaint, requiring drugging with Luminal. I am very grateful for your advice and quite realize that the errors of years cannot be put right in a few weeks."

A month later he wrote:—

"I have not had a *real* dose of migraine since commencing your treatment four months ago."

On the 6th March he sent me a bad report, telling me of "a very severe attack of migraine, but on the opposite side," and he concluded, and apparently correctly, that this was not one of his old migraines but an influenzal headache, as he felt weak and shaky. I thereupon sent him some Eupatorium perfoliatum 1X for influenza, and, after a while, some Sulphur 3X to deal with its after-effects. Both medicines suited him well and he rapidly got better. He rebuilt his constitution and by simple commonsense measures, which it would take too long to describe, one weakness after the other was eliminated. On the 5th October, 1929, he wrote:—

" It is now a year since I started following your excellent advice, and, looking back over that period, there is not the slightest doubt that the improvement in my physical well-being has been remarkable. Set-backs there have certainly been, but, taking the long view, the results are very gratifying and I hope permanent. I may not be ' just perfect ' as you once put it, but as time goes on I may even attain that stage."

Apparently the man was permanently cured. He wrote to me on the 14th February, 1933; four and a half years after I took him in hand:—

" I am very glad to say that, thanks to your skilful treatment of migraine, it is so long ago since I had an attack that I have forgotten when it was. I have had one or two exceedingly slight suspicions of it when I have had a worrying time or have neglected my diet for a period, but I don't know now what the old-fashioned attacks were like. For all this, please accept my grateful thanks. I have built up my method of life, as you suggested, eat plenty of vegetables both raw and steamed, use dairy produce instead of meat, and live a quite happy life instead of being the chronic invalid I was gradually becoming. If ever I should be in health difficulties, I should like to feel that I can rely on your skilful co-operation."

Success on the part of a prescriber, medical or lay, depends partly on his determination to cure the patient, partly on the determination of the patient to get well and to co-operate whole-heartedly with his adviser. Mr. J. C. was an ideal patient and his cure was largely due to his co-operation.

On the 18th March, 1932, I was visited by a lady 56 years old, Miss M. C., who explained to me that she was a cook, but not an ordinary cook. She was a great artist and told me that she had to give up work in consequence of her ever-increasing sufferings. Most great cooks whom I have known have been great sufferers. I suppose it is one of their professional risks. Artists must love their art if they wish to succeed. Good cooks love good eating.

The lady informed me that she suffered the most atrocious headaches, which ran along the top of the skull on a thin line, obviously along a nerve. When the pain got particularly severe, it crept down the right side of the face towards the right nostril and right ear. In addition to this neuralgic headache, she had also bilious headaches which had prostrated her periodically since childhood. The use of the right arm was apt to bring on the headache. She had the sensation of insects crawling over her, of cold water trickling down the back of the head. The attacks were becoming worse from month to month and were aggravated by stomach upsets.

It was significant that, before the attacks, her urine was clear, but it became cloudy during and after attacks. The same urinary symptom frequently occurs before, during and after attacks of epilepsy, gout, etc., and it indicates that bowels and other organs do not function properly, and that poisonous materials are periodically thrown into the blood stream, producing headaches, gout, epilepsy, etc. The lady had been treated by numerous doctors and specialists for the names of her complaints. Not one of her advisers had ever enquired into their causation and Miss M. C.'s method of living.

I discovered that 33 years previously she had fallen very severely. Her chin struck a tiled floor, she had broken eight teeth, lay unconscious, and had experienced great pain when chewing during the next two years. Since then she had also suffered much from violent sneezing fits. I concluded that that injury was largely responsible for her troubles. She took large quantities of salt and mustard which undoubtedly had injured her liver and kidneys, was constipated, had varicose veins, worse on the right leg, which proclaimed that the liver, which is situated on the right side of the abdomen, was not functioning properly, and this assumption was confirmed by the fact that she disliked thick butter, cream, eggs. She felt a sinking at eleven o'clock which suggested Sulphur, felt always worse in the afternoon, which suggested Lycopodium, could not empty her bladder if people were near, which pointed to Natrum muriaticum, had the sensation of a hair in the throat which made one think of Silica.

As she was stout and flabby, I gave her a reducing diet, and told her that she would have to live largely on porridge made of whole wheat and bran, of which I showed her a sample. I shall never forget the expression of horror with which she looked at it: " Take it away, take it away. I cannot bear to look at it." The soul of a great cook rose up in indignation. I replied: " I shall not prescribe for you until you have eaten the portion before you." After eloquent protests she ate it.

I gave her Natrum muriaticum 30, 3 night and morning because of her chilliness, and huge intake of salt, Nux vomica and Carbo vegetabilis combined three times a day before meals to help her digestion and excretion, and Arnica 3X, a dose three times between meals for the shock and injury produced by her fall 33 years ago. Her bowels were activated by bran, reinforced by liquid paraffin if necessary.

On the 28th March she reported: " The neuralgic headaches, though still recurring nightly, pass away quicker, lasting from 3 to 4 or 5 hours. I certainly feel less tired after my day's work. My weight is 10 stone 5½ lbs." On the 10th April she wrote: " I am taking my case seriously because you have given me hope for good health, and I had begun to despair of ever having health again, having tried so many doctors. The neuralgia has been less severe this week and the indigestion also. I feel stronger. I weigh 10 stone 2 lbs. 2 ozs." On the 18th April she said: " I weigh 9 stone 13½ lbs., feel stronger and more able to face the day's work." I sent her Colocynthis and Magnesia phosphorica for her headaches. On the 25th April she wrote: " The biliousness seems a lot better, Magnesia phosphorica has helped me a lot with my headaches, I weigh 9 stone 13 lbs."

On the 6th May the lady came to me and I wrote to her: " You looked very ill, depressed, hopeless, when you came to me a month ago and thoroughly unwholesome. To-day you were smiling, had a beautifully clear skin, bright eyes, glossy hair, red lips, had lost a stone, walked with springy steps, and have vastly improved all round and further improvement is bound to follow." As she complained of rheumatic pain, worst in bed and relieved by movement, she was given Rhus tox. 3X in alternation with Arnica.

On the 23rd May she wrote: " The rheumatism has been much less severe and I have had very little headache. I weigh 9 stone 10½ lbs." Then she developed catarrh of the bladder and was given Cantharis. Then came pain in the kidneys and back and she received Berberis, mother tincture, in alternation with Arnica for her old injury. On the 8th June she wrote: " Pain in side of head is nothing like as severe as it was." On the 15th June she told me: " Berberis has benefited me greatly and also Arnica. I weigh 9 stone 8 lbs." On the 27th June she wrote: " I am feeling ever so much better. I shall recommend the homœopathic treatment to every one of my friends."

On the 11th July she complained of a new symptom: " I notice that very often when the pain in the head is bad, mucus seems to break at the back of the nose and then I get relief." I sent her Sticta pulmonaria, and that trouble cleared up. Then I was informed that she was apt to wake at three o'clock in the morning with a headache and very naturally I sent her Kali carb., and she wrote a fortnight after that that medicine had been extraordinarily helpful. On the 1st November she wrote: " I am feeling very well. It is really wonderful to me to go on week after week with no bad headache and no sickness."

Her last letter to me was dated 19th December: " I feel so much better that I am able to earn my living again." She had lost the terrific neuralgic head aches, bilious headaches, pains in back and kidneys, rheumatism, catarrh, and all her other troubles which had made life unbearable, and had become a healthy, strong, joyous woman once more. She tastes now the dainty food which she cooks but does not eat it. She has learned better.

Nausea and vomiting with Headache : (Amenorrhoea) –

– Nux Vom 1000

CHAPTER IV

Some Show Cases—Diabetes, Disseminated Sclerosis, Cancer, Sarcoma, Enlarged Prostate, Paralysis, etc.

MR. B. J. a clergyman, 64 years old, living in Wales, wrote to me on the 30th June, 1934, that he had been suffering from Diabetes for two and a half years, that he had been continuously under Insulin, and that he was injecting about fifteen units of Insulin a day, regulating the quantity by analysis of urine, which he made himself several times a day. I replied promptly that I did not care to undertake his case as I had found that Insulin never cured diabetes, but made the patients slaves to that dangerous drug.

He insisted upon having my advice, and, very much against my wish, visited me in London on the 13th July, 1934, and gave me all the details of this case. The doctors and specialists who had treated him had carefully analysed his urine, blood, etc.; they had given him the usual diet and the usual Insulin and had treated " the disease " without investigating the individual needs of the individual patient, as is usually done. I told Mr. B. J. quite frankly that I was not at all interested in the analysis of his blood and urine and his standardized diet, but that I wished to find out the cause of his trouble which to me was all-important. He could not enlighten me, but careful enquiry elicited the fact that he had had a great trouble twenty-seven years previously which I considered the cause of his disease. I wrote in my directions: —

"The most striking fact which came out in your interrogation was that in 1906-7 you were deeply disappointed in love and have been terribly depressed ever since. There is evidently a deep psychical injury."

Very frequently increase in the sugar content of Mr. B. J.'s urine coincided with the deepest depression caused by thoughts of his old love and by an overwhelming sensation that the lady of his choice was near him or was suffering. Ignatia is a great medicine for grief and sorrow. As the trouble was of such long standing a high potency was needed. I gave him immediately at my house a single dose of Ignatia in the 1,000th potency, told him to take a single dose of Ignatia 200th potency rarely as needed, and gave him Diluted Phosphoric Acid containing a little Ignatia of which he was to take ten drops after meals. Mr. B. J. looked very sceptically at the tasteless sugar pills and the colourless drops which he was given.

Improvement was instantaneous both in the man's illness and in his mind. Three days later on the 16th July he wrote: "Analysis of urine shows that this morning the urine was sugar-free, although I injected Insulin only once yesterday instead of twice as before." On the 20th July, after seven days' treatment, he wrote: "My depression is certainly less severe than when you saw me. I feel considerably better. I am awfully glad I came to see you. Life has already taken a brighter and more gladsome aspect." On the 27th July, after a fortnight's treatment, he wrote: "You will rejoice to learn that my reaction to your treatment continues to be most satisfactory. During the last five days there was not even a trace of sugar in my urine." Three days later on the 30th July, he wrote full of joy: "Henceforth I shall test the urine only three times a week and after a few weeks' time only once a week."

Mr. B. J. wrote one joyful letter after another. He then went to Shrewsbury, and to his dismay sugar reappeared in the urine. I discovered that he had taken considerable quantities of mushrooms, to which he was unaccustomed. I forbade him eating any more mushrooms, and urine became rapidly normal, although he did not resort to Insulin. On the 25th August he wrote: " My urine is still free—sugar free —and the depression is quite gone." On the 15th September, after two months of treatment, he stated: " My general health has much improved since my visit to you. Your medicine has worked quite a miracle. I have put on weight."

Shortly after he complained about his eyesight. It is a well-known fact that diabetics are liable to cataract. I thought a blood-clearing medicine indicated, and sent him a few doses of Sulphur 6X, which led to an improvement in his eyesight. My patient took doses of Ignatia 200 more and more rarely. On the 1st December, 1934, he wrote: " I have not taken a single pill since the 25th September." And he wrote on the 4th December: " The measure of my gratitude to you is inexpressible by the language at my command. There is no combination of words that can tell all I feel for what you have done for me."

On the 8th February, 1935, he wrote: " I am delighted with the success of your treatment of my diabetic affliction. It is really marvellous. Not for several years has my health been so good, and, as to the depression, it has all gone. When I am worried, there is a return of the depression for the period of the upset, but as soon as the worry ceases, depression flies away, and I am in the pink of good condition. Under God's gracious blessing I am indebted entirely to you for the present good state of my health. You will, I am sure, be interested in the following fact. Until about three weeks ago I prayed as usual: 'Oh Lord, heal me of my diabetes.' Whilst on my knees in my morning devotion I made the above request, and the Lord replied immediately: ' Why pray for that which

E

you already possess.' Since then I have ceased to pray for a cure. If the old request forms itself on my lips, as sometimes it does, I fail utterly to give utterance to it. The form my prayer now takes is: ' I thank thee, Lord, for directing me to homœopathy, and enabling me to give up Insulin,' and I invariably conclude my prayer with the words. ' Bless Mr. Ellis Barker.' " On the 12th February my patient wrote: " You are my most kind friend and greatest benefactor. During my journey through life I made many friends, but not one benefactor whom I can compare with you. As Jesus Christ stands alone as a physician who has healed the disease of my soul, so you stand alone as the physician who has healed the greatest disease from which my body has suffered—the disease which orthodox physicians declare to be incurable. I never cease to thank God for having led me to consult you."

Successes like this diabetes cure and the sensation that one has helped a splendid man who has suffered greatly in body and mind make life worth living, and the satisfaction derived from such a cure is the greatest reward of every true doctor.

On the 1st November, 1934, I received a letter from the Regional Benevolent Agent of the British Legion Relief Fund at Leeds with regard to a Mr. J. T., who suffered from disseminated sclerosis—in plain words, from creeping paralysis. The patient had appealed to Sir Herbert Barker, Sir Herbert Barker had advised Mr. J. T. to consult me, and I wrote to the agent, that I would gladly see the man, but added: " Disseminated sclerosis is a very difficult complaint to deal with. It is incurable from the orthodox point of view, but I have had occasional successes."

On the 21st November, Mr. J. T. came to my consulting rooms. He was a gardener, 43 years old, had been married eleven years, and was childless. He had suffered from paralysis since childhood. When he was 13 he had been operated upon for appendicitis, and eighteen months afterwards he lost control of the muscles of the face. When serving in Mesopotamia in 1915 his legs became paralysed and then other members were similarly affected. He could not keep his balance with his eyes closed, he found it impossible to touch his nose with his eyes closed. He stumbled when trying to use his legs, his eyelids fell down, and he had to lift them up with his fingers if he wanted to see. He had been given the usual routine treatment with the usual lack of success, and he was in despair.

I discovered that he lived on a ghastly diet, strong black tea, white bread and butter, large quantities of meat, sanatogen, etc. He had been vaccinated frequently, and at the first vaccination the vaccine had been taken from another child. In 1917 he had received a severe blow on the head by a bullet striking his steel helmet.

I gave Mr. J. T., who was toothless in consequence of his wretched diet, a diet rich in bran, wholemeal bread, raw fruit and salading, and forbade flesh, fish, fowl and all heating foods. For medicine I gave him Sulphur 6X as a blood-clearing medicine, Causticum 3X for the paralysis, which he had to take daily, and for the probable causes of this paralysis I gave him a dose of Thuja 200 as a vaccination antidote every Sunday, and a dose of Lueticum 200 every Wednesday. To supple his limbs he was to be massaged by his wife with unrefined cod-liver oil, with which I had done veritable miracles in the past.

On the 9th December, after two and a half weeks' treatment, his wife reported: " The eyelids have been quite all right this week and have not dropped. I really think there is an improvement." He then was given Fluoric Acid 6 and Thuja 3X. On the 22nd December his wife reported: " My husband's eyelids have been normal for about 12 days," and on the 30th December she reported, to my joy: " My husband has had an extra good week. He is improving wonderfully. He sleeps and walks much better." On the 3rd January the Honorary Secretary of the British Legion at Fence reported to me: " There is no doubt whatever in the matter that the man Mr. J. T. is decidedly improving, and we are hoping under the circumstances that your further efforts may result in a permanent cure after some time."

Of course there were ups and downs, but the man did wonderfully well; and then he was given a few doses of Lueticum 1,000 and Aurum 6X twice between meals.

On the 15th March, after three and a half months' treatment, his wife wrote: "My husband is walking very well indeed, and you would be surprised how many people have called to see him since starting your treatment. They think it is wonderful to see him looking like his old self again." Then his wife told me his walking was normal, and the 15th April, 1935, she joyfully told me that her husband had walked a mile.

On the 16th April the Honorary Secretary of the British Legion wrote: "There is no doubt whatever that the man is improving. Mr. J. T. still has his bad days, but they are at longer intervals, and he recovers more quickly. He can walk very much better; in fact, he has improved in every way. He goes to his panel doctor monthly for his insurance certificate, and he told the doctor he was going to get better. The doctor replied: 'We shall see.' 'There is no seeing about it,' said Mr. T. The case is causing considerable interest in our district. The treatment will have to be continued by hook or by crook with your consent. The Committee tender hearty thanks for your work to date."

On the 10th May Mr. J. T. visited me for the second time. He had changed beyond belief, he looked the picture of health, energy and happiness, and, instead of shuffling and stumbling along with the help of his wife, he walked with springy athletic steps. Standing at the side of the table, he put first the right foot on the table, standing on the left leg, and the left foot on the table, standing on the right. He touched his nose with tightly closed eyes, which he had never been able to do when examined by the specialists. He told me that he could walk miles, that his eyelids had not fallen down for months, that he could work hard in the field or garden. He and his wife had not desired children because he had been afflicted since before their marriage, now they hoped to have children.

I have a patient in the eastern district of London, a Mrs. L., a highly intelligent woman about 50 years old, whom I treated for gallstones and various other complaints. Occasionally she had told me that her mother was very stout, that she ate incredible quantities of meat and other heating foods, took strong tea, large quantities of condiments and alcohol, and that the old lady was sure to suffer in due course. Her fear came true. The lady developed a tumour in the breast, it was declared to be cancerous, an extensive operation was made, and microscopic examination proved that the growth was malignant. As the doctors had not given any instructions as regards her diet, she continued to eat and drink the most irritating foods, disregarding the warnings of her daughter.

Before the operation the old lady had developed jaundice and had lost weight. As happens frequently, after the operation she gained flesh and felt quite comfortable, but in due course there came trouble. Ominous swellings developed in and about the operation scar, the old lady became deeply jaundiced, and then came discomfort, and at last pain unbearable and outrageous.

In autumn 1934 the daughter of the cancer sufferer told me over the telephone that she had just been with her mother and she was suffering terribly. She concluded: " Do you think you can help her? " In these cases the doctor has no treatment, except pain-killing morphia, which does no cure, but which injures and poisons the patient. The after-effects of morphia are comparable to the after-effects of a debauch, only they are very much worse in the case of morphia. Homœopathy is wonderfully resourceful in such cases. One has to enquire carefully into the character of the pain, and prescribe infinitely small doses of a medicine that gives the same kind of pain if taken in large doses.

The old lady had two different kinds of pain. There was in the first place a terrible pain of constriction in and about the operation scar, a pain comparable to that caused by winding wire tightly round the chest. The second kind of pain was a terrible burning sensation which was accompanied by extreme restlessness. As the burning pain was relieved by heat, the choice of the remedies was obvious. I sent the old lady Cactus Grandiflorus in the 30th potency for the constricting pain, and Arsenic in the 200th potency for burning pain and restlessness. The patient was to take whichever medicine was indicated by her symptoms, and doses were to be taken only when necessary.

To my surprise and delight both medicines gave the most wonderful relief. The pain disappeared completely. The old lady lost her jaundiced looks; she declared herself cured, and she developed an enormous appetite.

During the eight months following the prescription of these medicines there has been steady progress. She has become stouter than ever. Her daughter had wished to bring her to me in her motor-car, but the old lady has become so enormously stout that she can no longer go by car. I advised her daughter to bring her to me in a furniture van.

In summer 1934 Miss S. of Hendon told me casually that her mother was in bed with pain in one of her legs. I thought it a matter of little importance, and sent her Bryonia, which she was to take if the pain was aggravated by movement, and Rhus Toxicodendron, which she was to take if the pain was relieved by movement. Neither medicine helped. I tried various other remedies, and at last I went to see Mrs. S. I discovered she had been in bed for months, but she looked the picture of health, had a milkmaid's complexion, bright eyes, was vivacious, and could not explain the character of her pain. She was obviously not a very observant woman. She could not even tell me whether the pain was felt in the muscles, in the nerves, or in the bones. At last the daughter told me casually that the pain was always aggravated if the mother took a meal. Pain in the leg aggravated by eating is a rare and unusual symptom. I discovered that symptom in Kent's *Repertory*, and against it there was only one remedy Kali Carbonicum, plain carbonate of soda. Reference to the *Materia Medica* showed that this remedy was likely to be helpful. I sent her Kali Carbonicum in the 6th decimal potency. She took a millionth of a grain of carbonate of potash three times a day with excellent result. The pain disappeared, but it came back again. I tried Kali Carbonicum in lower, higher and very high potencies, but they only helped for a time. There was obviously some very serious factor in the way which had to be discovered.

An X-ray photograph of Mrs. S. disclosed the terrible fact that she suffered from a large sarcoma seated at the bottom of the spine. Sarcoma is classed with cancer, under the general heading of malignant diseases. Both are equally deadly. Orthodox medicine has no treatment for sarcoma except operation, which was out of the question, as the lady was well over 70, and was determined not to be operated upon.

Her case resembled that of the mother of Mrs. L. There was burning pain, relieved by heat and restlessness. I therefore resolved to treat Mrs. S. with Arsenic. She received that medcine in various potencies from the third centesimal to the thousandth potency, and she reacted most satisfactorily. Her pain disappeared, but she could not leave her bed. She remained cheerful, and enjoyed every day of her life. At last the bladder ceased to function, either because the growth was pressing on the nerves controlling the bladder, or because the bladder had been invaded by the growth. The urine had to be drawn off with a catheter and it was very foul. Berberis and Chimaphila, both in mother tincture, gave some relief, but Arsenic in various potencies was her great standby.

At the beginning of May, 1935, Mrs. S. was losing ground rapidly, her colour became ghastly, she looked very ill, and on the morning of the 17th May she died peacefully without pain. For months and months Mrs. S. had been the victim of one of the most painful diseases known to medicine, but she died without pain peacefully and without morphia. Homœopathy can give wonderful relief in cases where a cure is not possible.

In a special chapter I have described a number of cases of enlarged prostate in which improvement occurred with the usual slowness after months of treatment. Occasionally cases of enlarged prostate, declared incurable except by operation by the orthodox doctor and specialist, get well in a few weeks; but these cases are exceptional, they are true show cases. An enlargement which has been caused in the course of ten or more years cannot be expected to disappear except after many months of patient endeavour.

On the 13th December, 1934, I was visited by Mr. W. C. G., a retired accountant, who looked in poor health, had had a nervous breakdown in 1913, and his doctor had told him there was no treatment for his enlarged prostate except operation. Being nervy he worried much about his prostate, which had troubled him for many years. I gave him an appropriate diet, an abundance of liquid to make his urine less acrid and started him on Sulphur 6X to be taken night and morning, and a combination of Ignatia 3X and Carbo Vegetabilis to be taken before meals. As he had a weak chest, he was given Bacillinum in the 30th potency once a week. After a week's time I replaced Sulphur by Arsenic 3 because of his restlessness, and gave him a 100th of a grain of thyroid before meals as he did not have much appetite.

He improved with surprising rapidity. On the 15th January, 1935, a month after the beginning of the treatment, he wrote to me: " I am glad I was prevented from writing to you yesterday as I had intended, for I saw my doctor. He told me I was looking much better, and then I said that I was cured of my complaint, and he thought it was marvellous. He was much interested in my case and says that although the inflammation is gone, the prostate still remains enlarged. At the back of his mind there was the thought that the symptoms may return. Be that as it may, I am delighted to inform you that I have no swelling, pain, or discomfort, and can pass water naturally and easily, even at night. Apart from this, I feel better than I have for many years. My brain, which I used to think was shrinking, has swelled out again and is functioning properly. So I really think you have rejuvenated me. Many thanks for what you have done." Six weeks after, Mr. W. C. G. wrote. "It is six weeks since I wrote to you. I am glad to say there has been no return of the symptoms."

In a single month the man considered himself cured. A moderate increase of the prostate reduces the holding capacity of the bladder, it is very frequent and of no particular seriousness. On the other hand, an inflamed prostate causes pain, an intolerable urging, difficulty of holding and making water, with great anxiety. That condition can readily be cured by non-heating and non-irritating diet, and a few homoeopathic medicines, a treatment which is unfortunately unknown to the orthodox members of the profession.

Malaria is a dangerous and an exceedingly pertinacious disease. It is treated as a rule with large doses of Quinine, which is harmful to the blood, and many of those who have taken much Quinine will remain jaundiced for life, while others become deaf. People who have been in the tropics and who have contracted Malaria have frequently regular recurrences which undermine the health and they are kept in check by large doses of Quinine. Homoeopathy has had wonderful successes in dealing with acute and inveterate Malaria and Quinine poisoning which goes hand in hand with that disease.

One of the most valuable remedies for dealing with Malaria and Quinine poisoning is ordinary table salt

in infinitely small doses homœopathically prepared
and potentised. The homœopaths call this remedy
Natrum Muriaticum. I have devoted a special chapter
to this wonderful medicine, superscribed " Miracles
done by Table Salt " in my book *Miracles of Healing
and How They are Done*. Hahnemann, the founder of
homœopathy, wrote with full justification: " Pure
common salt, dynamized, like any other homœopathic substance, is one of the most powerful
medicines; it is a heroic and mighty remedy."

On the 11th September, 1929, I was visited by an
emaciated lady, a veritable skeleton covered with
jaundiced skin, with deeply sunken eyes. She told
me that she was a missionary from West Africa. She
had always been anæmic, she felt terribly weak, and
she suffered from daily attacks of Malaria which were
kept in check by Quinine, taken in doses of 30 grains.
Her liver, gall-bladder and spleen were greatly enlarged, she had huge vaccination marks, she complained about bearing-down pains, always felt chilly,
and had a sinking feeling about eleven o'clock in the
morning. These symptoms pointed clearly to Natrum
Muriaticum as her remedy.

I gave the lady a mixed diet with an abundance of
vegetables, vegetable water, wholemeal bread, 3 pints
of Milk, 3 Eggs a day, and recommended plenty of
bitter vegetables, sultanas and raisins because they are
rich in iron and prescribed for her fever and chilliness,
Natrum Muriaticum in the 30th potency, which means
in doses of a decillionth of a grain, and Arsenicum by
the millionth of a grain. She was to take three doses
a day and to change every day from one medicine to
another. I told her not to take any Quinine unless
she was compelled to do so by an actual attack of
Malaria.

I have a photo of Mrs. C. L., taken on the 30th
September, 1929, in which she is a picture of emaciation. She immediately started putting on weight at
the rate of two or three pounds a week. She wrote
on the 11th October, a month after the beginning of

the treatment: " I have gained three pounds in weight again this week. I have felt much better, and am eating and sleeping better. I have not had any fever until this week. After my sister's sudden death, I felt very poorly, knowing that liability to fever is greater when one's condition is low. I had a sudden attack on Tuesday evening. So I took Quinine. This is the only Quinine I have taken since seeing you exactly a month ago." The next letter, written on the 18th October, told me: " I have gained three pounds 3 ozs. this week." On the 22nd November she wrote: " I feel remarkably fit. I have gained five pounds nine ozs. in the last three weeks, have not taken any medicine at all, my appetite is splendid, I can take walks and do my housework, and the sharp spell of frost we had did not leave me miserably cold as has usually been the case when I have been in England for the winter. I think you will agree I am not in need of further treatment."

Mrs. C. L. visited me some time afterwards, and I did not recognize her. She had become a magnificent woman, she had gained 30 pounds, and had had no further fever attacks. She told me that she would let me know if she needed further help. As I did not hear from her, I can only assume that her fever was permanently eliminated by a few infinitely small doses of Table Salt, reinforced by Arsenic in doses of a millionth of a grain.

Peculiar and unusual symptoms frequently point out the remedy that will cure. Among the peculiar symptoms indicating the use of Natrum Muriaticum is the inability of urinating in the presence of other people. I had been very fortunate in treating a Mrs. L. She sent me her husband, who also needed help. Mr. G. L. had been extremely poor in his youth. He then was tall, very slender, a magnificent runner, excellent at many sports and games. He had become wealthy, he had abandoned bodily exercise, and, like many former athletes, he had become extremely stout, and he complained of a poor digestion and weak chest.

He was apt to contract bronchitis, pleurisy and pneumonia and dreaded exposure to the fresh air.

I asked him if he could tell me of any unusual symptoms, and he told me that he was quite unable to empty his bladder in a public lavatory if anyone else was present. That symptom, his chilliness, the watering of his eyes, and his great liking of salt, clearly indicated that he needed Natrum Muriaticum, and I prescribed for him that medicine in doses of a decillionth of a grain. A week after his wife told me excitedly over the telephone: " A miracle has happened with my husband's eyes! " " He never spoke to me about his eyes," I replied. " Of course he did not mention his eyes because you are not an oculist." Mrs. L. told me that her husband had been quite unable to read in artificial light. He had consulted numerous opticians and oculists who had prescribed glasses, but they had not helped him. He was a very domesticated man. So he sat in the evening at the table shading or covering his eyes. " But now he can read in the artificial light without glasses! It is wonderful! " About a year afterwards Mr. G. L. called on me and told me that his stomach and chest had greatly improved. " Can you still read without glasses in artificial light? " I asked. " Yes, I can." " And what about your little trouble in going to the lavatory? " " That has completely disappeared as well." Natrum Muriaticum is a wonderful medicine.

Early in 1933 I was consulted by a professional lady practising in the Harley Street quarter. She complained about indigestion and constipation. She looked jaundiced, had dark eyes, dark hair, a dark skin, was extremely irritable and was very fond of highly spiced food. All her symptoms clearly pointed to Nux Vomica. I prescribed for her Nux Vomica in doses of one thousandth of a grain. A few days afterwards I saw her and she angrily enquired, " What was the name of the medicine you gave me? It poisoned me! " I immediately told her, " I have

given you Nux Vomica." "Never again give me
Nux Vomica!" It came out that the medicine had
totally upset her and had led to something like a
brain storm.

Homœopaths can antidote an unsuitable remedy
by the same medicine in a very high potency. The
fact that Nux Vomica in a small dose had so badly
upset the lady indicated that this was the right remedy,
but that it had been given in too large a dose because
the lady was ultra-sensitive. A few days afterwards
I met the lady once more, and I handed her three
sugar pills moistened with Nux Vomica in the 200th
potency, and told her that the medicine would antidote
the effect of the previous dose which had upset her so
badly. Happily she swallowed the dose without
enquiry.

She started improving rapidly. Her constipation
disappeared completely. She became gentle and
sweet-tempered, and she was amazed when she was
told that the same medicine which had made her so
ill had benefited her so greatly. She was given a few
doses of Nux Vomica, she has been taking a dose every
two or three months, and she has kept perfectly well
ever since.

Mrs. L. A., living in Sussex, came to me on the 1st
May complaining of disseminated sclerosis. The lady
was 49 years old and hobbled along with difficulty
with a stick. The trouble had started when she was
19 years old, and was therefore of 30 years' standing.
Mrs. L. A. looked desperately ill and weak, and had
been treated for disseminated sclerosis by doctors and
specialists who had told her frankly that the disease
was incurable and that it could only get worse. Indeed,
it had been doing so from year to year.

In addition to being physically incapacitated through
the weakness of her legs, Mrs. L. A. looked ill, and
there was obviously some other very serious trouble.
She had a poor chest and difficulty in breathing, and
had been in a sanatorium for tuberculosis, which
disease was still upon her. Further, the position was

complicated by the fact that there was obviously a grave inherited taint. The patient's teeth had been black and crumbling, she had terrible nights, and suffered most then. There was obviously a combination of taints which had to be combated.

I gave her Sulphur 6X night and morning, and a combination of Nux Vomica and Carbo Vegetabilis before meals to antidote the numerous medicines and injections which she had previously received. In addition, I gave her once a week Bacillinum 200 and once a week Lueticum 200. She had no appetite. She was given a blood-clearing and eliminating diet with an abundance of vegetables, fruit, milk, eggs, cheese, wholemeal bread, and bran, and I raised her hopes by telling her that I liked her stick and wanted to have it and that before long she would be able to do without it.

After a week, Mrs. L. A. wrote: —

"It is with much pleasure that I can write my first week's report. I started the medicines and diet, and got a real good night's sleep, peaceful and without pain. I cannot tell how long it is since I had a good night, but not of late years. I wake up fresh and feeling better. Ever since I came to you I continue steadily to gain ground, and am fully conscious of it. Legs are stronger and steadier. Headaches have now ceased, these were continually with me in the past. Bowels are acting normally, and the pain and bleeding have also stopped. I feel ready for my food and quite enjoy it. My spirits are brighter, and I find it is good to be alive. A very short time ago I felt that death would be welcome."

After a fortnight, the lady wrote to me:—

"It is with deep thankfulness and pleasure that I send you my second week's report. I am experiencing just a big steady increase of strength and vitality through my body. My legs are less heavy and much more under control. I am once more starting a few foot and leg exercises, without getting too weary. I am sleeping much better: no uneasy dreams, no pain."

The third weekly report stated:—

" My legs are most surely getting stronger. I started going out for walks *alone* this week. I did not use my stick at all heavily, as I have been doing for the past two and a half years, and I find my legs are very much stronger and that I can now walk without help. In fact in every way I am ever so much better. In myself I really feel better than I ever remember being. It is just wonderful, and I am deeply thankful."

The fourth weekly report proclaimed:—

" I can walk better, ankles and knee joints are getting looser, knees do not suddenly give way now, numbness in legs is disappearing. I am gaining confidence, and am getting on now without the support of a stick. General health is ever so much better in every way. I have gained 5 lbs. in 3 weeks. The flesh of my body is firmer, my skin is a better colour, I feel entirely different from what I did when I came to you. I can face difficulties without getting upset. I am so thankful, words are difficult to express what I feel."

On the 7th November, 1934, I was consulted by Mr. J. J., a retired government official, 61 years old, who had had several attacks of paralysis which had affected the right side. The right leg was heavy and awkward, and the right arm was weak, while three fingers of the right hand did not function. The patient had a high blood pressure, was very tremulous, and felt very unsafe about himself. Mr. J. J. was far too stout. He had had two serious infections and looked apoplectic, and it was of the greatest importance to bring down both his weight and his blood pressure. I gave him a reducing diet, absolutely forbade flesh, fish, fowl and everything made of them, alcohol, coffee, strong tea, spices and condiments, and he cheerfully and manfully embarked upon the adventure of rebuilding his body.

For medicines he was given Sulphur, Thuja, Pulsatilla—the latter because he wept easily—and

Syphilinum 200, a dose once a week. The man improved rapidly and greatly, and after six months he
came to me. He had lost 2 stone of his overweight,
was walking absolutely normally, his crippled right
hand was crippled no longer, and he was able to do
heavy work in the garden with it. His giddiness had
gone, and he looked and felt many years younger and
stronger.

On 18th March I was visited by Mr. E. W. H., of
Wembley Park, who brought me his eight-year-old
daughter and told me that she had been seen by a
doctor who had declared that her tonsils were in a
very bad condition and that they should be taken
out immediately.

I am of the opinion that tonsils are not redundant
pieces of tissue which are of no particular use and
which are an encumbrance, but that they are valuable
organs of elimination. Moreover, I believe that swollen
and septic tonsils are by no means a local trouble, but
are a local manifestation of some constitutional disorder which should be treated constitutionally.

The little girl looked pale, weak, frightened, and
altogether in a poor condition. She was one of three
children, and the other two had also had much trouble
with tonsils and ears. Apparently, one had infected
the other. I chatted with the little girl for a few
minutes to get her confidence, made a few jokes, and
then asked, to the great surprise of the girl and that
of the father: " Will you please take off all your
clothes, including shoes and stockings? " " But only
her tonsils are out of order! " " That may be, but
I want to see the child as a whole."

When the little girl had taken off her clothes I
noticed that her limbs were not straight, she had a
poor chest, very flat feet, her ankles and in fact all
her joints were weak, her body had a poor colour. I
also noticed that there was a rupture in the right
groin, her teeth looked very soft, and the child looked
highly toxic, and on closer inspection I noticed a rash
all over the body. She had a temperature of over 103.

I told the father that I hoped that this rash would not develop. Meanwhile, I gave her some Aconite, doses to be given in quick succession, sent her to bed and gave directions that I should get frequent reports over the telephone. The position was obviously obscure, possibly dangerous.

Before the child left I looked into her throat. Her tonsils were slightly swollen, and the right tonsil was distinctly the larger, which suggested Lycopodium. In view of the poor condition of her bones, ankles, teeth and ligaments, I gave the child Calc. phos. 3X to be taken night and morning, and Lycopodium 12X, a dose between meals, providing the fever should go down.

At first the temperature subsided, then it rose again, then it went up to above 105° and the child was delirious. The parents sent for their local doctor, who had no advice whatever to give except that the tonsils should have been taken out long ago. As the rash had not become worse, he attributed no importance to it. The child had pain in the right ear. There was obviously some septic material which had produced the high temperature. I therefore prescribed Pyrogen 6, a dose night and morning, and Mercurius biniodatus 3X, a dose every few hours, to act on the tonsils and right ear. In twelve hours the temperature was normal. During the two or three days when the child had fever, she had refused food and had been fed on lemon juice, orange juice, barley water, etc. About twelve hours after the first dose of Pyrogen the child cried out for food and ate a large meal.

Pyrogen is a very interesting medicine. Pyrogen, also called Sepsin, is prepared from putrid meat which has been allowed to stand in the sun for a couple of weeks. In accordance with the principle of similarity, small quantities of this septic material, highly potentised, are apt to cure septicity. Pyrogen is invaluable for blood poisoning. A billionth of a grain given twice a day obviously saved the situation in the case of this child. The orthodox practitioner had no advice to

F

offer except the taking out of the tonsils, although that operation would by no means have improved the child's flat feet, weak ankles, narrow chest, anæmia, soft teeth, rupture, etc.

This small incident should be a lesson for all those who are told in a tone of authority: "The tonsils must come out." The practitioner who attended this family, told Mr. and Mrs. H. that the whole trouble came from the tonsils, and that the child would be better as soon as the tonsils were cut out. Of course, nothing could be more absurd than that assertion. Weakness of the tissue, ligaments and bones and the general inadequacy of the body were probably in existence from birth or from before birth.

On 1st April Mr. H. came to my rooms again and brought me his little girl. She looked a totally different child. She had a brilliant compexion, bright eyes, red lips, was vivacious, very happy, and looked the picture of health. I heard to my delight that the child had an enormous appetite, played all day long, was full of energy, and that her tonsils gave no trouble. The pain in the right ear had disappeared. Last, but not least, and this is the most interesting thing of all, the rupture in the groin had practically disappeared as well. The doctor who had treated the child before she was brought to me had also been shown the rupture, and he had explained that nothing could be done for it except an operation.

Homœopathy saved the little lady from two operations. If the tonsils had been cut out and if the rupture had been treated surgically in the usual way, these two evidences of constitutional mischief would have disappeared and the doctor would have been satisfied with the work carried out, and possibly the parents would have been short-sighted enough to be satisfied as well. By the surgical treatment of tonsils, right ear and hernia, the constitutional condition of the child would not have been improved.

The resourceful homœopath can deal without lengthy

diagnosis with any case, however obscure to the orthodox physician and specialist, by matching the leading
symptoms of the patient with a drug which produces
the identical, or similar, symptoms when taken in large
quantities. He can deal with cases of extreme seriousness which are incurable from the orthodox doctor's
point of view, or which are considered to be purely
surgical, such as cancer, sarcoma, enlarged prostate,
etc. Even minor cases, such as enlarged tonsils, yield
readily to homœopathic treatment, and cures are
occasionally produced at a speed for which there is no
parallel in orthodox treatment.

The complete disappearance of pain in cases of
cancer and sarcoma with very rare doses of homœopathic medicine in infinitely small quantities, the cure
of enlarged prostates without operation, and the rapid
improvement of cases of paralysis or disseminated
sclerosis declared absolutely incurable are examples in
point. It is remarkable that Mrs. L. A. recovered the
use of her legs in four weeks after years of deterioration under the treatment of distinguished specialists.

CHAPTER V

Nerve and Brain Cases

SOME years ago there was a lively controversy in one of the medical papers, between Sir William Willcox, the leading English poison expert, and Sir Maurice Craig, one of the leading nerve and brain specialists, anent the use, or abuse, of drugs of the Barbituric group, Veronal, Allonal, Luminal, etc. The expert on poisons pointed out the great danger of these medicaments, describing numerous cases in which ruin and death had resulted from their use, while the nerve specialist stoutly maintained that these drugs were indispensable in the treatment of his patients.

All the sleep-inducing and pain-killing drugs known to orthodox medicine are poisonous. They soothe, give sleep or eliminate pain, although in some cases they fail to act. Occasionally one can give wonderful relief to a patient with an infinitely small homœopathic dose when Morphia in large doses has failed. However, orthodox doctors do not believe in infinitely small doses and dislike the trouble which their use would entail. They prefer a potent drug which can be employed on all their patients, and which will give them sleep or freedom from pain by overwhelming their nerves and brain.

On the 9th January, 1934, Sir William gave an address on drugs, of the Barbituric acid group, in which he said:—

" The actual danger to the public of this country at the present time from addiction to these drugs is greater than from any other group. The risk of death from accidental or purposeful over-dose is a very real one.

" I have seen a large number of cases of suicide or attempted suicide among people who have been taking these drugs for a long period. They take an over-dose often because their minds are so confused that they do not care what may happen, and hope for the worst. It is essential that the public should not have access to them, except on a medical prescription which should be retained by the pharmacist and not repeated, except under medical orders. The medical profession should exercise care in the prescription of these drugs and not order a total quantity on prescription which, if all were taken at once, might be a fatal dose."

Sir William then mentioned some of the dangerous derivatives of Barbituric acid, such as Veronal, Medinal, Soronal, Dial, Quadronox, Herbal Luminal, Sodium Luminal, Sodium evipan, Proponyl, Neonal, Phanodorin, Evipan, Nembutal, Ipral, Allonal, Veramon, Gardenal, Cibalgin, Somnifaine, Beatol Amytal, Pernocton.

His warning was tragically confirmed a few days after. Towards the end of January, 1934, Dr. William Harris Houghton, of Brighton, an exceedingly promising man, of 34, committed suicide, after having been ruined by the very drugs against which Sir William had warned. Before ending his life, Dr. Houghton wrote a letter to the coroner which he wished to have published for the benefit of posterity:

" I am committing suicide because I am frankly a Morphinist. Indeed, I have been one since 1930, when I developed the habit, following a mastoid operation, but during the intervening time I underwent several ' cures,' some at the hands of so-called ' specialists ' and others under my own supervision. Both were equally futile.

" It was under the care of a specialist that I learned the use of Luminal in the treatment of Morphinism. Since that time I can honestly say that I have never known a happy day. Of all drugs, that and its fellows in the barbituric group are the ones to be studiously avoided. Please make that quite clear for the benefit of posterity."

Thousands of unfortunate men and women are done to death every year by the reckless and criminal prescribing of habit-creating poisons, which give temporary relief. There are doctors and specialists who make a living by supplying unfortunate individuals with these dopes. They ought to be expelled from the medical profession. Among them are some so-called specialists who treat the great majority of their cases with nothing but Luminal, Bromides, Morphia, Cocaine, etc. These men are infinitely more dangerous than the wretched keepers of Opium dens.

The great drug houses provide the medical profession with a large number of dangerous drugs which are alike in their evil effect, but which bear widely differing and very attractive names. If a patient who has been taking Veronal for six months hears of a case of Veronal poisoning and rushes to her doctor, she will be reassured and will be told: " Take instead Medinal which is quite safe," and if she has heard bad accounts of Medinal then she may be recommended one of the less known substances with a seductive name, such as Beatol, which suggests beatitude, or Somnifaine, which suggests sleep.

I have been consulted by numerous people who were completely ruined by Veronal and Luminal, given to them under an open prescription which enabled them to take large quantities.

Many patients, especially wealthy ones, expect their doctor to rid them immediately of their nervousness, sleeplessness, pain, etc. Doctors without a conscience will readily prescribe a pleasant poison instead of telling their patients: " Take a light dinner and a sharp walk before going to bed, and cure your nervousness by cutting out strong cigars and cocktails."

The modern doctor goes about with a large quantity of poisons with which he can immediately allay pain, give sleep, soothe the nerves. Occasionally their medicine cases are left behind or are stolen. The possibility arises that a child might swallow some of the sweet pellets and die, and a frantic appeal to return the receptacle is made by wireless, and the newspapers. These cases had become so frequent that Lord Trenchard, the Commissioner of the London Police, found it necessary to send through his secretary an appeal to the General Medical Council, the disciplinary body of the medical profession. He wrote on the 24th March, 1933: —

" I am directed to inform you that the attention of the commissioner has been called to the number of 'thefts and losses of cases containing dangerous drugs, serums and bacteria. I am therefore to ask whether your Council would be good enough to consider the possibility of drawing the attention of the profession to this matter."

In innumerable cases drug addiction is due to the light-heartedness with which Opium, Morphia, Cocaine, Heroin and other dangerous drugs have been prescribed. Orthodox doctors and specialists readily give the most dangerous benumbing drugs to their nerve and brain patients. They are resourceless and do not know how to cure these unfortunate beings. For instance, the textbooks tell them that the drugs for epilepsy are Bromide and Luminal.

Some years ago a business man from Sheffield consulted me because of epilepsy from which he had suffered for more than twenty years. A number of the leading Sheffield doctors and specialists and some London specialists as well had either prescribed Bromide and Luminal or—Luminal and Bromide. So the poor fellow thought that there was no alternative. Many epileptics end their days in the lunatic asylum, brought there by Bromide and Luminal. I saw the man, and enquired: " Did any of your specialists ask you any questions about your diet? " " No one ever did." He told me that he took salt, pepper and mustard by the tablespoonful, huge quantities of meat, drank tea "as black as ink and as hot as hell," smoked 2 ozs. of strong tobacco a day, and consumed incredible quantities of alcohol. For twenty years the wretched man had been kept under Bromide and Luminal until his brain had given way. He rapidly improved under dietetic and homœopathic treatment.

Homœopaths use Opium, Morphia and many other dangerous drugs, but they use them in infinitely small quantity and then they are not benumbing but have the opposite effect. Veronal, Opium and similar drugs produce sleepiness, stupor, coma. In cases of overwhelming sleepiness, stupor and coma, in diabetes, after an apoplectic stroke, etc., the experienced homœopath will give Veronal, Opium or Morphia by the millionth or by the billionth of a grain instead of an injection of Strychnine or Camphor or some other violent stimulant.

The homœopathic practitioner does not carry with him a case full of poisons. Some homœopathic doctors do not carry a subcutaneous syringe. My old friend, Dr. John H. Clarke, did not possess one. One of my patients, Mrs. N. A., who had been operated upon for cancer of the bowel, was dying. She had been kept free from pain for years, but she was terribly restless. Her family wished for a doctor. Dr. Clarke was sent for. The poor woman was tossing about on the bed in confusion and murmured that she could not find her legs.

An orthodox doctor would have given a Morphia injection. The symptoms clearly indicated Baptisia. We read in Boericke's *Pocket Manual*, under " Baptisia ": " Mental confusion, delusion of divided personality, thinks he is broken or double, and tosses about the bed trying to get the pieces together, delirium, wandering, muttering." Dr. Clarke had with him a pocket case of 150 medicines. It contained Baptisia. He took out a few pilules, dissolved them in water, and poured a little down the lady's mouth. Later on I saw the lady's daughter, who said : " Dr. Clarke must have given my mother a very potent sleeping medicine. She fell asleep and died peacefully."

Homœopaths have numerous medicines for sleeplessness. In Kent's *Repertory of the Homœopathic Materia Medica* 230 are enumerated. At first sight selection from 230 drugs for insomnia seems impossible. It is quite easy as long as the prescriber remembers that he must deal with the most prominent symptoms. In summer, 1933, a wealthy lady came to me in despair. She had taken Veronal in increasing quantities for years and it did not act any longer. Careful enquiry elicited the fact that her sleeplessness was due to the over-activity of her brain at night. Every tyro knows that strong coffee produces that kind of sleeplessness. I sent her some sugar pilules moistened with ordinary coffee, a thousandth of a grain to the dose. She wrote after a week that she had stopped the medicine. She was frightened. It was far more potent than Veronal. She had slept better than she had done for years. I told her that she could safely take the medicine by the hundredweight.

For several years I had been treating a great lady, a Miss B., after orthodox medicine and surgery had failed. She was grateful and occasionally told me about her best friend, a Miss H. J., who was nervously afflicted. I had suggested that she should bring her friend to me, but she had always declined. She was treated by the leading nerve specialists of Harley Street, and when her friend took her to the Continent, she was treated by the leading foreign specialists, regardless of expense.

On the 29th June, 1931, Miss B. came to me about her health. When our conversation was drawing towards an end, I asked: " And how is your friend Miss H. J.? " With tears in her voice Miss B. replied: " It is terrible, terrible. She has rapidly gone down hill. I tried in vain to keep her at my house. I had to put her into a private institution for the mentally deranged. I wish I had brought her to you years ago." I answered: " There may be still a ray of hope. Possibly I may be able to prescribe on her symptoms." I asked a number of questions, and it appeared that Miss H. J., who was 62 years old, had become deranged after the change of life, that her condition was worse after sleep, that she was extremely talkative, had violent throbbing of arteries, could not stand any pressure round throat and abdomen. These few symptoms pointed with the utmost clarity towards Lachesis, the poison of the Surukuku snake of South America, a grand climacteric medicine. No homœopath could have prescribed anything else for her. Further, I discovered that Miss H. J. did not perspire. That symptom suggested Sulphur. I resolved to employ Lachesis and Sulphur in high potencies in alternation.

I asked: " Can you give any medicine to your friend? " " That is quite impossible. There is always at least one nurse in the room." " Can you go to the institution at teatime? " " I can." " Very well. Go there at teatime twice a week, let us say Wednesday and Saturday. I will give you two boxes with 12 sugar pilules in each. One box will be marked ' Wednesday ' and the other ' Saturday.' Hold between finger and thumb 3 of the medicated sugar pills, and when the tea for your friend is poured out, ask the nurse or the nurses: Is it raining, or is that my car? and while they are looking out of the window, drop the pilules into your friend's cup where they will dissolve immediately." I warned her that, if Lachesis should be the right medicine, her friend might have violent aggravation, which should not alarm her because it was a thoroughly favourable sign.

In order that no mistake should be possible I immediately dictated the following letter: —

" DEAR MISS B.

" You have told me that your friend is very talkative, worse after sleep, perspires little, cannot stand pressure round throat and abdomen, and that all her troubles began after the change of life. I give you for her two boxes marked—Lachesis 30 (Wednesday) and Sulphur 30 (Saturday).

" Give her every Wednesday 3 pilules from the one box and every Saturday 3 pilules from the other box, and watch with the utmost attention the effect of these two remedies. A considerable aggravation after the first dose of Lachesis 30 would be a most promising sign. The medicines can be taken dissolved in water or any kind of drink. As I told you, it is quite possible that we may be able to cure her, and that, before long, she will be able to leave the institution."

On the 2nd July Miss B. wrote to me:—

" The first dose of Lachesis has been given to Miss H. J. The result was that, roughly about one hour afterwards, she became very excited, but in about an hour and a half or two hours she calmed down and was quite quiet for the rest of the day, but confused."

Every experienced homœopath knows that an initial aggravation, particularly when a medicine in a high potency has been given, is extremely favourable. On the 30th July Miss B. delighted me by a letter:—

" I am giving Miss H. J. the medicine myself. I put it into her tea. I must tell you there has been gradual improvement for a week. She is not yet quite clear, but much clearer than she was. You will, I know, be as glad to hear this as I am to tell you. She has been having much better nights, sleeping right through from 11 till 6 or 7 a.m."

On the 4th August Miss B. wrote to my delight:—

" You will, I know, be glad to know that Miss H. J. has come through and is wonderfully better. I am bringing her home on Saturday."

On August 9th Miss B. wrote:—

" I have Miss H. J. at home. She is wonderful. I have told her she has been taking your medicine for the last five weeks."

The leading nerve specialists of England and various continental celebrities had completely failed benefiting Miss B.'s friend during several years of so-called treatment, in which the unfortunate woman was given nothing but benumbing dopes, which naturally made her condition worse. They had employed all the scientific methods of diagnosis known to medical science, examining the patient scores of times. By the use of homœopathy I succeeded in five weeks where they had failed, although I had never seen her.

Miss B. brought her friend to me and I found her perfectly rational and normal, but her physical condition was very unsatisfactory. Her kidneys did not function properly, owing to the incessant doping which had been done during a number of years. Yet, not one of the great specialists had thought it worth while to give her a non-heating diet, which she needed, especially in view of the condition of her kidneys. Dopes and violent laxatives were given and the poor woman was allowed to eat and drink what she liked, to her hurt. Not unnaturally she suffered from arteriosclerosis. She was apt to have violent attacks of throbbing arteries, especially in her head. She suffered badly from insomnia and had been given the usual poisons, such as Veronal. As her sleeplessness was due to over-activity of the brain, I sent her Coffea 3X and for her attacks of throbbing arteries Belladonna 1X. On the 13th August her friend wrote:—

" It has not been necessary to give Miss H. J. any medicine for sleeplessness as she has been having very good nights. Yesterday afternoon she had a sharp attack of throbbing in her head, neck and stomach. I at once gave her 3 Belladonna pilules for this, repeated the dose after a quarter of an hour, and gave her a third dose after an hour. After this she became quite normal and it was not necessary to give her another dose. I am sure you will be very pleased to hear the result of your treatment, as this is the first time she has ever been relieved. These attacks have usually lasted for days and have even gone into weeks."

Before she came under my care, the poor woman was given the most powerful medicines in maximum doses which did not help, whereas the small doses of homœopathy helped immediately. Yet the great lights of the profession who know nothing about homœopathic treatment treat with contempt the new science of healing. On the 27th August Miss B. wrote to me that her friend had suffered from sleeplessness and that, instead of giving her Morphia or Veronal, she had tried Coffea:—

" I find Coffea 3X excellent for Miss H. J. About five nights ago she felt that she was not going to sleep, so I gave her a dose and it worked beautifully. I have given her more of these and shall want some more."

On the 17th April, 1931, a patient of mine brought me his best friend, Mr. A. J. A., a young man of 24, who had been deeply depressed for months and was contemplating suicide. The young man looked at me with wild eyes, felt totally collapsed, could not speak. I had to give him a glass of strong wine to enable him to answer my questions.

Five or six months previously, at Christmas, 1930, the trouble had begun. He had felt very irritable, he had fainted at the end of January, 1931, and, when he recovered consciousness, he was violently sick and rambling. He went to the doctor, was advised to take a holiday, and in February it was noticed that he walked about as in a trance, mumbling and wild-looking. He had been given the usual sedatives without any effect. I discovered that, some time previous to the first attack, he had received an extremely severe blow on the nose which had deflected the septum and had caused a permanent disfigurement. When Mr. A. J. A. was four and a half years old he had had rheumatic fever, followed by heart disease, and had been attending hospital regularly for eight years. He had not been allowed to take part in games, was afraid of exercise, felt worried about his heart. He had been studying recently with the greatest concentration.

The young man looked weak and ill, he wore a strangulation collar, interfering with the blood supply to the brain, he was in the habit of taking fantastical quantities of salt. He lived on a very faulty diet. I gave him a régime rich in milk, eggs, cheese, vegetables, wholemeal bread, and, as I considered his condition largely due to salt-poisoning, I gave him Natrum Muriaticum 30 to be taken in alternation with Anacardium 3X. Anacardium is excellent for those who complain about weakness of memory and lack of pluck. Besides, it is valuable for those who complain about indigestion improved by eating.

On the 23rd April he wrote: " My memory has certainly improved, but I find it still difficult to concentrate and my brain gets very confused at times. I am suffering from giddiness. I have gained 1 lb. in weight." His next letter was dated the 1st May: " I am very glad to say that I have brightened up very considerably and am gradually getting down to the work again. I now begin to feel hopeful." His letter dated the 8th May told me: " I am getting into the work more and more." On the 12th May he informed me: " I am very glad to say that the very violent headaches have gone. It seems that they may have something to do with my stuffy nose, as they hardly ever occur when the nose is clear. When my nostril gets blocked, I get dull and depressed."

The injury done to his nose by the heavy blow seemed to have had some effect on one of the nasal cavities which possibly was filled with pus and in some way the brain might have been affected. I gave him Arnica 3X for the old injury and Kali iodatum 2X for his stuffed-up nose. On the 18th May he came to me and I was surprised at his appearance. I wrote to him: " You look wonderfuly well, have improved far more than I had anticipated from your letters. You look a different man. Instead of looking wild-eyed, anxious and very ill, pale-faced, pale-lipped, you had to-day bright eyes, red lips, a pink complexion, looked settled and healthy, memory and power of concentration are vastly better, and your physical troubles have completely disappeared." I then gave him Sulphur 30, a dose to be taken once a week, and told him to continue with Anacardium and Kali iodatum.

As his moods were apt to change easily, I gave him Pulsatilla 3. On the 29th June he wrote: " My head pains are almost negligible, my moods have been almost consistently normal." As Pulsatilla suited him particularly well, I kept him on Pulsatilla for some considerable time. On the 20th July he wrote: "I am very conscious of the debt of gratitude I owe you. I am now feeling my old self. My head pains have completely gone and so have my nose troubles, indigestion is non-existent, I sleep well." I alternated Pulsatilla and Anacardium, and later on gave him Ferrum phosphoricum as a tonic and Hydrastis to enable him to put on flesh.

On the 21st December he took leave of me, telling me: "I am feeling very well. I am afraid that I have not yet attained to the eloquence of a Cicero and that any words of gratitude I might express must sound weak, but I would like to say how very grateful I am to you for all you have done for me in pulling me through and for your sympathy and encouragement." Orthodox treatment had done nothing for the young man. He had gradually been going downhill and the fear of his best friend that he might destroy himself might have come true.

On the 23rd December, 1933, I saw Mrs. P., a lady of about 40, one of three children. The other two were magnificent, but she had always been in a very poor condition. She had always been in the doctor's hands, and was treated by most of them as a neurotic. When I asked "Were you injured at birth?" she made me feel deep grooves on both sides of the skull under the hair which were created at her birth and which never disappeared. When one comes across many of such cases, one comes to the conclusion that most doctors should not be allowed to possess either forceps or a subcutaneous syringe. Both are abused with equal recklessness. In innumerable cases mother and child are injured for life by a doctor who is in a hurry or is clumsy. Some time ago a lady came to me and asked me whether anything could be done for her daughter, aged 35, who suffered from such terrible epileptic fits that she could not leave her house. It appeared that 35 years ago, when the child was born, a doctor used the forceps with such brutality that he injured the mother severely and the baby was born, a mass of black bruises, with a dent in her skull. Epileptic fits started there and then and had continued ever since. Mrs. P. improved rapidly under my treatment.

On the 12th September, 1927, Mrs. B. W. wrote to me from Bury, in Lancashire:—

" Will you help me back to health? I have been so ill that I did not think that there could be any happiness in this world. I have not been well for years, first one thing and then another. My nerves have been dreadful for a long time. I used to have such terrible headaches that I never could go out like other people, and, since the beginning of this year, I have had such dreadful fits of depression and exhaustion till at last I collapsed altogether. All this time I had been under specialists and my doctor, who literally drugged me to death, and, whilst I was in bed, I thought it was all wrong, and at last I wouldn't touch any drug or medicine whatever, much to my doctor's consternation.

" I had read your book *Good Health and Happiness* and I asked him what he thought about it and the question of diet, as you said in your book that most diseases were due to faulty living. He replied: ' That is all bunkum.' My nervous prostration is such a terrible thing to recover from. It has affected my eyes and head so badly that I could not read for five minutes, and I am just beginning to be able to stand anyone talking to me. For years I have not had an ordinary excretion. My colon, one specialist said, was irritable. Do forgive this long letter."

I asked her to send me further information and her photograph. She then told me that her circulation was very bad, that she did not perspire at all, had bad dreams at night and that a nerve specialist had informed her that she had a cardiac murmer, information which naturally alarmed her. She had had a large fashion business, had to give it up owing to her illness, felt too nervous to go out, play tennis, etc.

As her photos gave me the impression that her thyroid did not act sufficiently, I sent her some Thyroid 2X to be taken with meals to start with, and gave her by letter all encouragement I could. On the 14th October she wrote:—

" I had a furious headache, but I feel very much better altogether. I do not ever remember a headache going away like that before. My complexion is clearer than it was, I have no trouble about my excretions, my spirits are very good and I don't get depressed at all now. I used to go to London very often alone on business. Do you think I shall ever be able to do it again?"

She complained of both headaches and sleeplessness. I then prescribed for her one of the best sleeping medicines I know and one of the cheapest—a brisk walk or run before going to bed. It was difficult to induce her to carry out that prescription but I succeeded, and on the 26th November she wrote: " I am so pleased to be able to tell what a very good week I have had and how much better I feel. I haven't even a bad headache to report, and during the last few nights I have slept about 6 hours each night and I only woke up once. So I am improving very much." On the 28th January, 1928, she wrote: " I am getting stronger every day. I feel I want to laugh all day. I am beginning to feel that the world is a good place to live in after all."

For some considerable time her letters were written with a shaky uneven hand and with faulty alignment, usual in bad nerve cases. It improved gradually. On the 7th May, 1928, I wrote to her: " The firm clear handwriting, alignment and style of your letter of the 5th proclaim that you have vastly improved." She began to go to dances, took part in operatic performances, etc., played tennis, became normal. On the 24th May she wrote:—

" My soul is filled with joy. To-day I have been playing tennis. It is two years since I played. I could not realize that it was myself standing on a court. You know these things feel as yet quite unreal and I feel as if I might wake up and find it was a dream. That is how I felt. Now the funny thing was, I was playing one of the doctors who had attended me during my long illness, and he said ' You know, I think it is marvellous the way you have pulled up after being so ill. I didn't think you would ever play

G

tennis again. What have you been doing?' I answered 'It's that wonderful treatment you and Dr. H. gave me; all that Bromide and plenty of under-cooked meat and chicken.' He was quite honest about it and said 'No, I do not think it was that, but won't you tell me?' I replied: 'Well, I will tell you some day.' I thought this encounter amusing, but their treatment of my case was not at all amusing. Anyhow, Mr. Barker, I am rapidly forgetting the past."

On the 26th September she wrote me another delightful letter:—

"I felt I really must write to you to-day, whatever happened, for this is a sort of birthday. It is a year ago to-day that I commenced to rebuild my constitution with your help. I feel a perfectly different person from what I did a year ago and next year this time I hope to be perfectly strong and robust. I am feeling very well now and I look as if I do. Almost every day someone tells me how much better I look. I have such a feeling of well-being that I never had before and I feel that in a very little while I shall be stronger than I have ever been in my life. I am quite anxious that you should see what you have done for me."

I am glad to say that Mrs. B. W. got perfectly well, perhaps less owing to my treatment as to her being no longer doped with daily doses of Bromide and other benumbing poisons and "strengthened" with poisonous doses of Arsenic, Strychnine and other so-called tonics.

A lady patient of mine had often told me that her widowed sister had been in a mental institution, and begged me to take her in hand. On the 8th February, 1933, I was visited by Mrs. M. W. of Coventry. The poor soul was terrified. Her daughter had dragged her into my house with the greatest difficulty and there she was, like a hunted wild animal, and wanted to run away. It was a typical case of melancholia and general prostration. In the introduction to my directions I summarized her condition as follows:—

" You are 66 years old, and have come to me complaining about deep depression and melancholia, general weakness and stiffness of legs for which you have been given arthritis treatment, and you complain that your brain refuses to work. You are constantly indulging in self-reproaches without justification and have led a life of unremitting toil.

" You look in poor physical condition, have a yellowish complexion, sleep well, feel best at night, feel poorly all day, particularly on waking, had 2 years ago and 10 years ago a very severe nervous breakdown. You have always had much rheumatism, are always cold, feel best in the heat, complain of palpitations on the top of the head, motions are regular, urine is smelly and dark, your teeth chatter, you are very thirsty, and my impression is that all your troubles are due to the change of life. You live on a very unsuitable diet, taking just what comes handy, take much tea, have the feeling of a ball rising from the stomach."

She had been given Bromide and Medinal to numb her nerves and brain. I kept the prescription, and absolutely forbade these dangerous poisons. Apart from them she had been given nothing.

As her trouble had come on after the change of life, I gave her Lachesis 30, a priceless remedy for the troubles of the climacteric, a single dose to be taken every Saturday, Sulphur 30 for clearing up her system, a single dose to be taken every Wednesday, and Ignatia 30, marked " Nerves, deep sighs," a dose to be taken at odd times when she felt nervy or was sighing much. Nerve and brain cases do best when given medicine in high potencies and in infrequent doses.

I regulated her diet. Flesh, fish, fowl, strong tea, coffee, overmuch sugar, packeted and tinned foods, shop jam, and other artificialities were forbidden. She was to live on bran porridge, an abundance of vegetables and fruit, milk, eggs, wholemeal bread and butter, unbleached sultanas and pea nuts with their skins.

On the 16th February her daughter wrote: " My mother is continually complaining of a very bad thumping in her head and the pit of her stomach, but she does not cry so much, her bowels are working properly, and she has just said to me ' I believe I feel a bit better.' " I sent her Belladonna 30 marked " Throbbing in head and stomach, to be taken as needed."

A homœopathic prescriber must change his remedies with changing symptoms. He cannot sit still in idleness after having given Bromide and Medinal, to put the patient into a continual stupor. On the 23rd Mrs. M. W. to my surprise wrote to me herself: " Those pilules you sent for the throbbing in the head and stomach seem to have relieved both. I do not feel so depressed, but feel very irritable and cannot sit still. My brain seems too active." The new symptoms called for new remedies and I sent her some Arsenic 30 marked " restlessness " and Coffea 30 " overactivity of brain, keenness of senses." On March 2nd she told me that Sulphur 30 did her most good. Needless to say, she did not know what she was taking. On the 9th of March I was told that she still was weeping so much. As she was very affectionate, I sent her Pulsatilla 3, a dose to be taken three times a day, which helped her.

On the 14th March, five weeks after the beginning of the treatment, she visited me with her daughter. She had vastly improved. I wrote to her: —

" I am extremely pleased with your appearance. You look years younger, have clearer eyes, glossier hair, redder lips, a clearer complexion, do not burst into tears, have learned to laugh, have a normal expression instead of looking wild, and you have vastly improved all round, and I feel confident that further and greater improvement will show itself presently. I have every reason to be satisfied with you."

She was delighted with that letter and, unless I am much mistaken, read it scores of times. Such a letter is an invaluable medicine in nerve cases. Often patients of this kind tell me that they read my letters every day, and that they are the finest tonic for them.

When she was at my house she had told me of new complaints. She could no longer concentrate, her memory had gone to pieces, she felt physically and mentally utterly fagged. I gave her there and then a single dose of Lachesis 10,000th potency, and two boxes of pilules, one containing Anacardium 3X, marked concentration and memory, and the other Arnica 3X (fag, physical and mental), which she was to take in alternation. In addition, I told her daughter to massage her mother, especially her legs, with olive oil, because she could walk only a few yards, and was unable to walk up the slightest incline. She told me later on that the dose of Lachesis 10,000 " gave me more pain in my head." This was a proof that her head symptoms were largely due to the climacteric and that Lachesis was the right medicine. She developed new symptoms which called for new remedies. She was given Helonias 1X for backache and tiredness, which obviously came from her womb, and Phosphorus 3 for confusion on waking in the morning.

Her daughter wrote to me on the 28th June: —

" I certainly see an improvement in my mother. She does not cry out as she did, nor is she so hysterical. She talks more and can mix with her friends once more without feeling so depressed. She now is determined to get better and gets up early and about her work. She says she often notices relief after taking a little food."

" Improvement when eating " is a key symptom of Anacardium. So I sent her some Anacardium 3X. On the 7th November she visited me once more in London, and I found her practically normal mentally and vastly improved physically. I wrote to her: " I was amazed and delighted by your appearance, and your improvement is all the more notable as you have been without medicine for many months."

CHAPTER VI

Some of My Failures

A S I am an ordinary mortal, I am not invariably successful, although the proportion of my successes has been high. A good prescriber will learn much from his successes and from his failures, and from the successes and failures of others. I therefore think it only fair to my readers to tell them of my failures. A doctor should at the end of the day review the events of the day and ponder on his successes and non-successes, giving himself praise and blame according to his deserts. Medicine is an art, and a wise artist will criticize his work unsparingly.

Success or failure in treatment depends largely on the personality and will power of the practitioner. He must be determined to make his patients well, and he must be able to arouse that determination in his patients. Very frequently at the end of a lengthy interview I tell a patient: " I am afraid I can do little or nothing for you." and I see the immediate effect of my words in an expression of the face with which I am very familiar. And, after a cruel minute, I add quickly and with a tone of determination: " But you can cure yourself. My work is of little importance. I am merely the architect. I draw the plan, but you have to do the building and rebuilding." A patient addressed in this way may show immediately by his reaction to my words whether he is likely to be a real help in the treatment or not.

There are many causes which prevent one succeeding. The text-book notion of incurability need, of course, not be considered. One does not treat an abstraction called a disease, but a human being according to his or her individual needs. I have not yet come across an incurable disease, but I have certainly met incurable patients. There are patients whom nature is determined to kill. They are going downhill and they will not react to treatment, however carefully chosen. The so-called disease may not be a serious one. According to the textbooks it may be comparatively trifling, but the patient does not react, whatever is done, and nothing will stop the downward course. Health is merely a question of reaction. I explain this to despondent patients who have been declared incurable by the highest authorities.

There are two classes of patients who are my despair. They are those who do not react. The exact opposite are the people who react powerfully and badly to every medicine, who say truthfully: " Every medicine upsets me." Most of them have been over-drugged with orthodox medicine and they react splendidly to homœopathic drugs. On the other hand, there are patients who are upset even by the smallest homœopathic doses.

A man came to me complaining of psoriasis. His symptoms pointed to Sulphur. He told me that he had been given Sulphur by his doctor, but it had upset him. As he had been treated with Sulphur in large quantity, I sent him sugar pills medicated with Sulphur in doses of one millionth of a grain. It would have taken him a thousand years to absorb a single grain of Sulphur if he took three doses a day. I never told him what the sugar pills contained, but he bitterly complained that I had sent him Sulphur notwithstanding his warning. There are people who are so sensitive that they will detect by their manifestations Sulphur or some other drug if given by the billionth of a grain and by the decillionth of a grain.

A splendid old nurse visited me complaining of paralysis agitans (shaking paralysis). She had been treated by a number of the leading physicians of the orthodox school without success and told me that every medicine upset her. I tried to cure her with sugar pills medicated with very small and infinitesmal doses of medicine and I found that her assertion was perfectly true. I then sent her unmedicated sugar pills which had exactly the same taste as the medicated ones. They had no effect whatever. I then sent her to my friend, the late Dr. John H. Clarke, who taught me homœopathy. He tried his luck with low, medium, high and very high potencies and failed every time. She was incurable.

About the same time a lady came to me from Church Street, Kensington. She was about 45 years old and suffered from a combination of abdominal, gastric and mental symptoms. Doctors of the past would have declared her troubles hysterical and would have bled her profusely, possibly with great success, but bleeding is no longer fashionable. She could not take any other diet than the faulty diet to which she had been accustomed, and she could take no medicine whatever. I tried the indicated homœopathic medicines on her in small and infinitely small doses and was told every time after a dose or two that she had been " terribly upset." I then sent her some unmedicated sugar pills. They upset her worse than the medicated sugar pills, and that was the end of the treatment.

Among the most difficult cases are people of great position and of great wealth. They are accustomed to be attended by fashionable courtier-doctors, whose main aim is to please the patients. Years ago a well-to-do business man told me that his wife had a terribly ulcerated leg. " Is she under treatment? " " Yes, the doctor comes every day." " What has he prescribed? " " A medicine containing Arsenic and an outward application with Arsenic in it." " Has he regulated her diet? " " No." " And what does your wife live on? " " She gets the best of everything." " Is she stout or thin, does she take exercise or no exercise? " " She is extremely stout, cannot take exercise and cannot bear the open air." It came out

that the wife ate three dinners a day. Her breakfast
consisted of 2 eggs, meat, tea with plenty of cream in
it, large quantities of bread with thick butter, honey
and so forth. In every form she took about 6 eggs
a day and had meat or fish three times a day. I told
the husband that the only way to cure the woman
would consist in starving her, that ulceration was the
safety valve of nature in her case, that if the doctor
should succeed in stopping ulceration with Arsenic,
the disease would strike inward and would probably
produce cancer.

A few days later I met a consultant friend of mine,
and I expressed my indignation at the doctor who
called every day and gave the poor woman nothing
but Arsenic. My friend said with a cynical smile:
"What else can the poor devil do? The stout lady
lives for the pleasures of the table. If her doctor
should dare to recommend a reduction of her diet,
she would dismiss him and get another man. Well-
to-do people do not like to have their diet interfered
with. That is well understood by every doctor."

I have experienced the same trouble with many of
my patients. I was consulted by Mr. H., of Park
Lane, He was a fat, greasy man, with an unhealing
wound following a serious operation. I received his
complaints, and discovered that his real disease was
over-eating. He listened to me with a frown, explained
to me that he had to eat seven-course dinners either at
his own house or at his friends', and that was the end
of the treatment. Another wealthy man told me that
he was quite willing to live sparingly himself, but the
difficulty was the cook. His cook was a wonderful
artist, his dinners were celebrated in town, and he
would certainly leave him. Besides, he could not sit
at the table of his wealthy friends and refuse the
choice and over-rich dainties prepared by other cooks
of the same type. He tried for a few weeks to live on
a greatly simplified diet, but although he benefited
greatly, he gave up.

Some years ago a doctor in Harley Street told me

that a patient of his, Lord ——, wished to see me professionally. He suffered from an obscure disease. He had a swelling, possibly cancerous, in the right side of the abdomen. Besides, he was suffering from diverticulitis, which was in his family.

I saw Lord —— at his town house, and he showed me the swelling in his abdomen, which I did not touch. I think it is a great mistake to finger swellings in which nature tries to isolate disease matter. Clumsy manual examination is apt to spread the disease all over the body. I have had women come to me who told me that they had noticed a swelling in their breast and that they had massaged it away. They had converted a local breast cancer into a general systemic cancer in every case, except one in which there was cancer *en cuirasse*. As the man had been constipated all his life and had been living on a devitaminized diet which is apt to produce diverticulitis, which means, in plain English, the formation of numerous pouches or sacks of the soggy bowel wall which fill with hard excreta, I recomended a diet rich in those vitamins and mineral elements of which he had been deprived all his life by his excellent cook.

Fearing that the swelling was cancerous, I put him on a strict, non-flesh diet, forbade alcohol, etc. In order to make sure that my directions should be carried out, I went to the kitchen and interviewed the cook. She was stout and magnificent, looked like the typical stage cook, and, like all the men and women doing high-class cooking, was very seriously troubled with her digestion and excretion and had to rely on numerous and varied medicines to carry on. After a few days I learned that his lordship was "sick of those damned vegetables and fruit," and had ordered fish, flesh, and fowl, potted meat, and other unsuitable things. Besides, he had drunk iced champagne which had made him very ill. When remonstrated with, my patient told me: "I never could eat that damned rubbish and won't eat it now."

Medicinal treatment was as difficult as dietetic regulation. I was told: " I never take any medicine unless I know what it is." Of course, if I had told the man " You must leave yourself unreservedly in my hands and take the diet and medicines prescribed because otherwise you will die of cancer," I should have killed him. I succeeded with homœopathic medicines in improving his condition. He learned to prefer Carbo vegetabilis 30 to charcoal biscuits which he had taken hitherto in large quantities. The charcoal had been forming black knobs of pure coal in the bowel pouches. His terrible cough and expectoration disappeared under the indicated remedies, but it happened that he refused to take an important cancer medicine because he did not fancy it. Every prescription was checked by him by means of the *Materia Medica*. Sometimes he refused medicines because he thought they did not suit his complaint. Others he would not take because he did not like their name. After a struggle which I carried on in the hope of saving his life—he was a charming and highly intelligent man—I had to withdraw, telling him quite frankly that he had made my task impossible. Six months after he died of cancer. He had worn out a great many doctors.

His case reminds me of that of Prince Bismarck. Bismarck had led a very wild life, eating and drinking fabulous quantities at Gargantuan meals, smoking to excess, etc. In the course of his life he had been treated by about 100 doctors, the heads of the profession, and had terrified them all. He had dictated treatments to them with very unfavourable results. Dissatisfied with the celebrated professors whom he had ordered about, he sent one fine day for an unknown youngster, Dr. Schweninger, who was interested in nature cure and homœopathy and who had no belief in orthodox drugs, given in large quantities.

Like a good homœopath, he asked Bismarck numerous questions, especially about his diet, which no one had ever asked before. At last the prince got angry and told the young doctor that he was getting tired of being questioned. With extraordinary presence of mind, Schweninger replied " If you do not want to answer questions, you ought to have sent not for a doctor but for a veterinary surgeon. He never puts questions to the animals he treats." The prince got red in the face and rang the bell to have the impertinent doctor thrown out. On consideration he was impressed by his courage, patted him on the back, and told him to go on with the interrogation. Schweninger had defeated Bismarck and he remained Bismarck's doctor for many years till his death, to the envy of the great but servile German consultants. A practitioner who wishes to succeed with his patients must dominate them. He must be the master, but he must be a reasonable master. Only a Bismarck will submit to a doctor like Schweninger, after having treated all the celebrated doctors as if they were mere lackeys.

Another nobleman, Lord ——, asked me to help him. He had a most excessive watery catarrh, resembling hay fever, which had plagued him for half a century. He did not want to know anything about his complaint or treatments. He was willing to do anything he was told. He had readily submitted to numerous operations which had aggravated the position. I never could get an adequate account of his symptoms. He reminded me of an old lady in the country, who wrote to me: " I feel funny inside. I am sure you know what I mean. What do you recommend? " I tried three or four homœopathic remedies on him, for he told me he could not be bothered with a diet, and as his complaint of half a century's standing was not cured in three or four weeks, he gave up. It never occurred to him that it was unreasonable to expect that I should be able to cure his trouble in a few weeks without being given adequate facts.

Some years ago Sir H. H. called on me. He was a stout elderly man, well-to-do, and had been treated all his life by the heads of the profession. A friend of his, a celebrated titled surgeon, had recommended him to consult me about his digestion. A short interrogation made it quite clear to me that the man suffered in all probability from gastric and duodenal ulcer, produced by the ministrations of a high-class cook. I told him that I suspected ulceration, gave him a simple natural diet, and the indicated homœopathic remedies. He took the diet for a few days, hated it like poison, and declared that it made him worse. Then he rushed to a doctor and complained that I had diagnosed ulceration. " Is that true? I am sure it cannot be true! " " Of course, it is not true," said the diplomatic medico. I received a strong letter that my diagnosis of ulceration was absolutely wrong, and Sir H. H. went back to his refined cuisine. The idea that men's minds are governed by brain or will is mistaken. In many cases the governing factor is the palate.

On the 4th December, 1931, I was consulted by an elderly peer. He had been a man of magnificent physique, a great athlete, and he had lived well, as do most athletes. With increasing years his strength declined, exercise was discontinued, but the diet was left unchanged. Lord —— complained about the condition of his heart, lungs, arteries and he had been told by his doctors and consultants that nothing could be done. I impressed upon him the fact that his trouble was due to over-nutrition, and sent him my directions. He had to abandon flesh, fish and fowl, to which he had been accustomed, and leave off alcohol which he had taken at every meal in considerable quantities. I told him that I should replace alcohol by unobjectionable tonics. He violently objected to tonics, he did not care for the restricted diet. I endeavoured in vain to give him ease and comfort by homœopathic medicines.

A well-known soldier, General ——, consulted me some years ago. He was over 70, and complained of utter weakness. His doctors had braced him up first by means of powerful tonics given by the mouth, and then by injections of tonics of a very dangerous character. He was somewhat obese, had an excellent cook, took practically no exercise, and lived on concentrated food, for which his system had no use. I explained to him that his weakness was largely due to the poisonous tonics with which he had been doped. He saw the reasonableness of my diagnosis, tried to follow me for some time, and then gave up. It is very difficult to cure habitual dope-takers.

A Cabinet Minister wrote to me from Ireland that he was unutterably weak, and asked for my advice. His case was identical with that of the old general. He benefited greatly, but after a time went back to his injections.

The Hon. Mrs. ——, a wealthy woman, came to me in 1933. She had been weak and ill all her life, she had employed scores of doctors and consultants, had undergone all the most fashionable and the most expensive treatments and was in a worse condition than ever. Her children were weaklings. Not one of her numerous advisers had endeavoured to change her way of living . At last she had discovered the worthlessness of the previous treatments and came to me for help. I tried my best, but failed utterly. She was a Society woman, she had to go to luncheons and dinners every day and she " simply could not refuse the good things put before her." On the other hand, a famous lawyer, Sir ——, overcame this difficulty by dining frugally at home when invited to dinner and toying with the food on his plate when nominally dining with his friends.

Some patients die because they get well too quickly. Too rapid a recovery is extremely dangerous, because patients feel so well that they take risks which otherwise they would not dare to take. Some years ago an old friend of mine, a French lady, 70 years old, sent me a message that she was dying of Hodgkins' disease and that the doctor had given her no hope. I got into the car, rushed over to her house and found her in bed. She seemed to be in a dying condition. Her face was yellow-white, her nose was pinched, her eyes had lost all sparkle and were sunken, she had lost her hearing, could hardly speak, but her glands were only moderately swollen. There was a nurse in the room. "Has the doctor said anything about diet?" "Not a word." She was fed on the most unsuitable food, as if she was a healthy woman, and digestion and excretion were secured by powerful medicines. "What have you got in that bottle?" "Fowler's Solution of Arsenic. I have to give her so many drops per hour." I turned to my friend: "Will you allow me to treat you?" "I beg your pardon?" I shouted the words into her ears and then wrote them on paper. She whispered a feeble "Yes." I immediately forbade ordinary cooking, meat extracts and such-like rubbish on which she had been fed. She was to live exclusively on extremely weak China tea, with plenty of milk, sweetened with an abundance of honey, honey water, lemon water sweetened with honey, bran decoction with lemon juice and honey, orange juice in any quantity, raw pineapple juice, grape fruit juice. She was given Kaylene to deal with bowel toxins and Aconite to deal with her fever, and her doctor was informed that she did not require his services.

In a week's time she was vastly better, and had regained her hearing, to the amazement of her doctor who had called "as a friend." He had found her out of bed and had told her: "Next time I call, you will probably see me off to the front gate." Mrs. L. had always been exceedingly susceptible to draughts. When she sat down to dinner, her servants had to put a folding screen around her. I told her that Nature would probably cure her and she was enthusiastic. On a rather chilly day she told the nurse: "I am going to sit on the balcony." The nurse protested in vain. The old lady insisted, felt chilly, asked for additional wraps and rugs, but stayed on the balcony. The nurse was wringing her hands. The next day she was down with pneumonia, and shortly after I attended her funeral.

One of my most brilliant heart cures was that of Mr. J. B., whose case I have described in the beginning of this book. When I took him in hand, he had been lying in bed by doctor's orders for I do not know how long and his wife had to turn him round in bed. He was well over 60, had lived only too well all his life and had never taken any exercise. By gradual training I enabled him to walk from 10 to 12 miles at a stretch in the Scotch hills. Feeling better than ever in his life, he took risks recklessly. If anything went wrong, he asked the chemist for advice or consulted a cheap doctor. He did not listen to my warnings.

He had had an attack of influenza, the local doctor had put him to bed, and had given him a very feeding diet " to keep up his strength," and when he got out of bed he had gained a stone. I had previously reduced him by about 4 stone. I advised him to go back to the old diet and to reduce his weight by about 2 lbs. per week. He thought my advice too cautious, took a strict fast during a whole week, combined with heavy exercise, and lost a stone in a few days. He felt very weak, confessed his folly and told me that he was deeply depressed. The mental symptoms are infinitely more important than the physical symptoms. If he had told me that all his organs were functioning badly and if he had concluded with the words: " Notwithstanding all my physical troubles, I feel in high spirits " I should not have minded. I told him that he should come up to London at once. He made excuses. His wife had arranged for a holiday in the Scotch wilds. Afterwards both would come to London. He arrived at his holiday destination, felt unwell, the local doctor was fetched, he was given Digitalis, and died.

Nearly all cases which come to me have been pronounced "absolutely incurable" by physicians, surgeons and specialists. Under these circumstances one would imagine that the percentage of my failures should be high. In reality it has been low, except in certain diseases, such as epilepsy, diabetes, Hodgkins' disease and cancer. These diseases are difficult to handle in themselves, but the worst is that patients suffering from them usually come to me after doctors and surgeons have spoilt them completely. The epileptics have been doped for years with Bromide and Luminal and are poisoned through and through. Diabetics are as a rule utterly indifferent to their fate and unhelpful. Besides, their condition has been aggravated by Insulin. Patients with Hodgkins' disease have been filled with Arsenic and cancer cases come to me when surgeons and radiologists have done their worst. Notwithstanding this great handicap I have succeeded in curing a number of cases pronounced to be cancerous.

Admiral W. was suffering from cancer of the œsophagus. His wife asked my advice. The doctor had recommended radium treatment. I warned her that I had never known radium do any good, that it was apt to destroy cancer locally by spreading it all over the body. Orthodox medicine gained the day, as happens frequently. Admiral W. underwent radium treatment, the disease spread all over the body, and his end was terrible. Other cancer patients who, against my advice, underwent radium treatment, operations, lead injections, etc., had the same fate.

On the 3rd May, 1932, I was visited by Mr. J. S., a well-to-do printer. He had lost his voice, had lost much weight, had pain in the throat, had consulted a number of doctors and specialists and had been advised to undergo an operation. He told me that he was quite determined not to be operated upon. His brother had died of cancer of the tongue, he had been treated with radium and his sufferings had been atrocious. " Did any of your doctors or consultants give you any dietetic directions?" " None."

Interrogation revealed the fact that he had four meat meals a day, the last before going to bed, that he took the strongest and hottest tea, alcohol, large quantities of salt, pepper, mustard, pickles, he smoked cigarettes all day, took snuff, which dropped from the back of the nose into the throat, was constipated, took no exercise. The doctors and specialists had looked at his throat. I did not look at the throat at all.

H

It was unnecessary. I explained to him that for years he had over-heated his system most atrociously, that an outbreak was bound to come and that, not unnaturally, it had come in the throat which he had abused with boiling hot drink, tobacco, etc. He agreed with my view and promised to change his ways.

I put him on a mild diet, forbade smoking and snuff-taking, alcohol, boiling hot drink, etc., and asked him to take physical exercise. He grumbled, but obeyed. In a short time he gained 10 lbs. in weight, got rosy cheeks, and his voice improved. Soon afterwards he grew weary of his diet. I heard from his friends that he was eating, drinking, smoking as before. Aggravation followed, he underwent radium treatment, like his unfortunate brother, and died at the Cancer Hospital.

I do not want my readers to think that I am a superman who fails in curing the most difficult cases only because patients have previously been treated unsuitably, are unwilling to carry out my directions, or have become reckless through too rapid a recovery. I make mistakes, like everyone else. I am keenly aware of the inadequacy of my knowledge although I have spent a fortune on medical literature and have studied it intensively for many years.

I divide my patients into two categories, those who are willing, helpful and enthusiastic, and those who are indifferent, sceptical and obstructive. Of the patients of the first category, the large majority get well; of the patients of the second category, the large majority do not get well. The two most powerful medicines I know are the determination of the practitioner to effect a cure by orthodox or unorthodox means, and the determination of the patient to help the practitioner intelligently.

The largest contingent of my failures is furnished by patients who give up treatment too soon. They do not realize that diseases which have been in existence for many years cannot possibly be cured by treatment during a few weeks or months, or by a prescription or two. It is quite understandable that people do not want to look upon themselves as chronic invalids. I remember how I hated to go to the doctor when I was a desperately sick man. Unfortunately people with chronic diseases cannot grasp the fact that patience and long-continued co-operation on the part of practitioner and patient are needed to effect a cure. Many of the cases described in this book were under my treatment for two years or longer. Samuel Hahnemann declared that the cure of a chronic disease would take at least two years. Of course, during the years of treatment there ought to be continuous improvement, accompanied by occasional set-backs.

The orthodox medical man believes that chronic diseases are incurable and he does not attempt to cure them. He may tell the patient that he must try to get accustomed to the fact that he suffers from such-and-such disability and make the best of life. He will give him a prescription to allay his pain, or to relieve his cough, or to promote bowel action, or to soothe the irritation of the skin, or to enable him to sleep, etc., and when the tonic, laxative or sedative prescribed acts no longer, another prescription is given, which will cure as little as the first.

The average doctor adopts an unfortunate attitude towards his patients. He treats them not with human sympathy, but with a certain aloofness and coldness which may be very scientific and which is the proper attitude of a laboratory man who watches his cultures and microscopes. I rejoice with those who are getting better and suffer with those who do not do well. If a patient is not responding to treatment, I may telephone every day and enquire, although he may be poor. The average doctor acts more or less like the ticket clerk at the railway window who hands over with indifference a ticket in exchange for the appropriate cash. That is a most regrettable attitude.

The laboratory has de-humanized the medical profession. I know doctors whose voice and smile are as good as a medicine, whose very presence warms and cheers the patient, and there are others whose gloomy looks and sullen ways make people shudder. A good presence and the right spirit are invaluable factors. Hippocrates wrote 2,300 years ago that no one can be a good doctor unless he loves the art of medicine and loves mankind. Medicine should not be a profession, but a calling. No one can be a good doctor unless he feels the divine call. Unfortunately many young men enter the medical profession not because they feel an irresistible urge to heal their fellow beings but because they hope to make an adequate income. Medicine is not a science but an art. An artist is born, not made. There are born doctors and surgeons and there are those who can never become doctors or surgeons, even if they have been in the "healing business" for decades.

CHAPTER VII

Gall Stones and Kidney Stones

GALL stones and kidney stones are extremely frequent among those advanced in years. Women are particularly prone to gall stones. In many cases small stones in gall bladder and kidneys cause no discomfort and they are discovered only when the organs are opened up after death. Unfortunately gall and kidney stones are apt to cause occasionally the most excruciating pain. The pain is so terrible that the patient cannot move. If his medicine is on the other side of the table he may sit in agonies for hours, unable to reach over or get up. The pain is created by a stone passing through a narrow duct where it is held up, causing violent inflammation. People usually notice that they have gall bladder trouble only when they are driven frantic by unendurable pain.

When the orthodox doctor is for the first time in his life consulted about gall stones, he may open his textbooks in order to find out what he should do. If he opens the classical textbook *The Principles and Practice of Medicine,* by Osler and McCrae, of which more than 300,000 copies have been sold, he will find under the heading " Cholelithiasis " a number of pages devoted to the origin of gall stones, of which nothing certain is known, to their physical character, size, shape and chemical composition, to the symptoms which they cause, etc., and, after having patiently read through pages of irrelevant matter, which will enable him to talk learnedly to his patient, he will read under the heading " Treatment ": " In an attack of biliary colic the patient should be kept under Morphia, given hypodermically in quarter grain doses. . . . The patient should be given laxatives and should drink copiously. . . . The diet should be regulated. . . . Various remedies have been advised to dissolve the stones within the gall bladder, none of which are efficacious."

As usual, the orthodox doctor is resourceless. The only thing he is recommended to do is to give temporary relief with injections which allay but do not cure and, if the trouble gets intolerable or the gall bladder gets too large, getting filled with stones or pus, an operation is advised. Similar information is to be found in the other textbooks.

It is clear that the orthodox doctor can do nothing to cure gall stones. If the leaders of the profession would study homœopathic literature, or discuss the subject with homœopathic doctors, they would discover that gall stones and kidney stones can be dissolved in numerous cases by homœopathic and dietetic means and that Morphia and other benumbing poisons are not necessary. Unfortunately the investigation of homœopathic treatment is refused and the public is deprived of treatments which cure. Countless sufferers are handed over to the surgeon without need.

I have been fortunate enough to relieve and cure numerous cases of gall stones although I have never talked to my patients about Cholelithiasis and the chemical composition of their stones. Most gall stone patients come to me and other homœopaths in the hope of escaping an operation which their instinct tells them may be unnecessary. Their instinct often is right. Unfortunately gall stone patients are frequently hounded to the surgeon by the hint: " You had better not delay an operation, for otherwise there may be cancerous developments."

On the 5th March, 1928, Miss A. G. wrote to me from Bedfont, Middlesex: —

"I am called upon to make what is to me a rather important decision. I am advised by the doctors to have my gall bladder removed. They say that, owing to certain malformation, there is a deposit in it, and it can be cured only by an operation.

"I am utterly ignorant of matters medical, but, even so, I cannot conceive that a mutilated human being can ever be perfectly normal and, if at all possible, I would like to avoid the operation.

"I have had the pain for five years, but I have had not much recently. I have had a great deal of treatment for it. I am told that if I do not have the operation, I shall go from bad to worse and become a nervous wreck, as the continued pain will wear me out. If you think anything can be done to avoid this contingency I should be glad if you would give me an appointment."

I saw her on the 13th March. She was in the thirties, looked prematurely aged, worn, jaundiced, and was walking with difficulty and was sitting with an arched back. She explained to me that the gall bladder trouble had caused a distortion of the spine, interfering with her walking.

After listening to her account, I came to the conclusion that the trouble might be due in part to auto-intoxication because she had always been constipated. As a pupil and admirer of Sir Arbuthnot Lane, I attach the greatest importance to a well-functioning drainage system. Only I go farther. I am interested not only in the perfect functioning of the bowel but also in that of the skin. I explain to many patients that they are in the condition of a house where the drains are clogged and the windows, the pores, do not open.

After listening to Miss A. G.'s complaints and putting numerous questions, I came to the conclusion that nothing could be done for her and that the surgeons were right. I did not care for the responsibility of undertaking her case. I was well aware that gall stones, if not dealt with in time, are apt to bring about

cancerous and other developments which may en-
danger life. I told her of my hesitation, but she
pleaded so hard with tears in her eyes, that at last
I consented. She was delighted, but I felt greatly
troubled. I had not the heart to tell the poor creature
frankly and brutally what I thought.

In accordance with my promise, I sent her a diet
sheet. She was to take about 3 pints of milk, 3 eggs,
grated cheese, an abundance of vegetables, potatoes,
fruit, and absolutely no flesh, fish, fowl or anything
made of them, no pastries, chocolate, cake, little butter,
no cream. Her bowels were to be regulated with
liquid paraffin. She was to take Vichy water three
times a day before meals and Kaylene to absorb bowel
toxins. The organisms of putrefaction in the bowel
are starved out if the patient is fed on a fleshless and
fishless diet. That is a powerful recommendation for
vegetarianism.

To my great regret she reacted poorly. The pain
in her back became worse, but with splendid courage
and faith in me—I thought there was not the slightest
reason for her having any confidence in my ability—
she went on and refused to be discouraged. On the
17th March she wrote to my surprise: " The pain has
lessened and my stomach feels very much more comfortable than it has for a long time past." On the
21st March she wrote: " I feel much better generally
and the pain is not nearly so acute." On the 26th March
she told me: " I am still progressing satisfactorily
and all my people say how much better I am looking.
But, most important of all, when I awoke this morning,
the pain in the gall bladder was absent, although there
remained, of course, a certain amount of soreness.
I have been almost entirely free of pain during the
day. Hitherto it has always troubled me most first
thing in the morning." On the 29th March she wrote
me a letter comparing her condition when I took her
in hand and her then condition after three weeks'
treatment : —

"When I came to you my complexion was very sallow, I had bags under the eyes, no colour in the cheeks, but now it is much clearer with faint pink, and the bags have disappeared. My back felt very weak and ached dreadfully at the least exertion. It is now much stronger and the pain has disappeared. Three weeks ago I had always headaches after meals, but this symptom has gone, and my urine, which was always very cloudy, is now quite clear. The pain in the stomach which plagued me from morning till night is now only intermittent, and my circulation seems much better than it was."

On the 3rd April she wrote that she was more than satisfied with herself, and went to Torquay for a holiday. She wrote from Torquay on the 19th April: "I have felt better than ever before." On the 7th June, after three months' treatment, I saw her again, and I wrote to her: "I am more than delighted with our interview. You have put on 8 lbs., you look ten years younger, you hold yourself straight, you walk with an elastic step, and you are cheerful instead of being utterly depressed. We must now start a new chapter in your rebuilding."

During the first three months of the treatment I had not given her any coarse roughage because I suspected ulceration in stomach and bowel. I had also not given her any medicine whatever. I now gave her bran porridge, told her to leave off Vichy water and replace it with decoction of Wormwood, or with water in which potatoes had been boiled, a wonderful anti-acid. She was to have her back massaged with olive oil and she was to take Sulphur 3X to purify her blood, cleanse and activate the skin, etc.

Further progress followed. She wrote on the 18th June: "I do not get headaches any longer." On the 4th July she reported an attack of sickness: "It was not anything like as violent as the attacks I had months ago. I am gaining in strength and buoyancy. The soreness in the region of the gall bladder is getting less and less." On the 10th July she reported: "I am perspiring now on the very slightest provocation and

I get no headaches. When I look back I realize how very different I am now to what I was four months ago when I came to you. I thank my lucky star I did not get carved up! The Wormwood decoction gives me wonderful energy."

Sulphur had re-established perspiration which had been absent for many years and the Wormwood decoction has acted magnificently. Sulphur, which is used by homœopathic practitioners on the great majority of their patients, is practically not used at all by orthodox physicians. It is not sufficiently "scientific." If they use Sulphur at all, they use it in the colloidal form, preferably subcutaneously, when it does much mischief. The modern physician knows nothing about herbs. Herbal lore has been killed by the drug houses, which provide doctors with scientific extractives and combinations of dead chemicals, although nature has produced the most wonderful combinations of live remedies in her herbs.

Occasionally Miss A. G. received homœopathic medicines, such as Sulphur, Carbo vegetabilis 3X, Lachesis 12 to regulate menstruation, Hydrastis, which acts magnificently on bowel, liver and gall bladder, and so forth. Menstruation improved also. She became completely changed, was able to dance all night long, and considered herself completely cured. Years afterwards she told me that she felt perfectly well.

In this, and in numerous other cases, I have found than one ought never to take a pessimistic view. There is an unlimited power of repair within the human body. It is most inhuman to tell a patient " nothing can be done." One can always do something and can at least relieve suffering, not necessarily with poisonous benumbing drugs. The most violent pain can, as a rule, be eliminated with an infinitely small dose of some homœopathic medicine which produces the same pain in large doses. The terrible burning pain of cancer of the stomach can usually be relieved with Phosphorus or Arsenic in infinitely small doses. A physician who readily sends his patients to the surgeon does not understand his business. He should always try his hand and he may be gratified with numerous successes, such as that of Miss A. G. It is true, the surgeons had told her that she could only get worse if not operated upon, but then surgeons take a purely mechanical view of the human body and treat it with that lack of respect with which housebreakers demolish a beautiful building.

On the 6th February, 1929, I was visited by Lady L., who complained about gall stones. Like all gall stone cases, she suffered from numerous troubles, and the existence of gall stones was only the most urgent one. She was 51 years old, looked anæmic, her eyes had no sparkle, she slept badly, had an irritable bladder, an enlarged stomach, a prolapsed bowel, her kidneys were weak and her liver did not function. She looked toxic, had dark stools, had always been constipated. As a child she had suffered from ringworm badly, a condition which is usually associated with a tubercular tendency, and tuberculous mesenteric glands were cut out years ago. She could not digest fat, had lost all her teeth through pyorrhœa, had noises in the right ear, easily got influenza and complained particularly about deep depression and lassitude. She was a great salt eater and felt chilly. Her whole system needed rebuilding.

I gave her liquid paraffin to regulate her bowels, advised a lacto-vegetarian diet with an abundance of bran—and gave her Hydrastis 1X night and morning to activate liver and gall bladder and Thyroid 2X before meals to improve her appetite and to detoxicate her system. On the 24th February she reported: " I am glad to say I am feeling better. The indigestion has gone. I have still a bad taste in my mouth on waking, and my son, who has not seen me for over a month, said I was looking very much better." I then gave her Berberis, a valuable gall bladder remedy, and as she started complaining about her diet, I asked her to visit me. She arrived on the 13th March, and I wrote to her: "I find you wonderfully improved, notwithstanding your insufficient intake. You no longer feel and look flabby." I gave her further helpings of Berberis and sent her Magnesia phosphorica in case of pain.

In April improvement came to a standstill and I sent her Sulphur 12X to stimulate her power of reaction. On the 12th May she wrote: "I am feeling very much better, am sleeping better, my bowels are acting twice a day, I have had one attack of gall bladder pain, but it did not last very long, nor was it so severe." On the 26th May her husband wrote to me that he was much encouraged by her progress and very hopeful.

In view of her tuberculous tendency, I was anxious for her and gave her Tuberculinum, etc. Then she became impatient and she wrote to me on the 8th July: "It is now five months since I started on your treatment. I feel a great deal better, and if attacks occur, there is a longer period in between. *I think now I will try to go on without any medicine.*"

Lady L., who had been a sick woman since her birth, imagined that she might be cured of her gall bladder trouble and all her other defects in five months, and she became restive. She was desirous of treating herself or to try treatment elsewhere. I persuaded her to allow me to help her along. She resumed treatment and I gave her, according to indications, China 1X as a tonic and liver and gall bladder medicine, Calcarea renalis for kidney stones, Podophylline for her liver. On the 6th September she wrote: "I have had no gall bladder pain since the beginning of July." Then came still further letters reporting improvement, but on the 26th August, 1930, her husband wrote that she definitely wished to give up. I wrote in reply:—

"Lady L. came to me complaining principally about her gall bladder. As she has told me that she has had no gall bladder pain for many months, I am inclined to conclude that the gall bladder trouble is cured. Occasionally she wrote to me about other troubles, such as attacks of influenza, septic throats, etc., and I dealt with all those troubles rapidly and I think effectively. However, ever since the beginning of the treatment I found some reluctance in your wife to keep me informed. In my original directions I pointed out to her that there might be a chest weakness. Hence her liability to influenza, etc. Unfortunately I have never been able to give to this factor as much attention as I would have liked to. Lady L. wishes to be treated only for those symptoms which inconvenience her at the time, a perfectly understandable attitude, which, however, is very undesirable from my point of view. Co-operation was made difficult by her reluctance to see me. During the 18 months I looked after her I have seen her only three times."

Lady L. required not merely curing of her gall bladder, but rebuilding throughout, and this needed not 18 months, but from two to five years. She had improved vastly, but she broke off too early. Chronic and firmly established disorders are incurable to orthodox medicine. Homœopaths can cure such disorders, but time is needed. If I had been given adequate time, I might have made Lady L. perfectly normal.

An orthodox doctor, if consulted by a lady suffering with the troubles described, would have tried Belladonna plasters and such-like things to relieve the terrible gall bladder colics, and if this should be ineffective, would have used Morphia to deaden the pain. He would probably have recommended an operation and his opinion would have been confirmed by a consultant. The orthodox physician is guided by the maxim that "chronic diseases are incurable" and he limits his ministrations to relieving the most urgent symptoms with sedatives, sleeping draughts, etc.

On the 19th September, 1927, I was visited by a Mr. W. S., a business man, living at Skipton, Yorkshire. He arrived with his wife. Both seemed extremely anxious. The husband had been operated upon for gall stones in 1924 and 1926 by Lord Moynihan, the foremost abdominal surgeon. The operations had cost several hundred pounds and he had been told that henceforward he would enjoy good health. In some cases the excision of the gall bladder is easily borne. In others the patient's health is ruined for life. Thé same unevenness of results may be observed in men who had their prostate cut out and in women who had their sex organs taken away. Some do well and praise the surgeon and others curse the day when they were operated upon. The excision of organs is a very speculative undertaking.

Mr. W. S. looked hopeless, deeply jaundiced, a tottering old man, although he was only 56. Body, nerves and brain had suffered greatly. He was no longer able to look after his business, could not add up figures, was terribly nervy, and he got once a week the most atrocious attacks of rigors, which started with icy chills, followed by fever. They wore him out and drove him to despair. His weight had gone down from 12½ stone to 10 stone, his eyes were sunken, he looked like a victim of malaria. The liver did not act properly. Doctors and consultants had failed to benefit him. He had also tried a cure at a sanatorium without success. I was his last hope.

The liver and gall bladder play a very important part in the digestion of food and particularly of fat, which of course includes butter and milk. Liver and gall bladder are also of very great value in the process of excretion. Before all, it was necessary to activate liver and bowels, and improve the digestion. The alimentary mechanism of the pig closely resembles that of human beings. I told him to take, with every meal some pig-bile tabloids to replace the missing secretion, gave him liquid paraffin as a bowel lubricant, and a fat-free diet. On the 23rd September, after three days of the new treatment, his wife wrote: " Mr. S. is feeling wonderfully well to-day, the best day in all the week. His bowels freely move and he feels better in every way in consequence. He is so bright and happy to-day. To-day is the first morning that his urine is clear. His normal colour of skin is coming back, his eyes are clear and not sunken."

Three days later, on the 26th September, she wrote: " He is taking his medicine most regularly and is full of jokes about it. He is ever so bright and is eagerly looking forward to his dietary table. I know one thing, his appetite is better."

Mr. W. S. had made a most auspicious beginning, a thing of inestimable value. Unless striking improvement comes soon, patients of this type lose heart. His was a very obstinate case, for the body would not adjust itself to the absence of the gall bladder.

Presently I gave him large quantities of bran and as he had occasionally violent diarrhœas, he was given Kaylene. As the liver did not function properly, he was given liver soup of my invention made as follows: 6 or 8 ozs. of raw English liver were to be run through the mincing machine three times, to be dropped into boiling water or milk, and after a minute of cooking the soup is ready. I found this the most satisfactory way of giving liver to patients. His dietary was greatly improved and he had a glass of wine at every meal to give him an appetite and help digestion. On the 7th October, after nearly three weeks, his wife reported: " Mr. W. S. has an excretion three times a day, urine is clear, and with all the food he is having, he never complains of indigestion. His tongue is no longer coated as it used to be. His eyes are bigger and brighter and his skin is not yellow but is very pale. My husband does business more easily and is again able to concentrate his thoughts."

He went ahead nicely, putting on weight, and he flourished greatly. On the 1st November, Mr. W. S. wrote to me: " My weight at the present time is 10 stone 13, 11 lbs. more than I weighed a month ago." I then gave him cod-liver oil and malt and assisted the process of digestion and excretion with Thyroid 1X. This medicine was replaced later on by Thyroid 2X. When he developed flatulence, I sent him Asafœtida, which is excellent both for nerves and flatulence. Later on, hearing that his complexion still remained pale and yellowish, I sent him Hydrastis 1, which benefited him greatly. On the 16th August his wife told me that her husband occasionally suffered from turns of sickness, accompanied by dark yellow, foaming urine. This pointed to Chelidonium and he was given Chelidonium with marked benefit. Then symptoms appeared which seemed to demand Cholesterin, and he was given Cholesterin in alternation with Chelidonium. Cholesterin did him a particular amount of good.

On the 9th October, 1928, a year after the beginning of the treatment, he came to me and I wrote to him: "I am more than delighted with your appearance. As I told you, you look 10 years younger, and it is a pleasure to look at your pink complexion, red cheeks, ruby lips, sparkling eyes. You have been rejuvenated."

On the 2nd June, 1930, I received a letter from his wife, who told me that her husband was still taking the Pig Bile tabloids, which he had found indispensable. She wrote: —

"I am sure you will be pleased to know that my husband is keeping in splendid health. He is never without the Cholesterin tablets and the Pig Bile tabloids. He does not make a habit of taking them. He only takes them when he needs them. He is very active and he is splendid. We are very grateful because you have helped him more than any other man ever did."

CHAPTER VIII

Gastric and Duodenal Ulcer

ULCERATIVE degeneration of the stomach and of the duodenum, the part of the bowel which adjoins the stomach, is exceedingly frequent. It is a disease of civilization. Sir Arbuthnot Lane and many other eminent physicians and surgeons have told us that this trouble is unknown among primitive races, and their opinion has been confirmed by numerous doctors and surgeons who have been practising for years among the natives of Africa and elsewhere. The ulcer-free natives rapidly become subject to this trouble if they live on the white man's food. General Sir Robert McCarrison, the head of the great Pasteur Institute, at Conoor, Southern India, Professor Plimmer, of London, and many other investigators, have produced numerous cases of gastric and duodenal ulcer, appendicitis, colitis, etc., in animals of every kind, and in birds, by feeding them on the over-cooked, devitaminized, and demineralized food of the civilized.

The causation of ulcerative degeneration of the alimentary tract is obvious, and the cause points to the cure. Nevertheless, we find that the great textbooks of pathology consider the cause of these ulcers as a mystery, and scientists whose vision is limited by the walls of their laboratory are searching for the causative micro-organism of this complaint.

The leading textbooks on treatment give, as usual, a lengthy description of the disease, in which a great

I   117

amount of space is dedicated to the "morbid anatomy," to the appearance of ulceration after death, while the space given to treatment is scanty. In *The Principles and Practice of Medicine*, by Osler and McCrae, 8th edition, we read that such cases should be treated with absolute rest in bed and a carefully regulated milky diet, and then we are told: "Medicinal measures are of very little value in gastric ulcer, and the remedies employed probably do not benefit the ulcer, but the gastric catarrh." The principal remedies recommended are Bicarbonate and Bismuth, as an anti-acid, and Opium, Morphia, etc., in case of pain. Operation is advised in chronic and severe cases. In the *Index of Treatment*, by Hutchison and Sherren, 7th edition, we read: "If there is pain, we may give the anti-acid mixture, containing Bicarbonate of soda, Bismuth and Magnesia." In Letheby Tidy's *Synopsis of Medicine*, we read under the heading "Treatment": "As regards the ulcer, all drugs are useless, except Bismuth and alkalies," and the Bismuth, Bicarbonate and Magnesia mixture is recommended as the only medicine. I could quote twenty similar recommendations, given in other standard works.

Busy doctors who do rush work do not consult the ponderous textbooks which run to a thousand pages or more. They consult little pocket-books, such as *The Consultant's Appointment Book*, issued by Burroughs and Wellcome, and various other diaries, published by the other great drug houses. In the Burroughs and Wellcome diaries we find under the heading "Peptic Ulcer" the recommendation of Calcium Carbonate Compound, which contains the usual three anti-acids. Also mentioned are Belladonna and Atrophine. The latter is an extractive of Belladonna. The orthodox treatment of gastric and duodenal ulceration is primitive, resourceless, and, needless to say, ineffective. At the hospitals and dispensaries people who complain of their stomach or of indigestion, are mechanically handed "the white mixture," and if after months of its use, there is no improvement, the sufferer is told that there is nothing to be done except an operation.

If we now turn to the homœopathic treatment of gastric and duodenal ulcer we enter a different world. The homœopath has no stock mixture for all ulcers and other stomach complaints which he hands out to all. He carefully studies all the symptoms, local and constitutional, of the patient, and then prescribes the remedy. In the little *Pocket Manual of Homœopathic Materia Medica,* by Boericke, 31 remedies are enumerated under the heading "Ulcers of Stomach." In its German equivalent Balzli's *Taschenbuch,* 37 remedies are named.

Many orthodox physicians have learned that the "white mixture" relieves but does not cure. They may give it for a time to humour the patient. Some of the modern textbooks do not even mention the white mixture because of its uselessness. For instance, in Gould and Pyle's *Pocket Cyclopedia of Medicine and Surgery,* only a milky diet and operation are recommended.

I have been consulted by a large number of patients with gastric and duodenal ulcer, who had suffered from this complaint for years and who had been treated by many physicians and specialists without success. In every case nothing had been done, except giving them a milky diet, rest and the white mixture. In not a single case I heard that the doctors had enquired into the diet of the patient which had caused ulceration, and had completely reformed it, replacing the devitaminized and demineralized foods on which the patient had been living and which had caused the complaint, by natural foods rich in those essential elements.

Mr. E. W., a boilermaker, of Middlewich, Cheshire, wrote to me on the 16th July, 1929:—

"I underwent an operation for chronic appendicitis in 1926, followed by another one for gastric ulcer in 1927. I have been living on a diet since then, but I have not made much progress and still have pains in the stomach. May I come and see you?"

On the 9th August I was visited by the patient. He was 29 years old. Ever since 1921 he had been suffering from severe pains in the stomach which gradually became worse. He vomited much, the surgeon found at the operation of 1927 an ulcer near the outlet of the stomach, and he made what is called a gastro-enterostomy, an artificial connection between the wall of the stomach and the bowel. After the operation the poor fellow had pneumonia.

The patient looked thin, weedy, washed out, emaciated, consumptive, and he told me that his weight had gone down from 12 stone 6 to 8 stone 5. There was a pronounced tenderness in the gall bladder region. He had always been constipated and was kept regular by tablespoonful doses of Cascara, a much used but injurious bowel irritant, and, to neutralize his gastric acidity, he had been given for years the usual Bismuth and Magnesia mixture. Naturally, large quantities of so-called anti-acids are injurious to the system. He had been living on white bread and butter, meat, eggs, etc., as if he was a healthy man. I have a photo showing his emaciated frame at the beginning of the treatment.

I forbade flesh, fish, fowl and everything made of them, spices, condiments, alcohol, strong tea, coffee, and put him on a diet consisting chiefly of milk, eggs, honey and water in which vegetables had been boiled without salt or soda, fruit juices, etc. As the stomach pain was relieved when taking food, I gave him Anacardium 3X, indicated by that symptom, to be alternated with Kali bichromicum 3X because the pain was felt on a small spot. He was given Carbo vegetabilis 6X as an anti-acid. It is better to give a patient a millionth of a grain of charcoal than the notorious Bismuth and Magnesia mixture by the tablespoonful.

His first weekly report of the 19th August told me: "My appetite has been better. I have gained 1 lb." The next report of the 26th August said: "I have gained 1¼ lbs. and I am very pleased at gaining instead of losing weight all the time. I have started to go to

work again." Then came a standstill, followed by a
set-back, possibly caused by his going back to work
too soon, possibly by his eating 11 ozs. of honey per
day. On the 14th October he told me: " I have
gained 1½ lbs. last week, have felt much better, have
not had the gnawing pain." On the 28th October my
patient told me that he had gained 2 lbs. On the
11th November he wrote: " I have gained 1 lb., my
stomach seems to be behaving itself. I only wish I
had come to you sooner." Next week he told me:
" I have gained 2 lbs."

Medicines were changed in accordance with changing
symptoms. He was given Argentum nitricum 3 for
great acidity and violent stomach flatulence, Phosphorus for burning pain, etc. Then he got a very bad
cold and, as he looked tuberculous, I gave him Tuberculinum 12X once a week, and Spongia 1X for his dry
cough, and I was gratified to be told: " The medicine
you sent me did a world of good." His stomach got
occasionally upset and medicines had to be changed.
On the 7th April he wrote: " It is quite seven months
since I came to see you, and I am both satisfied and
grateful for what you have done for me. My parents
and friends cannot express their thanks to you. They
were spending so much money in doctor's treatments
and I was no better for it."

Ulcers of long standing are difficult to cure, even if
they occur on the surface of the skin. Many old men
and women have had an ulcerated leg for 20 or 30
years. Internal ulcers are equally stubborn. They
are apt to skin over and break open again. I have
found that it is necessary for ulcer patients to follow
a careful diet for years. The case of Mr. E. W. was
particularly serious because he had undergone two
big operations and a large part of the stomach surface
was destroyed by the ulcer and cut away. Hence his
nutrition was extremely difficult. In course of time
I added mashed vegetables, then entire vegetables, to
the dietary, fruit, roughage, etc., carefully feeling my
way. Then the poor fellow got into trouble because

employment fell off and he was too independent to accept gratuitous treatment. On the 16th February, 1931, his correspondence stopped, and he told me that he weighed 9 stone 6½ and had gained a full stone since I took him in hand. He knew what to do and was given a stock of medicines to go on with. During the end of his treatment he was given medicines in higher potencies, such as Carbo vegetabilis 30 in which potency it is an excellent remedy for stomach flatulence and acidity.

Most patients who have been benefited by treatment never afterwards inform the practitioner. Possibly they imagine that a busy professional man is not interested in their further progress. On the 3rd January, 1934, two years after his last letter, Mr. E. W. wrote to me to my great delight:—

" I expect you will be surprised to hear from me after so long. I am still out of work. Unemployment is very bad in this part of the country. I still keep to the diet that you put me on, and I am a wonderful lot better than I used to be. I still get occasional trouble with my stomach, but not like I used to have. Sometimes it will be all right for three months. My weight now is 10 stone 4 lbs. When I came to see you the first time, it was 8 stone 5. So you will see how much I have gained since the first time you saw me. My parents and friends say that I am a living wonder. I have only you to thank and no one knows it better than I do."

I sent him some further medicines in a high potency, which I hope will complete the cure. I wonder what would have happened to him if he had undergone a second operation for ulceration. I do not think that he would have survived it.

On the 27th February, 1929, Mrs. M. K., the wife of a poor agricultural labourer, living at Warmsworth, near Doncaster, wrote:—

" I have suffered from indigestion since I was 15 and am now 53. Nine years ago I had a breakdown and heart attacks. Two years after that I had an operation for displacement of the womb, from which I had suffered ever since I had my third child, 19 years ago. Nearly five years ago I was taken bad and had two more heart attacks. Now I seem as bad as ever. My food doesn't seem to do me much good, and I get hunger pain which sometimes is better when I have had food, but the pain seems to get all round my body and heart and left breast, and I have to double up with it. I had X-rays taken nearly three years ago, as my doctor thought it might be an ulcer."

Relief of stomach pain by eating points to Anacardium, which happens to be an excellent remedy for ulcer of the stomach, and Colocynthis produces, in large doses, and therefore cures in small doses, abdominal pain relieved by doubling up. So I sent her both medicines in the third decimal potency and told her to live provisionally on a milky diet and to sleep with her abdomen well raised with a small mattress, a favourite method of mine for causing prolapsed abdominal organs to return to their rightful position. I also told her to take paraffin for bowel regulation, requested full details of her medical history, and asked her to send me a photo as she was too poor to come up to London.

On the 15th May she told me that she had been improving and getting stronger all the time. On the 10th June she wrote: "I am still getting better and stronger, and I am able to walk more than I have done for some time." At that time I got her photo. She looked weary and completely worn out, the type one associates with Sepia or Secale. She rapidly gained on weight. On the 25th August she wrote: "I am feeling still stronger, and I gained 4 lbs. in a fortnight." On the 10th January, 1930, she wrote: "I am feeling a lot better, in fact I am feeling a lot stronger than I have done for years." I then alternated Anacardium with Calcarea carbonica, because she had chilly, clammy feet, gave her Ceanothus because of pain under the left breast, with dragging and aching, possibly coming from the spleen.

She had received the same old mixture week after week from her local doctor who had done her no good.

For the first time in her life she was given individual treatment and discovered to her amazement that one trouble after another became less and then disappeared. In her joy she asked her married daughter to write to me. She was very much like her mother, was married, 25 years old, suffered with goitre, had been operated upon for appendicitis, had terribly profuse and painful menstruation and floodings, one of her ovaries was diseased, and she was told that the only cure consisted in the excision of womb and ovaries. She suffered, according to the doctors, from abdominal tuberculosis and salpingitis, was a bleeder. Before I had time to take her in hand she had to be rushed to a hospital to undergo an operation because of active tuberculosis about the sex organs.

The mother faithfully clung to me. Of course, my diet had to be adapted to her exceedingly slender means. Her digestive troubles became less, her heart became stronger and gradually her system was rebuilt. Many new troubles were mentioned. Like so many poor country people, she had rheumatism which was improved with Rhus toxicodendron, her liver caused trouble and she received Hydrastis, there was violent flatulence in the bowel and she was sent Raphanus.

I then discovered that she could not digest fat, cried easily, was better in the open air, had had irregular periods. If I had seen the woman at the beginning of the treatment, I should probably have given her Pulsatilla there and then. I sent her Pulsatilla for a few weeks, which did a miracle. Then she complained about sore spongy gums, for which she got Mercurius. She discovered that Pulsatilla was her best medicine. So I gave her Pulsatilla once more. Then she complained to me about " a nasty pain as if my womb was to come down, as if something would drop out." Of course I gave her Sepia and, as usual, success was marked. Thus we went on co-operating year after year. On the 22nd September, 1932, after three and half years' collaboration, she wrote to me : —

"I have been to the seaside for a few days" (I believe this was her first holiday since her marriage) "and I was so pleased with myself as I could go out and do more walking than I have done for years. I averaged about 6 miles a day and I could walk uphill without feeling any worse for it afterwards. I felt a bit out of breath, of course, but each day I could manage it better. I had not been able to go away from my home for years, but, thanks to you and to your medicines, I felt able to stand the journey."

I then tried high potencies on her and found that she reacted splendidly to Pulsatilla 30 and to Pulsatilla 200 in rare doses. On the 10th July, 1933 she told me:—

"I do not know what to do with my feet. They have hurt me a lot and I hardly know how to walk. I felt as if I was walking on stones. I am very flat-footed."

Calcarea carbonica is a great medicine for strengthening the bones and ligaments and it is excellent for flat feet. I sent the poor old lady a large box of Calcarea carbonica 6X, two tablets to be taken night and morning, and she told me in two or three letters that her feet were vastly better.

A little while ago she sent me her photograph. The picture taken when I took her in hand and the recent picture are on her file side by side. There is hardly any resemblance between the two. On the first picture Mrs. K. looked aged, worn out, misery personified. On the second picture she is happy, smiling, looks healthy, is a completely different woman and she looks twenty years younger, although she was six years older than at the time when the first picture was taken. For years I have heard nothing about her digestive troubles, probably due to ulceration, and her heart, for which she came to me originally. Apparently she has forgotten these things, although she had suffered from stomach and heart since childhood.

On the 24th August, 1933, I was visited by a Mr. F. T., 33 years old, single, working as a clerk and chauffeur, living at Hampstead, who told me that he suffered from violent pain in the stomach and abdomen, accompanied with nausea and sickness. This complaint had been with him for years, and he had been informed by various doctors that he was suffering from a duodenal ulcer which had first been diagnosed early in 1932. The discovery was due to his losing early in that year a large quantity of blood by way of the bowel. The pain was sometimes of a burning character and at other times of a dull aching character. It was not relieved by eating. It was aggravated by bending and improved by straightening up.

These pains had plagued him since 1925 or 1926, and it seemed therefore likely that ulceration had been in existence for at least seven or eight years. He had a great deal of heartburn after meals. For years he had been under treatment. He told me his doctors had given him " gallons " of the white mixture. Bismuth and other alkalies neutralize acidity if mixed in a laboratory vessel. From this fact arises the notion that the alkalies are a cure for acidity of the stomach. If the glands of the stomach which excrete acids are dosed with alkalies, they excrete an increased quantity of acids. Hence the white mixture, while momentarily relieving the patient, actually increases acid production. He also complained of lack of energy, loss of brain power, and of memory and replied slowly to my questions.

Mr. F. T. had been going to various doctors and he had faithfully swallowed gallons and gallons of the white mixture which had temporarily benefited him. None of the medical men had condescended to study his case. As soon as one bottle was exhausted another bottle was given, and the temporary benefit had kept Mr. F. T. going. He came to me because he had become alarmed. The white mixture did no longer act. During a fortnight he had been prostrated by violent pain in the abdomen, which was with him day and night. He had been told that an operation might be necessary, and he dreaded the surgeon's knife. He had lost a great deal of weight.

It was quite unnecessary to examine the man. The recital of his symptoms made it quite clear to me that the diagnosis was correct, and the large size of the spot where the pain was felt made it clear that ulceration was extensive and that there was the danger that the ulcer might eat through the bowel wall and that at any moment he might be prostrated with most dangerous peritonitis. I frankly told him that the position was serious, and that, if he felt violent pain, he would have to be rushed off to the hospital for operation. However, I gave him every encouragement and told him that the progressive loss of weight which he had suffered was only natural under the circumstances, and that he would regain it soon.

Homœopaths are guided not by pathological findings and exact diagnosis—there are hardly any exact diagnoses—but by the symptoms of the patient. As a rule patients with colic, gastric and duodenal ulcer, appendicitis and other abdominal complaints, are relieved by doubling up and pressure. The fact that Mr. F. T. was relieved by holding himself absolutely straight and that doubling up or bending was unbearable enabled me to " diagnose " the remedy at a glance. I took a few tiny sugar pilules medicated with Dioscorea villosa (Wild Yam), dissolved them in a cup of hot water, and asked him to sip a teaspoonful. The water was tasteless. The patient smiled at me sceptically and said " I am afraid you are trying the faith cure on me." " No, I am making an experiment which will show whether I have selected the right remedy." In ten minutes he said " The pain is distinctly less." " Take another teaspoonful." He took a few more teaspoonfuls of tasteless warm water and in half an hour his pain was gone. It was quite clear to me that Dioscorea was the right remedy for him. I had cured duodenal ulcer before with that medicine and I felt confident that it would cure my patient.

I gave him a box of Dioscorea 3X to take with him and told him to take 3 pilules three times a day, between meals. I also gave him Sulphur 6X, a dose to be taken night and morning, and some Carbo vegetabilis 30th potency to be taken at odd times if troubled with acidity. He looked at the various tasteless sugar pilules with a dubious smile and thought that the pain had disappeared in my house through coincidence. A few days after I sent him my directions, put him on a diet with large quantities of ordinary bran, vegetables, potatoes, milk, eggs, but absolutely forbade flesh, fish, fowl and everything made of them, white sugar, white flour, white bread, jam, spices and condiments, and forbade the use of aluminium cooking utensils.

Orthodox medicine puts those who suffer from gastric and duodenal ulcer first on a milky diet and then on a diet free from roughage, which, on abstract and theoretical grounds, seems called for. An internal ulcer may be irritated by bran, pieces of coarse vegetable, etc. However, I did not attach much value to physical injury of the ulcer in this case. Mr. F. T., like his father before him, had lived chiefly on a diet of white bread, meat, fish, cheese, boiling hot tea, etc., a diet deprived of vitamins and essential mineral elements. I took the view that, considering the seriousness of the case, high vitamin feeding was essential, that the risk of mechanical injury of the ulcerated portions ought to be run, and that the orthodox method of feeding employed in all hospitals should be disregarded. I thought this particularly necessary because the patient was extremely anæmic, weak, had been suffering much with varicose veins, and from effusions of blood into the tissues, etc., and he had been kept in bed by the doctors for six months, and longer, at a time. These developments also seemed to me due to vitamin starvation. I felt I took a considerable risk in devising this unorthodox dietary, but I thought the risk was worth taking. In my directions I told the young man that he was to gain from 2 to 3 lbs. per week. He reported to me on the 4th September:—

"Weight 10 stone 4, a 2 lb. gain. I have not entirely got rid of the pain in the abdomen, relieved by straightening up, but had it not very badly. I am certainly feeling brighter. My memory is improving, also my eyesight is better."

He wrote on the 11th September:—

"Weight 10 stone 5, a gain of 1 lb., slight pain. I am not disappointed at the apparent lack of real headway as I realize that I cannot be cured in two weeks."

The next report dated the 19th September said:—

"I am 10 stone 6, a gain of another lb., pain has been nagging, but not serious. I am convinced that there is a gradual improvement in my general health, and once or twice I have felt more fit than I have done for a long time."

His letter of the 26th September said:—

"Am 10 stone 7, have gained another lb., had during the week only one of two spasms of pain lasting about 10 minutes. I can now happily and definitely affirm a genuine improvement. My head is clearer, especially on waking. No more of that awful drowsiness that further sleep would never cure. Also the food gives me better staying powers, and I do not now experience that feeling of exhaustion in the evening which was a common occurrence some while back."

On the 10th October the patient wrote:—

"I endeavoured to go along without medicine as I was feeling so fit. All went well until Wednesday, when I had an attack of heartburn. Over the last week-end I had occasion to take only once a couple of heartburn pilules, Carbo veg. 30. Yesterday I had a slight return of pain, stopped by taking a couple of Dioscorea pilules. I remain much improved in quick thinking and remembering."

Several weeks afterwards Mr. F. T. called at my house. He looked a completely different man. He had put on more than a stone, had grown out of all his clothes, had brilliant colours, was in the highest spirits, had had no pain whatever, felt better than he had ever done in his life, and told me that he thought that he could now do without medicine.

The experimental attempt to feed a patient with serious, extensive and long-standing ulceration on roughage had apparently proved a great success. This cure should be of considerable interest to all prescribers who have to treat cases of gastric and duodenal ulcer. It was a revelation to me. I had previously in such cases invariably given a smooth diet. As the patient had been kept by the doctors on a milky diet for many months at a time, I thought it would be utterly useless to give him again a milky diet, which is poor in mineral elements, especially iron.

CHAPTER IX

Chronic Rheumatism and Arthritis

CHRONIC rheumatism and arthritis are crippling complaints which are difficult to cure, especially if they have been in existence for a long time. Orthodox treatment is unsatisfactory. Everyone is acquainted with cases in which long-continued medicinal treatment and prolonged stays at various watering places have failed. There is no routine treatment. One must go into the causation of the disease. In many cases it is due to chronic constipation, to a faulty diet, to an infection or to an obscure hereditary factor. Every possible hereditary taint should be considered. In many cases Carcinosinum, the disease product of cancer, given in infinitely small doses at rare intervals, proves highly beneficial. In other cases Medorrhinum or Tuberculinum effects a cure.

Some years ago a very wealthy man applied to me for help. He had a castle in the country and an establishment in Park Lane. He was crippled by rheumatoid arthritis and so was his brother. Very likely some hereditary factor was at least partly responsible. He had travelled to numerous watering-places in Europe and to the hot springs in New Zealand, had daily massage from an excellent masseur and had spent more than £20,000 on treatments of every kind, but none of them had proved successful.

My sense of smell told me the cause. The man had suffered from delay in the bowel for decades and the toxins had produced the degeneration which had crippled him. Yet no one before me had pointed this out to him. I told him that he would have to replace his laxatives by ordinary bran. "Bran? Is that the stuff which I give to my pigs?" "Yes." "And you expect me to eat it?" "Certainly." "Do you want me to eat it from a trough?" "You can please yourself. I personally would prefer eating it from a plate." He rose in speechless indignation and wanted to leave the room. However, I told him earnestly that I might cure him with bran and he consented to try. He improved vastly in a few weeks, he learned to love his bran dishes, and his wife and masseur commented on the fact that the evil odour from his body had completely disappeared. He improved immensely but complete cure was impossible. His hip joint had become badly displaced years ago. That condition could not be put right either by diet or by medicine.

In spring, 1928, my wife and I were tramping in the South Downs. We admired the view from Chancton-bury Ring, and fell in with a young lady who was enraptured with the prospect. After a while she told us: "I left my mother at the bottom of the hill. She is an invalid. I have to take her about in a bath chair." I asked: "What is the matter with your mother?" "She is stiff with rheumatoid arthritis and has been incapacitated for many years." "Is she constipated?" "Yes." "And is she very stout?" "Yes, very stout." "Possibly she might be cured by reducing her weight and regulating her bowel." The lady became interested and on the 14th April she came to my house with her mother.

Mrs. McG. was an extremely pleasant looking lady over 70, stiff all over, with thick nodes on her hands, and one of her hips had been displaced long ago. The medicines she had been given by various doctors had done no good. I explained to her that medicine was a very secondary thing in her case while diet was extremely important. Besides, her over-weight—she weighed nearly 12 stone—was a serious handicap. She could hope to learn to walk only if there were less dead weight on her troublesome legs. The lady promised enthusiastically to carry out my directions.

I gave her a reducing diet. She was to take two small slices of very crisp wholemeal toast with the thinnest butter and an egg for breakfast, an abundance of vegetables, potatoes, and an egg and a couple of biscuits mid-day; vegetables, potatoes, fresh fruit and perhaps another egg in the evening, and in between meals she was to drink about six tumblerfuls of water in which potatoes had been boiled, and containing the potato alkalies, and two tumblerfuls of nettle tea. I drew her attention to the fact that it would take a long time to get her into order. She was to lose from 1 to 3 lbs. a week.

On the 7th May she wrote to me that her weight was 11 stone 4 lbs. 8 ozs. On the 14th May she wrote to me: "I have lost 4 lbs. I am doing my duty and am losing weight. The chemist thought the scales must be wrong. He tested them and found them correct." On the 25th May she wrote: "I am feeling wonderfully well." On the 31st May she told me: "My leg is certainly getting easier and is not so painful unless I get over-tired." On the 6th June she said: "I am now 10 stone 11 lbs. 10 ozs." On the 21st June came the news: "I feel a great improvement in every limb since I began your treatment, and have every confidence that you will eventually cure me." In order to accelerate her progress, her daughter was to rub her body, and especially her limbs, with olive oil, and circulation in the legs was to be activated by hot footbaths at night, strengthened with mustard.

On the 4th July, after six weeks' treatment, she came to my house. She had lost about a stone, looked far better, but felt weak. Weight reduction had been too fast. I recommended her to take a pint of milk per day and a little cheese and told her that weight reduction should only be from 1 lb. to 1½ lbs. per week. The old lady found that not only her legs worked more easily, but that also her breathing became more comfortable. Previously she had been troubled with

K

asthma-like difficulties. On the 10th September she wrote that she was wonderfully improved, and was going on a journey which previously she would not have been able to undertake.

On the 29th October she wrote to my delight: " My breathing is quite good and I can walk up a hill quite comfortably. The only trouble is, I cannot manage the stairs very well, unless they are very shallow." I discovered that her insteps had sunken down, so I prescribed foot supports, which helped her greatly. On the 14th November she came to my house and I found her vastly improved.

It was now time to start specific medication. So I gave her Sulphur 3X to be taken night and morning, and Xanthoxyllum 3K for her pains in joints, to be taken in between. Both suited her admirably. On the 26th November she wrote: " Whether it is from the effect of the little pills added to the other treatment I do not know, but my leg is decidedly better at present." On the 3rd December she told me: " My leg is decidedly better. I wonder where I should have been at this time but for your treatment."

People with a good digestion are apt to put on weight with surprising rapidity. On the 2nd January, 1929, the lady told me shamefacedly that during the Christmas holidays she had gained 3 lbs., but then she had had the normal diet. I told her that her rapid gain was proof positive that a very sparing diet was necessary for her, and she agreed. There were complaints about rheumatism, particularly bad in damp weather and when sitting still. For this she was given Rhus tox. with excellent results. Then her weight started creeping up, and I told her that, unless she kept it down, I should have to give her a strict fast once a week. On the 28th May, 1929, she wrote: " Every one has been telling me how much younger and how well I look, and I feel so." On the 19th June she wrote: " Ever and ever and ever so many thanks for all your goodness and kindness to me, not only for having cured me of my rheumatism." On the 11th December she told me: "I am thankful to tell you I still keep quite well, and free from rheumatism, thanks to your treatment."

On the 12th February, 1930, she called at my house and I found her tremendously improved. As her rheumatism was now better in damp weather, I gave her Causticum 3 which proved very helpful. On the 19th March she wrote: "All my friends who have not seen me for a time have asked what I had been doing as I look years younger than when they last saw me. So I tell them it is all due to you and that I feel as well as I look."

The old lady had abandoned her bath chair and had learned to walk about. One fine day she blithely trotted across the road and was smashed up by a motor-car. She was rushed to the hospital and her daughter came to me in despair. She told me about the accident and exclaimed: "She has broken a number of bones and she is sure to die. What shall I do? What shall I do? She is my only friend."

I told her: "It is true your mother is well over 70, but my treatment has rejuvenated her, and, for all practical purposes, she is a young woman. If there is nothing worse the matter with her than broken bones, they will mend in record time, but of course there is the danger of injury to an organ." I gave the daughter Arnica for the mother's bruises and shock, and Symphytum, a wonderful bone-mending medicine. Unfortuately they could not be used, because the hospital people knew nothing about homœopathy and forbade their introduction. Still, the old lady did wonderfully well and to the surprise of the doctors and surgeons her bruises disappeared, and the bones grew together in record time, and six weeks after the accident she was at my house, looking as cheerful and happy as ever, but she was completely deaf. She had been given a bed next to a window. Her protests that a cold wind was blowing into her face were disregarded. She was told that the window had to be kept open from 10 to 6. Happily the indicated homœopathic medicines succeeded once more and she regained her hearing.

Mrs. McG. has remained well ever since and she is happiness and cheerfulness personified, and she can trot about, but of course a displaced hip joint makes progress somewhat awkward.

On the 4th April, 1933, I was visited by a magnificent specimen of manhood, Captain A. M., who had been employed in Central Asia. He complained to me bitterly about muscular rheumatism, which had attacked him for no obvious reason five months previously. Besides, he complained about a tennis elbow. Curiously enough, a diplomat and various other Europeans were also attacked by similar and excruciating pains, which occurred somewhat anomalously in various parts of the body. They had been exposed to extreme fluctuations of temperature which might have been responsible. Further, all of them had drunk unboiled water from a grossly polluted pool. Captain A. M. had had smallpox which produces the most atrocious pain in the back and elsewhere, he had undergone numerous inoculations and had been using aluminium vessels. There were many possible causes for his complaint.

In order to deal with his trouble scientifically, which means causatively, it was obvious that symptomatic treatment of the so-called rheumatism with the indicated homœopathic medicines would not suffice, and that, in addition, the possibility had to be taken into account that the attacks of pain were due to contaminated water, subcutaneous treatments, smallpox, and aluminium. I resolved to deal with all the possible factors. As relief was experienced by violent movement, I gave him Rhus tox. 3X, which was clearly indicated, and in view of his tennis elbow I gave him Arnica 3X. He was to take these two medicines at the rate of 3 pilules three times a day, to change every three days from one medicine to the other and to observe carefully which of the two was more helpful. In addition I gave him Thuya 30 as a vaccination antidote, to be taken every Saturday, and Alumina 200, as an aluminium antidote, to be taken every Wednesday.

On the 12th April he wrote that there was some improvement and on the 20th he reported: " I feel vastly better and indeed could say at the moment that I feel entirely cured." I thought this statement premature, and asked him to call. He came on the 24th April. I gave him a dose of Rhus tox. 30 at my house, and a box of Rhus tox. 6, 3 to be taken night and morning. He told me, to my delight, that the first dose of Thuya 30, given as a vaccination antidote, had caused a violent reaction in the form of severe pain, which woke him up at night, and that the first dose of Alumina 200 likewise had caused an outbreak of pain. I therefore concluded that his troubles were partly due to vaccination or to his various injection treatments. to which Thuya would act as an antidote, and partly to aluminium poisoning. He was a very observant man, and he reported on the 16th May:—

" I did not take the inoculation antidote last time as I was away and did not wish to incapacitate myself. On Saturday last I took a dose of the vaccination antidote again and had only a very slight reaction. The reactions seem to be getting less severe each time. I feel almost entirely well and I propose continuing with the antidotes for a time until they have no effect."

As a rule I start patients with low or medium potencies and then go on to higher potencies. On the 27th May Captain A. M. wrote: " The antidoes still bring a slight reaction. It appears to me that the antidote medicines should be taken until no appreciable reaction takes place." I approved and, as there was still some rheumatism and as the elbow trouble broke out once more after a violent game of tennis, I sent him four doses of Rhus tox. 200, to be taken rather rarely, and a box of Ruta 1X marked " Periosteum," because that medicine is particularly useful on the periostal structure. He reported on the 9th June: " I took a dose of Rhus tox. 200 on Tuesday of last week, and the rheumatic pains entirely vanished until the following Monday when they returned to some extent." Obviously the patient did well with high potencies. On the 12th June I sent him Arnica 30 and Ruta 30 for his tennis elbow, doses to be taken very rarely, and a single dose of Rhus. tox. 1,000th potency. On the 2nd July he wrote: " My rheumatism has been very much better. I have had to take Rhus tox. 200 about once a week when I felt it coming on again."

On the 17th July he visited me with his mother and I learned from her that she also was troubled with rheumatism and the question arose whether his complaint was due to inheritance. On the 21st July he was given Thuya 200 as a vaccination antidote and Alumina 200 as an aluminium antidote, a single dose of each to be taken once a fortnight. On the 31st he reported: " On Monday I took the inoculation antidote and within three hours had a slight ache in every muscle that has ever been affected." It was therefore quite clear that vaccination had been a causative factor. But he reacted to the aluminium antidote as well, though less strongly, by pain in the muscles.

Orthodox doctors have their pet rheumatism medicine or medicines and they give them month after month, year after year, even if there is no effect. Homœopaths cannot afford to act in this mechanical fashion. Homœopathic medication depends entirely upon the symptoms, and if the symptoms change, medication must be altered as well. On the 4th September, Captain A. M. wrote that the character of his pain had changed. Instead of coming on when at rest and improving on movement, the pain was now aggravated by movement and benefited by rest. I therefore sent him Bryonia 3X, which is indicated in that form of pain, whether rheumatismal or not. As it did much good, I followed Bryonia 3X by Bryonia 30 and then by Bryonia 200.

On the 9th October he told me that he had had

another attack of pain, though slight, and he sent me a most important piece of new information.

" By chance I have heard in the last few days of two people who got severe rheumatism as an after-effect of scarlet fever, contracted after childhood. I do not know whether I mentioned to you that I had scarlet fever for the second time when I was 19. I did not notice rheumatic symptoms at the time, but my feet used to swell every evening, and it was many months before I got over the apparent effects. Perhaps something still lingers. If there is such a thing as an antidote for the after-effects of scarlet fever, perhaps you will send me some? "

This highly intelligent officer had happily drawn my attention to a new factor which had hitherto not been mentioned. I sent him a few doses of Scarlatininum 100th potency, a dose to be taken once a month. On the 1st November he wrote: " I took the scarlet fever antidote and felt a reaction in all the affected muscles next day, and am now infinitely better. This seems almost to have done the trick. I will, if you approve, take another dose of each of the antidotes at intervals of a week or ten days." Of course I approved. It was now clear by his reactions that his rheumatism was due to what bacteriologists might call " a mixed infection." His reactions showed that he was extraordinarily sensitive to medicines in ultra-microscopic doses. It was therefore not surprising that vaccination, aluminium and scarlatina had had each their share. He thought that still higher potencies would be useful, and as he had to leave for India, I gave him a supply of high potencies, among them Rhus tox. 100,000th potency and Bryonia 100,000th potency.

The account of the treatment of this splendid soldier shows that homœopaths can diagnose promptly and reliably many diseases which are not diagnosable in the orthodox way. Orthodox medicine ignores aluminium poisoning because experiments made on animals have not absolutely proved that aluminium is a poison. Of course animals react differently from human beings, but this important fact is disregarded by the modern scientists. A rabbit can eat a quantity of Belladonna, which would kill a human being. Furthermore, modern science denies that vaccination may act as a poison which is able to upset the normal functioning of the body for life. Homœopaths are acquainted with that fact and they know how to antidote vaccinial poisoning. Lastly, orthodox medicine does not believe that the evil effect of scarlet fever may appear 15 years later in the form of mysterious rheumatic pain.

Very likely Captain A. M. would have been laughed at, had he gone to a dozen of the most eminent consultants and had asked them whether his rheumatism could have been caused by vaccinial poisoning, aluminium poisoning, and the ancient scarlatina. I daresay that the foul water which he and other Englishmen drank in Central Asia or exposure to violent changes in the temperature were responsible for the primary outbreak in him and his friends. Very likely that attack stirred up in his case the other factors which I was able to detect and to antidote. Homœopathy takes note of the slightest indications and can make the finest tests, tests which are unknown to official medicine.

CHAPTER X

Chronic Constipation and its Sequels

THE civilized and the uncivilized die of two entirely different sets of diseases. Primitive men are normally healthy and they die suddenly from exposure, want, violence, and various infectious diseases which may be called dirt diseases, such as typhoid, cholera, etc., which are little known among the civilized. The civilized die of chronic diseases and are chronically ailing. Our health and comfort depend on our daily doses of laxatives, sedatives, tonics, etc. To most men and women, pills and salts are at least as important as is food.

The uncivilized live on natural food and they have a healthy alimentary tract from the mouth to the anus. They have excellent teeth, roomy jaws and throats, a good digestion and a perfect excretion without artificial means, while the alimentary tract of the civilized is weak, disordered and diseased. Dental decay, pyorrhœa, tonsillitis, adenoids, dyspepsia, gastritis, appendicitis, colitis and cancer of the food tract, are universal among us. They are practically unknown among primitive peoples.

Food, and especially animal food, putrefies in a stagnant bowel. It generates virulent poisons and these are absorbed by the bowel walls, especially if they have been weakened and injured by irritating laxatives and purgatives. These poisons enter the blood-stream, they circulate throughout the body, and they produce countless diseases and disorders and aggravate every malady known to medical science.

In the opinion of Sir Arbuthnot Lane and many other eminent medical men, chronic constipation is one of the principal causes of cancer. It is certainly significant that most cancerous growths appear along the alimentary tract, in the mouth, the tongue, the œsophagus, the stomach and the bowel. The health of every house depends on its drainage system. The health of human beings also depends on the efficiency of their drainage system, on the easy and natural working of the bowel and the rapid elimination of poisonous waste matter.

Natural instinct points out the danger to human beings and animals. Primitive men and women empty their bowels two or three times a day. So do all animals and they become anxious at the first sign of bowel irregularity. Our domestic animals refuse food' at the first sign of constipation but drink copiously. We have lost our natural instincts, and unfortunately official medicine is so much interested in textbook diseases, most of which are caused or aggravated by constipation, that it takes little notice of constipation itself, although it is the most fruitful cause of disease among the civilized.

In the great textbooks of medicine, constipation as a disease and as a cause of disease is scarcely mentioned. The standard volume of Osler and McCrae, *The Principles and Practice of Medicine,* treats chronic constipation and auto-intoxication as of no account. Referring to the teachings of Lane, Metchnikoff and others, the volume states: " The fad is passing." Unfortunately doctors are taught during their years of study countless subjects which are of no practical use to them or to their patients, and the all-important subject of wise nutrition and regular excretion is omitted.

The majority of doctors, if consulted about constipation, merely recommend Cascara sagrada or some other laxative, and, if pressed for more satisfactory advice, they often say: " Do not worry about your constipation. It is a matter of no importance. I myself am troubled in that way and I take such-and-such drug."

Chronic constipation and auto-intoxication are responsible not only for the numerous diseases usually mentioned in the advertisements of the pill makers, but they are also responsible for mental degeneration, nerve diseases, insanity. Hippocrates taught twenty-three centuries ago that insanity can frequently be cured by bowel regulation. Men and women who are constipated get depressed and that depression frequently deepens into melancholia and insanity.

The vast majority of doctors either do not know how to cure chronic constipation or do not care to do so. I shall show by a few examples that even the most severe cases can be permanently cured by diet.

In May, 1930, I received a letter from a Mr. G. J. B., a retired business man, who told me that he was 82 years old, that in the past he had always had easy bowel action, but that two years ago he became very constipated, so much so that he feared an obstruction. He visited several first-rate consultants in London. The X-ray plates showed that there was an obstruction in the pelvic colon. Besides, there was an enlargement of the prostate. He had also had hæmorrhoids, which had been eliminated by injections. He had read the books of Sir Arbuthnot Lane and my own, and had become a vegetarian. Not unnaturally I feared that the sudden development of constipation in his extreme old age was a very serious matter.

The patient visited me on the 21st July. He looked a very healthy man and told me that he relied on Senna pods and Taxols for regulating his bowels. I gave him Ferrum picricum 6X for his enlarged prostate and Argentum nitricum 6X for violent flatulence, of which he complained. As paraffin did not act in his case, I gave him Vichy water, a tumblerful to be taken three times a day, three-quarters of an hour before meals, and as his skin was very dry and harsh, I told him to rub himself all over with whisky, an excellent skin softener. For bowel regulation I relied, as usual, chiefly on bran and that wonderful food acted splendidly.

Very old people are difficult to handle. It is not easy to change their views and ways. Besides, they are apt to forget taking their medicine, etc. Still, with patience and perseverance I succeeded. Mr. G. J. B. improved. He wrote on the 23rd November:—

" I have a bit of really good news that I think will please you. You will remember that when I first came to you in May of this year, what I regarded as my most serious trouble was constipation, arising from the bowel condition disclosed by Dr. Jordan's X-ray photos, and seeming to indicate permanent use of laxatives. Be that as it may, it has been a great satisfaction and relief to find that now for a fortnight I have been able to dispense with laxatives entirely, and I am hoping now that this happier state of things may continue."

What is called constipation is not a state of affairs which can be put right by the free use of some laxative or other. That trouble may arise from many different causes. It may be due to a faulty diet, to insufficient liquid, causing the bowel contents to become hard and dry, a faulty posture during the act of excretion, loss of internal flesh and fat which causes the contents of the abdomen to sag down, shrinkage of abdominal muscles which may be corrected by appropriate exercise, or self-massage, or a surgical belt, etc.

The old gentleman not only found it quite easy to dispense with laxatives which he hated, but notwithstanding the gloomy prognostications of the ablest consultants, he became rejuvenated. I provided him with the necessary homœopathic remedies, to which he objected very strongly because they were drugs, and I had to explain to him that I was giving him habitually medicines in doses of one millionth of a grain so that he would get only one grain of medicine if he took any of my pilules for a thousand years at the rate of three doses a day.

Occasionally the old gentleman got in trouble, fell down on one of his long walks, or contracted influenza, but every time he came up smiling. On the 12th December he wrote:—

" I continue in splendid bowel condition without use of any laxatives whatever, save such as the food itself represents. In fact, if anything, my bowels are on the easy and copious side. I would not have them easier or more frequent, and I am rather surprised at the quantity of my excreta in relation to the amount of food consumed."

This phenomenon is frequently found in those who take plenty of bran. Bran is not only an excellent food, for it contains extremely valuable proteins and an abundance of Phosphorous, Iron, Lime, etc., but it acts like a sponge, absorbing liquid, thus keeping the bowel contents moist and loose, facilitating excretion. On the 20th February, 1931, my friend wrote: " I am feeling well, though lazy and procrastinating. My bowels, which I regard as the main thing, continue in order, and I am sleeping well, latterly only waking once in the midde of the night and again towards morning. I have gained a couple of lbs. or so."

On the 20th April, Mr. B. came to London. He looked ten years younger. The bladder condition proclaimed that there was improvement in his prostate, which was partly due to improved bowel action, partly to dietetic regulation, and partly to gentle homoeopathic remedies. The bowel trouble was apparently permanently cured, for up to the end of 1933 I have received no serious complaint from him.

I received a letter, date the 11th April, 1930, from Mr. A. W. E., living at Ratcliffe, London, asking me for an interview, because of mucous colitis. I saw the patient, a young man of 21, clerk in the London County Council, on the 17th April, and he explained to me tha. he had the greatest difficulty with his motions. They were ribbon-shaped at some times and at others of stony hardness. They alternated with liquid diarrhœas, which were apt to come on very suddenly, to his distress, and which had the most putrid smell. He also had violent bowel urgings without result, especially at night. He told me that he had been kept for several weeks at the Mile End Hospital for observation, and that the doctors had not been able to diagnose the case to their satisfaction, and had suggested that he suffered from a polypus blocking the passage and had talked of an operation.

I ascertained that he had not seen any blood, nor had he had black stools, suggesting blood. He had been sent away from the hospital without any useful advice. His trouble had begun a year previously, he had been always more or less constipated and had been living on a diet poor in vitamins and mineral elements. He was tall, red-haired, very pale, very thin, and he was alarmed by the fact that he had lost 2 stone during his illness. He thought that he might have cancer. He weighed 9 stone 4 lbs.

The case was obscure, and, although bowel cancer is very rare in people of his age, I felt seriously concerned about him. I naturally put him immediately on my anti-cancer diet, forbidding flesh, fish, fowl and everything made of them, strong tea, condiments, but I also forbade roughage of every kind, vegetables and fruit, fearing that any of these might lead to trouble if there was an obstruction. Bowel action was to be normalized with liquid paraffin. He was to live on a milky diet, and he was to have an abundance of bran in the form of bran decoction without the roughage, and, instead of vegetables, he was to take large quantities of water in which vegetables had been boiled. As a tonic he was to have boiled, unbleached sultanas, passed through the sieve, the skins to be thrown away. Before all, I put his mind at rest as well as I could. He was given Sulphur 6X every morning, Nux vomica 3X last thing at night, and Belladonna 3X two or three times in the course of the day between meals. Nux vomica was to deal with the terrible stool-urging which he experienced during the night, and Belladonna was to cure the inflammatory condition within his abdomen.

On the 26th April he sent me his first report: "Owing to heavy pressure of work, due to the holiday period, I have been unable to take meals at regular intervals. My weight this day is 9 stone 8½ lbs. This seems a very big step forward. I am going to stool three times a day. During the last three mornings I have had a sharp, painful, liquid stool." I wrote in reply: "You are a miracle, having put on 4½ lbs. in a week." A week later he reported: " I must be a miracle. My weight to-day is 9 stone 11 lb. 14 ozs. The burning sensation is of a much less frequent occurrence." I replied: "In two weeks you have put on 8 lbs., a large family joint, and you must have improved immensely in every direction." The next letter, dated 10th May, stated: " My weight to-day is 9 stone 11 lb. 10 ozs."

He came to see me for the second time on the 15th May, after four weeks' treatment, and I told him to continue the medicines as before, but I gave him in addition Belladonna 30. He was to find out whether that drug suited him best in doses of a thousandth of a grain or in doses of a decillionth of a grain. On the 25th May he wrote: " My weight to-day is 10 stones 4 lbs. 3 ozs., a gain of a stone since I came to you. I have found Belladonna 30 to be most efficient." I told him to take that medicine sparingly. On the 14th June he sent me some interesting new information: "While in hospital, I was given a barium meal for an X-ray examination, and the film showed that the bowel was very prolapsed, causing obstruction. The radiologist seemed puzzled, and was at a loss to know why the meal did not pass out in scheduled time." Possibly the trouble was largely due to emaciation and the sinking down of the bowel, forming one of the kinks, discovered by my great friend, Sir Arbuthnot Lane.

Gradually I improved his diet, but kept him on Belladonna 30. On the 8th July he wrote: " My weight is now 10 stone 6, and my appetite is excellent, one might say enormous. I long for my food nowadays." Previously he had been unable to eat. I now put him on vegetables, fruit and roughage, including bran, in abundance, feeling confident that these could not injure him. Apart from perfectly natural set-backs, often experienced during intensive feeding, he did well. I gave him on the 17th July, Sulphur 30 " in the hope of establishing perspiration." On the 3rd August he wrote: " I now perspire more freely." On the 17th August he reported: " I have already had to discard my collars and obtain a size larger, and 1 expect that I shall shortly have to put my present suits up for sale. I weigh 10 stone 7½ lbs., an increase of 18¼ lbs. since the beginning of the treatment." I wrote to him on the 25th August: —

" The most important thing for you to do is to forget your old fears. As doctors and surgeons were searching for ' a growth ' in your inside, they naturally filled you with alarm, feelings which are not exactly helpful to recovery. Your magnificent reaction to my treatment seems to indicate that there is nothing of an alarming nature in your inside."

On the 28th September he was 10 stone 9 lbs. 9 ozs. As he felt liverish and weak, I sent him Hydrastis 1X, partly to act on his liver and gall bladder, partly to act prophylactically if there should be a cancerous tendency. As a tonic, I sent him China 3, the two to be taken in alternation. His letter of the 7th October told me: " I am now 10 stone 10 lbs. 9 ozs., I am very regular and there are no signs of any of the old troubles." On the 5th November I sent him Collin-sonia 1X, a wonderful medicine for hæmorrhoids and other growths in the bowel, on the assumption that possibly there were some growths obstructing the passage, and gave him Crataegus mother tincture as a tonic. On the 10th November Mr. A. W. E. wrote: " My appetite has assumed gigantic proportions. I weigh now 10 stone 12, a gain of 22 lbs." On the 21st December he wrote: " My weight is now 10 stone 13, a gain of 23 lbs. I am looking forward to this Christmas more than any previous one. It is good to know that I can eat as much as I want, without any fear whatever.

On the 19th February, ten months after our first interview, he came to see me. I wrote to him:-

"When you came to me first you looked like a spectre, emaciated, desperate. To-day you looked the picture of health, your weight has increased from 9 stone 4 to 10 stone 13, and all your troubles have disappeared. However, I noticed on your scrotum a considerable number of fleshy growths, ranging from the size of a filbert nut to that of small peas, of which you have never told me, as you ought to have done."

It is always wise to examine the whole of the body of a patient, even if the complaint is only about a strictly local trouble. Examination of the scrotum clearly showed to me the cause of any obstruction in the bowel. I explained to him that if one has "a lump-forming tendency," one may get lumps not only on the outside of the body, but also in the inside, particularly in the bowel. Polypi and similar growths occur readily inside the body, especially in the bowel. Mr. J. Lockhart-Mummery, the well-known surgeon and cancer specialist, has found in a vast number of cases bowel cancer associated with polypi.

Of course I did not tell the young man of this danger, but I gave him Thuya 30, a dose to be taken twice a week, and the growths on his scrotum were to act as an indicator as to the position of similar growths existing probably in his inside. To reinforce Thuya, I later on gave him Sulphur 30 as well. Presently letter after letter stated that the fleshy growths had become very much smaller. On the 2nd April he wrote: "The bowel trouble seems to have completely disappeared. People envy me for my wonderful health." On the 17th April he wrote: "I have never enjoyed better health in all my life. My weight is now 11 stone 1." I replied "Bravo!" On the 14th May he called on me. He looked wonderfully well and I told him to continue Thuya 30 and Sulphur 30 in alternation. I now told him to leave off liquid paraffin which was no longer needed. On the 10th October he wrote: "I enjoy the finest health of my life. My weight remains above 11 stone."

That ended the case. I told him to take an abundant

L

amount of exercise. When I saw him last he was a magnificent man, a model of strength and of virility, whereas he came to me as a stricken and despondent man.

On the 2nd July, 1932, I was visited by a Mrs. C. R., who lived in a small town in Dumfriesshire. She was married to a well-to-do man. Mrs. C. R. was a very refined woman, a lover of music, an excellent amateur violinist, and she complained about chronic constipation, shyness and nervousness. Her whole frame trembled when she had to appear in public, and before any public appearance she got violent nervous diarrhœas. For years her bowels had never acted without drastic purgatives.

She looked the picture of self-poisoning, thin, strengthless, overwrought, with a yellowish brownish complexion and body skin, from which came a pungent odour. She did not perspire at all, was subject to the most terrible chills and colds, felt best in wet weather, disliked to be touched, was easily startled, hated consolation. Her worst side was the left side and she was a vegetarian. I had no need to put her on a vegetarian diet. Her health history was bad. When small, she had diphtheria very badly, followed by paralysis, and it took her a long time to get over it. She had always been anæmic, had been given much iron and quinine, her periods were scanty and very painful, she had influenza in 1927 badly, and once a year ever since. She was born in the Tropics.

People may be terribly constipated on an exclusive diet of vegetables and fruit, and on fruit alone. I ordered her to take per day 9 heaped tablespoonfuls of bran in the form of bran porridge, and bran puddings, and told her to improve the activity of the skin and increase her strength by rubbing a tablespoonful of olive oil every night into the whole body. She was to take from 2 to 3 pints of milk, 2 to 3 eggs, 2 to 3 ozs. of mild, grated cheese per day, and to gain about 2 lbs. of weight per week.

She listened to my suggestions and the promise of improvement with an incredulous smile. She thought it most unlikely that I should be able to cure her constipation of many years' standing and the condition of her nerves, which had troubled her all her life. Her constipation was apparently due to prolapse of the abdominal organs and that condition and the colour or her skin and other symptoms suggested Sulphur and Sepia. I gave her Sulphur 3X and Sepia 12X, and she was to change from one medicine to the other every three days, observing which of the two suited her best. As she hated sympathy, felt always chilly and had a craving for salt, I give her Natrum muriaticum which has these symptoms, first in the 3rd centesimal and later on in the 30th centesimal potency.

She started improving in body and nerves, and then she complained about her heart and weakness. I sent her Crataegus mother tincture, and later on Phosphorous 3X. On the 29th September she wrote: " I have been feeling definitely better the last few days. I do think you have put me on the right road." In view of the vagueness of her symptoms, I had to try many medicines such as Ignatia and Arsenic for her nerves and restlessness, etc. On the 11th October she wrote: " I am getting to feel a little warmer, especially out of doors. Menstrual pains were not so bad." Meanwhile her bowels had become absolutely normal. As she told me that her influenza attacks usually started with feelings of chilliness and bone pain, I sent her some Eupatorium perfoliatum 1X to keep by in case of emergencies.

On the 14th November, 1932, she visited me for the second time, and I learned of many new symptoms. Her bowels were absolutely normal, her body smelt fresh and sweet, skin and complexion had vastly improved, she had beautifully red lips, but she had not yet learned to perspire. She told me she was afraid of darkness, got nightmare when sleeping alone, had a pain in the left abdomen, got headaches improved by tight bandaging. As I did not wish her to catch colds and influenza during the winter, she was given once a week a dose of Bacillinum 30 and once a week a dose of Influenzinum 30. For the curious symptoms "diarrhœa when meeting people" she was given Argentum nitricum 3, the box being marked "nerves and stage fright."

Patients make it difficult to treat them adequately because very frequently they do not give one the information one needs at the first and second meetings. One may be told long afterwards of most important facts and symptoms which have been withheld. On the 25th November, four months after our first interview, she wrote to me:—

"At four years old I had diphtheria followed by temporary paralysis. My mother told me that I never regained the same look of health after that, and lost what had been a particularly clear complexion. When I was 7 I had another very severe illness, akin to typhoid fever. At 8 years old I went to a very hard school, most unsuitable to me, as all my tastes are artistic. As a child I had frequent severe colds and much trouble with my teeth. Then I was sent to school in Germany where conditions were bad. There was one lavatory for at least 20 of us, and only one of the girls was really well.

"When I came home I had attacks of appendicitis and chills and colds with high temperatures and frequent attacks of influenza. I became very thin. I saw various doctors, but they never seemed to help me. I developed a curvature of the spine for which I had massage. Then I was married and had an operation for appendicitis. It took me a long time to get over it. Last year I had an attack of rheumatic fever. My nerves seemed to get worse after that and then I had two motor accidents. I used to feel cold even in the heat of summer."

Obviously Mrs. C. R. was in a much worse condition than I had gauged from our first and second interviews. The letter disclosed to me the fact that her troubles had started with diphtheria. Naturally I sent her on the 25th November Diphtherinum in a box marked

" Diphtheria antidote." It was in the 30th potency and she was to take a dose once on the 1st day of every month.

Progress was slow though steady. She imagined that she had arrived at the top of the ladder and wrote to me on the 3rd January, 1933, after five months' treatment: " I am very grateful to you for the improvement in my health. I don't think I shall ever be any better than I am now, and I do not mean to be pessimistic. You have done much more for me than any one else has ever done, and I wish I had consulted you years ago. The freedom from colds is wonderful for me, as I could never go anywhere without getting colds, bad throats and coughs with very high temperatures, every time, and I seemed to spend most of my time in bed. My nerves are better. I can stand greater speed in motoring, for instance, but socially they seem much the same."

I had to explain to her that she was only on the first rung of the ladder and that she ought to go on. Her nerves became better. On the 23rd January she wrote: " Last night I conducted a choir quite successfully." On the 13th February her husband wrote: " She has improved definitely in many ways, has better nerves, up to date no colds with high temperatures."

As her troubles were chiefly left-sided, I gave her occasionally doses of Thuya. For her fear of the dark I gave her Stramonium, for her old diphtheria I gave her Diphtherinum 200. I used a large number of remedies, much to my dislike, but none of the polycrests served. I discovered that she did better with the higher potencies. The medicine which suited her best to overcome her nervousness was Gelsemium 200. She wrote: " It helped me more than anything."

She now could conduct large choirs at festivals. Instead of being a chronic invalid, she became healthy, strong, buoyant. She wrote on the 12th July, 1933: " I know I am stronger and better. I used to envy people in bed, and now I pity them and have no longer the wish to be there myself." She became vigorous, working hard in the fields helping with the haymaking, and finding the greatest joy in doing strenuous physical work which she had never been able to do.

On the 16th November, 1933, she informed me that she weighed 9 stone 9 lbs. She had put on 23 lbs. of solid muscle. When she came to me she was 8 stone and her tissues were flabby and watery. I am still looking after her and hope that she will go ahead still further. She is very enthusiastic for homœopathy and has urged all her friends and acquaintances to be treated by that wonderful method of healing which has helped her so much.

Mr. H. G. V. wrote to me from Portstewart, County Derry, on the 21st November, 1928 : —

"My wife, like myself, is in her 85th year. She had, till a short time ago, for over 50 years, never a motion without either medicine or enema. Some time ago I came across your book *Chronic Constipation* and I must express to you my very deep gratitude.

"After adopting the regime recommended in your book, she has now a natural motion every second day and sometimes on successive days, and she hardly ever needs either enema or medicine. I may mention that I myself used to be inclined to constipation and had not infrequently to take a teaspoonful of Cascara. Having adopted your regime, I have never taken any medicine and am perfectly regular."

On the 18th November, 1930, when Mr. H. G. V. was 87 years old, I received a second letter from him : —

"As I know you have the welfare of humanity at heart, I am sure you will be pleased to hear that your regime has become increasingly efficacious in the case of my wife, and has remained absolutely efficacious in my own case, especially since I am using a very low seat in the lavatory. Besides, the effect on my wife's general health of the elimination of constipation, this has been followed by an improvement in the state of her brain, thank God. She has suffered from a cerebral affection for 27 years, but she is getting continually clearer.

"In my case too there has been a further benefit, which I think was the result of the deliverance from constipation. In January, taking a wrong turn in the dark, I rolled head over heels down the back stairs which are very steep and banged my head severely against the wall at the bottom, scalping myself. That may have been a blessing in disguise. I had an excessively severe concussion of the brain. I was in danger for a little time and doubt if I should have survived at all but for the excellence of my bowels, for which I have to thank you. I only had to take one aperient since my accident, and it may not have been necessary. I don't know how to thank you enough for what you have done for my wife and also for myself."

On the 14th March, 1931, when Mr. H. G. V. was nearly 90 years old he wrote to me: "The effect of following the advice of your book on constipation continues most satisfactory and increasingly so."

In innumerable cases the most obstinate constipation which cannot be overcome by powerful purgatives, enemas, washouts, high colon irrigation, massage, surgical belts, etc., will cede rapidly and permanently to the logical remedy of that state of affairs and appropriate diet.

Mrs. J. D. wrote to me on the 13th November, 1928:—

"I would ask if you would grant my brother an interview, as I believe you could (I am not exaggerating) save his life. He is a boy of 23 and has suffered from nervous dyspepsia for many years so badly that he is unable to follow his occupation, and as he is the only son left at home, this affects my father and mother very closely.

"We have spent more money than we can afford at attempts to cure him. He has stayed at a clinic in Germany, attended hospitals, had physicians and heaven knows what else, but he is driving my mother frantic with continued attacks. He is really in a very serious condition and nothing seems to help him.

"We had a physician in last week who informed him that he had to have his appendix and something else (I don't know what) removed, and after that have twelve months' special treatment and so on. So far as we know, there is nothing wrong with his appendix. This is a desperate appeal to you for help, and I hope you will give it."

I agreed to see the young man. He was tall, lanky, terribly nervous, very abnormal in every way, and in looking at him I said to myself that he might become a mental case any day. It appeared that he had suffered since the earliest childhood from constipation in the most obstinate form, accompanied by the most extraordinary mental outbreaks, such as sudden terrors, extreme weakness, shrieking and crying fits, fears of sudden death, etc. I listened to his tale and sent him my directions. The poor fellow had had numerous and very serious diseases. I summarized his account as follows in my directions: —

" You are 24 years old, single, had some trouble in your right hip when you were 7 years old, declared to be tubercular, were kept in bed for two years, were operated upon six times, had scarlet fever and diphtheria when you were 9 and 10 years old, and began to suffer very seriously with indigestion, constipation, fits of giddiness, emaciation, etc.

" You look very toxic, have much flatulence in the stomach which you cannot get rid of, go without a stool for many days, have a flabby yellow tongue, have to take medicine every night, take an enormous over-quantity of salt, find it difficult to control your appetite, cannot stand hot weather, take little exercise, must always be chewing something, and last, but not least, vaccination did not take. Your body has an unpleasant smell."

Constipated people not only feel physically upset, but are often mentally abnormal, bad tempered, cannot collect their thoughts, are depressed, etc. It is my invariable rule to give a vegetarian diet to all who suffer from bowel stagnation. I forbade absolutely flesh and fish, and everything made of them, gave the young man a diet rich in vegetables, fruit, wholemeal bread and milk, and ordered him to take very large quantities of ordinary bran three times a day.

I gave him Valerian for his nerves, China for his weakness, and liquid paraffin for bowel regulation.

I felt very sceptical because the man was mentally unstable, and on the physical side there was the ancient tuberculosis, etc. I was not surprised to hear after a little while that he did badly and was too ill to report to me.

On the 16th June I received from his people a telephone message that he had had a most terrible attack of nerves, that he shrieked that he was dying and that they had sent for the doctor. On the next day I received a letter from his brother-in-law, who told me that Mr. S. L. had felt worse since I had taken him in hand. At Mr. S. L.'s dictation his brother-in-law wrote : —

" During the first two days of your treatment my bowels acted vigorously and during the third and fourth I felt much better, but in the evening of the fourth day I came over very queer and finished off with a bad attack. These attacks are rather different from the former ones. An attack starts with a slight puffy numby feeling in the head, and as it gets worse I get an overpowering dizzy, faint feeling until I feel I am about to lose my senses. I then find that I can only take short gasps of breath.

" One of the worst of these attacks came on Saturday night when my sister 'phoned you. I had to fight to keep my senses and swallowed some brandy in hot water. I never seem to be free from this puffy feeling in the head. The attacks invariably come on in the evening."

Obviously his trouble was very largely nervous. The young man got almost crazy when he had an attack and drove the others crazy by his behaviour. Hydrastis canadensis is an excellent disgestive medicine and liver stimulant, and it has a favourable effect on the bowel. I gave him Hydrastis 1X and changed his dietary. The young man reported improvement but produced new symptoms, such as throbbing of the arteries of the head, etc. He wrote : " If I walk for about ten minutes, I feel I cannot take another step, also if I concentrate on anything it seems to weaken me tremendously. Apart from this weakness, I had been feeling somewhat better the last few days."

Hydrastis had lost its power for good and liquid paraffin was quite ineffective. I therefore tried on him Opium and Plumbum. Opium and Plumbum are terribly constipating drugs, if taken in large quantities. In homœopathic doses Opium and Plumbum are excellent laxatives. I thought it high time to attend to his tuberculous tendency and gave him Tuberculinum, a single dose of 3 pilules to be taken once a week. I gave him every possible encouragement in my letters and suggested his going for a few days to the seaside. On the 2nd August he wrote:—

· " I am glad to report that your latest medicines have had a very good effect. I returned from Clacton-on-Sea last night, and I can safely say that during the five days I spent there I felt better than I have done for a long time. I am wondering whether the air of London still disagrees with me."

As the young man had many indications of tuberculosis, I reinforced the weekly dose of Tuberculin with Phosphorus 3X, a dose three times a day, which is valuable for patients who have a very fair, delicate skin, excellent colours, beautiful teeth, fair hair, silky curved eyelashes, very clear whites to the eyes, etc., and that medicine helped him greatly. On the 12th September he came to see me and I wrote to him:—

" You have changed very much indeed, and if you go on like that, you will be quite normal in a few months. Although your colour is much improved, you are still very anæmic, you feel terribly hot in bed, feel worst early in the morning, your skin is full of pimples and blotches, especially on the back, and your bowels are not working as promptly as they ought to."

I changed his diet and gave him Sulphur 6X for his impure skin, feeling of heat in bed, and aggravation on rising, and I gave Gelsemium pilules to be taken at intervals if he felt an attack coming on.

At last he was able to go back to his business. On September 17th he wrote: " I have been working a little harder." A week after he told me hopefully: " I am glad to say I am not losing ground." On the

9th October he stated: "I am glad to report that I am feeling much better." I encouraged him to go to Switzerland, believing that high altitudes would complete the case, and I was not mistaken. He wrote to me on the 28th October:—

"I have been splendid since being at Interlaken. I have been in Switzerland just over a week and have gained 3 lbs. in weight."

He wrote to me on the 18th November from London:—

"I am very glad to be able to report very great improvement in my condition all round. My weight is now 10 stone 3, which compares well with my previous weight of 9 stone 9. My bowels are now working much more vigorously, and I am looking and feeling heaps better. I feel very grateful for your advice and feel that my present condition is due to your treatment."

At last the young man had come physically and mentally under my control. His hysterical behaviour by speech and letter had come to an end. Admonition, a natural diet and the indicated homœopathic medicines had completely changed him physically and mentally and he had become a normal and useful member of the community. He went straight ahead. On the 4th February, 1930, he sent me a long letter in which he told me:—

"I am glad to say that I have been in much better health since November last year, when I returned from my holiday, and I have had no attacks. Also I very rarely am constipated, and I do not take any laxative whatever except liquid paraffin, one tablespoonful twice weekly. I attribute all this improvement to your treatment, as, until I came to you, I had been getting worse and worse and, honestly, I had given up hope of ever becoming a normal being again. I have kept strictly to your diet. I do not take any salt, pepper, sauces, etc., as per your instructions. People tell me I look better. I believe I am fuller in the face."

Mr. S. L. considered himself cured and became a steady hard-working business man, doing extremely strenuous work and glorying in it. Eighteen months after our last interview, on the 4th October, 1931, he wrote:—

"I still follow the diet you gave me, and it keeps me clear of constipation. I manage to carry on with my work, but if I have heavy extra work to do, I am completely exhausted. However, I try not to give way to it, and have not visited a doctor since you attended me, nor have I taken any medicine with the exception of rare doses of liquid paraffin."

Before the young man came under my charge, he had been subject to the most violent hysterical outbreaks. He had been treated by many doctors and specialists who had completely failed to cure him with sedatives, such as Bromide, and powerful purgatives, which had, of course, aggravated the mental and physical troubles with which I had to deal.

On the 30th August, 1933, I was visited by Mrs. M. S., the wife of a very successful professional man, who had gone to live in the West Indies. The lady was 68 years old. She had had a number of children and she complained bitterly about constipation from which she had suffered since she was 20. She was extremely nervous and irritable, suffered from sleeplessness and rheumatism. She looked very toxic, she had developed a large fibroid when she was over 40 and, probably quite unnecessary, not only the growth but the womb and ovaries had been taken out. She was in a very poor physical condition. Many doctors had tried to cure her with laxatives of every kind which, of course, had not effected a cure, but had aggravated the condition by irritating the bowel.

While her previous advisers had carefully examined her, I did not examine her at all, but submitted her to the usual interrogation, telling her that I was not much interested in the local condition. In the course of this verbal examination it came out that she took hardly any liquid, in all perhaps a pint a day, that she never was, and never had been, thirsty and that she drank just as little when in the Tropics, as she had done when in England.

I had to explain to her that she suffered not from any fault of the apparatus of excretion, but from lack of liquid which caused her motions to become hard and dry, and from a faulty diet. I prescribed for her a diet with an abundance of bran in it, for bran keeps the motions moist, told her to take much liquid between meals, prescribing exact quantities and gave her Sulphur 6X night and morning as a blood-clearing medicine and Nux vomica and Carbo vegetabilis combined, a dose three times before meals, partly to help her digestion, partly to antidote the laxatives which she had been taking for 48 years, partly to cure her irritability. She faithfuly promised to carry out my directions.

The lady called on me again after a few weeks and had vastly improved. She informed me that she had had regular natural motions for the first time for decades. Her complexion had cleared up beautifully, she felt far more energetic, her rheumatism was better, and she was far less nervous. Shortly afterwards she left for the West Indies.

On the 27th December, 1933, four months after the first interview, her husband wrote to me from the West Indies: "You will be interested to hear that Mrs. S. has maintained the improvement you noted before we left England, and since then she has improved further, increasing her weight to the best she has had in many years. Indigestion and constipation have disappeared."

For nearly half a century Mrs. M. S. had been continually ailing or ill. Constipation and auto-intoxication had caused outbreaks of boils, swelling of glands, rheumatism, and had probably produced the fibroid tumour of the womb which was "cured" by a barbarous and probably totally unnecessary radical operation. Her numerous doctors had done nothing for her trouble, except give her laxatives and deal with the consequences of her constipation by operating here and there. Thus her life had been a misery.

CHAPTER XI

The New Art of Diagnosis

I AM thoroughly acquainted with the orthodox methods of examination. I have watched many doctors at their work. I was a sick man for many years and I was examined by numerous doctors in England and abroad.

There are many excellent books on diagnosis. I have about twenty of them in my library. The leading treatises are huge volumes which cost two or three guineas. They are profusely and beautifully illustrated. They contain pictures of patients suffering from the various diseases, X-ray photos of their bodies, and specimens of the diseased tissues and of the various micro-organisms. They are filled with the lore of the laboratory and the mortuary. They are written by diagnosticians for diagnosticians and they are of very little practical use in treatment.

I suppose every one of my readers has been medically examined at some time of his life and he may have been greatly impressed by the thoroughness of the examination, by the numerous and very wonderful appliances used and by the scientific outfit of the consulting-room. The method of handling patients is a science and an art. It is studied carefully by every medical student and doctor, and special lectures are given on the subject. I have before me a volume entitled *Art of Practice,* published by the Post-Graduate Association of Cambridge. It is a reprint of a course of lectures. Chapter IV is headed " Influencing patients through the Reason." We read in it:

"A full equipment of diagnostic instruments will repay itself a hundredfold in the long run. Most patients have been to some other doctor at some time in their lives before coming to you. They will compare your use of diagnostic instruments with what they have before observed. A well-equipped outfit gives confidence. It will be reported in a way you hardly expect and a strong means of gaining reputation results.

"A pocket magnifying lens costs 1s. 6d. to 2s. It is a good plan to inspect all skin diseases with one. In percussing use a pleximeter. An ivory one can be had for 2s. or less. A Tucker Wise's cyrtometer for measuring expansive movements of the chest costs 10s. 6d., and has a good moral effect on patients anxious about their lungs. It is one of the commonest convictions of patients that their blood is out of order. A profound impression can be made by Hæmocytometers and Hæmoglobinometers, etc. These are a little costly, but in a good-class practice they are well worth having.

"Every instrument that you can afford should be in evidence. A microscope, ophthalmoscope, a frontal mirror, stethoscope, test tube stand, spirit lamp, and reagents may lie on the table. The medical journals may be there also."

The doctor is recommended to impress his patients by the appearance of scientific knowledge, as evidenced by various instruments. Percussion with the fingers is better than with the pleximeter. Chest expansion can be measured with an ordinary tape measure. A stethoscope is rarely necessary if the doctor has a good hearing. On the other hand, I know a doctor who is completely deaf who uses the stethoscope on his patients. There are many doctors who hope to obtain prestige by crowding their consulting-room with scientific instruments of which they do not know the use.

The practical hints with regard to diagnosis contained in *Art of Practice* are interesting and illuminating: —

"It is better to be sure, cocksure, even if occasionally mistakes are made, than to go through life expressing doubt. Mistakes will do harm, but much less harm than a hesitating manner. A doubtful diagnosis can be given in an emphatic manner. You can say, as if you were certain, as if every medical man would be certain that the exact nature can only be told by further observation.

"When examining a patient, don't say 'This looks strange' or 'that is curious.' Avoid saying 'I think the disease is so-and-so.' Say positively that it is what you think it is. If you have made a mistake in diagnosis or treatment, do not be too ready to admit it, say nothing.

"It is very unwise to diagnose where the diagnosis may turn out to be wrong. Errors of prognosis are often more dangerous than errors of diagnosis because the patient can easily check the error. When the time of recovery is indefinite, it may work to use indefinite language, to say that it will take 'some time' or that 'it depends on the vitality.' If asked whether a case will prove fatal, say that it will depend on the possibilities of complications. This leaves you a reasonable margin for uncertainty."

The extracts given show that diagnosis, as practised by thousands of doctors, and possibly by the vast majority, is undertaken not so much for ascertaining the disease and the way to a cure, but for impressing the patient. The volume mentioned recommends deception pure and simple. However, I think that the gullibility of patients is not so great as the anonymous author imagines. It is true I have heard people say: "I have been to Dr. So-and-So. He has the most wonderful array of instruments I have ever seen and he employed 14 different instruments in diagnosing my case." This kind of patient is an exception. People who go for the first time to a doctor may be impressed by weird and wonderful instruments, but when they find that the treatment which they receive is as poor in results as that given by the average panel doctor, they will become sceptical with regard to the so-called scientific side of medicine, as displayed in mechanical appliances.

I believe the anonymous author of *The Art of Practice,* perhaps it ought to be renamed " The Artfulness of Practice," is mistaken with regard to the psychological factors upon which he recommends medical men to rely. I have found that most patients, especially women, do not like the sight of scientific instruments which causes them to think shudderingly of the operating table. To them a consulting-room which smells of disinfectants and an outfit which causes them to think of mortuaries is most depressing. Most patients like to be treated like human beings, not like pathological specimens.

I have found scientific instruments unnecessary. I receive patients in an ordinary living room and I do not display the instruments which I possess and which I find useless for practical purposes and disturbing to the peace of mind of the sick and the sensitive. Patients should be seated on a comfortable chair against the light so that the practitioner can study unobtrusively the patient's looks and expression, while his own face is in the shadow.

From my point of view, the most important part of the examination is not a more or less superficial examination of the various organs, which usually shows nothing useful, but the interrogation of the patient. He should be encouraged to state his complaints in his own language and the practitioner should note down immediately the story, as told to him. When the patient has finished the account of his troubles, then questions should be asked which will bring out the necessary details.

Let us say a patient complains about a bad cough for which the ordinary doctor prescribes his usual cough mixture. The more conscientious practitioner will ask: "What is the character of the cough? Is it a barking, choking, convulsive, wheezing cough, is it dry or moist, is the expectoration easy or difficult to raise, scanty or abundant, and is it thin, lumpy, stringy, what is its colour, what does it taste and smell like, what time of day or night does it occur, what makes it better and what makes it worse?" Noting down all the replies, the homœopath will, by consulting his *Repertory and Materia Medica*, be able to discover

M

a homœopathic remedy which may cure the cough in a few hours or in a few days, although it may have been in existence for years and has proved incurable to a number of doctors and consultants.

A cough, like every complaint, is not merely a local trouble, caused by a swollen and relaxed uvula which tickles the back of the throat, or by inflammation at the back of the throat, deep in the larynx, or in the bronchies, but it is as a rule a constitutional complaint. It may be due to a foul blood stream and many other causes.

When all the essential cough symptoms have been put down, the practitioner should enquire into the patient's way of living. He should not be satisfied with the answer: " Oh, I eat and drink just the ordinary things." He should say: " Please tell me in full details what you eat and drink at every meal and in between," and he should put down everything in writing. Then he should ask: " Do you take much or little sugar, salt, pepper, mustard, vinegar, pickles, do you take your tea strong or very strong, hot or very hot, how much milk do you put in, how much sugar, etc.? " It has happened to me that patients who had assured me that they ate and drank only the ordinary things were amazed when I told them: " Are you aware that you are taking in the course of the day sixteen cups of boiling hot tea, each containing four pieces of sugar? You are taking a lb. of sugar in the tea alone."

If a patient says: " I like to taste my food and use some salt," the question should be asked, " How much salt do you take? " and a salt cellar should be handed to him for practical demonstration. It may then only be found that the patient uses a teaspoooful of salt with every egg, etc.

When the patient's diet has been ascertained and has been put down in writing, he should be asked what medicines he has been taking, whether he perspires much, little or not at all, what has been his medical history and inheritance, and no general statements should be allowed. A patient may say: "I come from a very healthy family," but on enquiry it may appear that there is much tuberculosis on one side of the family or the other.

It is necessary to enquire into smoking. Many health troubles are due to too much smoking. Inhaling should be forbidden. Enquiry must be made whether strong, medium or mild tobacco is smoked. Many pipe smokers smoke very filthy pipes and they should be taught to clean them with boiling hot water and soap. If there is any suspicion of nicotine poisoning, smoking should be curtailed and the patient be taught to plug pipe or cigarette holder with cotton wool to filter out the worst irritants.

Contraceptive methods should be enquired into. Frequently mischief results from their use and from the use of vaginal douches. An exceptionally healthy woman came to me suffering from cancer of the stomach. I could find no cause for her trouble until I enquired about vaginal douches. To my horror the lady told me that she had been douching every night during the last twenty years with Sulphate of Zinc, a virulent poison.

Some years ago I saw a man crippled with osteo-arthritis. He had been an officer, had gone through the War with distinction, had been pensioned, and the diagnosis osteo-arthritis had been made. When I entered his bedroom, I could scarcely see him for tobacco smoke. The place was strewn with cigarette ends. I learned that he smoked 50 cigarettes a day, inhaling, and took about 50 Aspirins. My diagnosis was poisoning from tobacco and Aspirin. Shortly after I was called to a financier with progressive paralysis. His disease also was due to incessant cigarette smoking and daily over-doses of Aspirin. Both patients had become enslaved by their drugs. In both cases my principal prescription was reduction by one cigarette and one Aspirin a day, but both lacked the will power to carry out my recommendation.

Enquiry about cooking utensils must not be omitted.

Vessels made of copper, brass and aluminium should be forbidden. A lady was brought to my house suffering from disseminated sclerosis. Everything had been done in her home to ensure good sanitation. The lady for very fond of porridge. I discovered that her porridge was made in an aluminium saucepan in the evening, was kept in it during the night and was warmed up in the morning. She complained that these aluminium saucepans went quickly into holes. The poor woman had absorbed enormous quantities of aluminium dissolved in her porridge.

Baths and exercise also call for enquiry. There are men and women with prolapsed abdominal organs who take vigorous physical exercise which makes the prolapse worse. Miss F. K. came to me with serious prolapse of the womb. She played tennis with the utmost vigour. After every game she felt prostrated with a dragging pain which lasted three or four days. It had never occurred to her that the violent exercise was doing her harm. She took cold baths every morning summer and winter, even when she was unwell. She was surprised when I forbade strenuous exercise and cold baths until the prolapse was cured.

Many ladies take hot baths every morning and they are surprised that they catch cold easily. I frequently tell them that they must either abstain from washing off the natural oil which protects their bodies or must replace it by rubbing olive oil into the skin. Many a woman takes a boiling hot bath, lies in it for a quarter of an hour, dresses in flimsy clothes and then exposes herself to the coldest wind. Those patients who are weak should take at most one warm bath per week.

Sleep should be enquired into, how many hours the patient sleeps, what postures he assumes, whether sleeplessness is due to brain activity, worry, late meals, insufficient exercise. Dreams should be enquired into. They are of great importance to the homœopath who knows that certain dreams call imperatively for this or that remedy.

The mind symptoms are very important, but patients do not like to discuss them. Still, the practitioner should ask: " Are you irritable, restless, morose, talkative, etc.? "

Last of all, the delicate sex question should be approached, and the patient should be encouraged to talk freely about that side of his or her life.

Only when the complaints of the patient, his way of living, occupation, medical history, medical inheritance, etc., have been acsertained, should a physical examination be undertaken. It may disclose the fact that the pulse is irregular, or that the heart gives cause for anxiety, or that the stomach does not function properly and is enlarged, etc. These things had been ascertained previously by numerous doctors and consultants who tested the various organs, but they did not trouble to enquire into the causes which produced the symptoms complained of. The practitioner who employs a thorough interrogation may be able to give a vastly better diagnosis than the greatest specialist. While getting replies to his numerous questions, he may visualize the true cause of the trouble, so that he need not examine the patient.

If a patient has admitted that he takes 14 cups of tea " as hot as hell and as black as ink " with four pieces of sugar in each cup, the practitioner may safely assume that the trouble of stomach or heart complained of is due to the tea. If he has been told that the patient takes large quantities of salt, pepper and mustard he will know what has probably caused the deterioration of kidneys and liver, and will know how to cure the patient, provided he is still curable. When he has been told that the lady before him has had terrible disappointments and has been trying to find solace by a gay life, he will know the cause of her nerve troubles.

Some time ago the wife of a manufacturer in the North consulted me about a mysterious disease. Doctors and specialists had failed. At last her doctor had sent her to Ruthven Castle for a thorough scientific diagnosis. She had been kept there for three weeks, she had undergone every test known to science, and the stay and the diagnosis had cost £97. She came to me with a bundle of documents, which she wished me to inspect. She had been told that she suffered from an exceedingly rare disease of the pancreas. I hardly listened to her account, nor did I look through the documents. I asked her some questions and discovered that she took boiling hot strong tea in large quantities and masses of the most pungent condiments. Besides, she lived on a diet devoid of vitamins and mineral elements. The cause of her complaints was perfectly clear. To my amazement, she told me that at Ruthven Castle she had never been questioned about her dietary.

An inspection of the whole body is frequently of infinite value. One may discover important anomalies which the patient did not mention. A young man came to me complaining about constipation. When he had undressed I found that he had a considerable number of stalked moles and other outgrowths on his body. It was therefore reasonable to assume that he had similar outgrowths, such as polypi, in his bowel. Another patient had given me a long catalogue of complaints and past illnesses, the causation of which was obscure. As soon as he took off his clothes I discovered the most fearful vaccination scars. He had forgotten that many years ago he was vaccinated and that he nearly lost his arm through septic developments.

It happens to me frequently that patients who have been to eminent doctors and consultants look around my room with surprise because they see no scientific instruments to impress them. However, after an interrogation I am very frequently told that none of their doctors and consultants had taken so much trouble to ascertain all the important facts relating to their present and past condition, their inheritance and so forth. This method requires time and patience.

The first interview needs an hour or more. However, it is worth while. Only by patient thoroughness can the true causation of certain diseases be revealed. Subsequent interviews may be relatively short, especially if the patient is doing well. If he is doing badly, another hour may be needed to elicit those facts which failed to come out at the first interrogation.

If the practitioner cannot get the information he needs from the patient, he should ask the companion, daughter, husband or wife. Occasionally the patient has forgotten important facts, or does not care to mention them.

Orthodox doctors keep case books or a card index system in which they enter their findings. The printed forms supplied to doctors by the trade are faulty. Much room is given to the scientific side, but there is little room for the all-important facts relating to the daily life and past history of the patient. The average doctor puts down the results of his organ examination, etc., and the patient has no knowledge whether the doctor has got the full facts. In order to make certain that I have fully grasped the condition of the patient, I place at the head of my directions a full summary of my findings. This gives the sick the certainty that the practitioner has taken full note of all his complaints. Besides, in looking over the statement of his case, a patient may notice that the doctor has misunderstood some statement of his, or that he himself has left out some point of importance. I frequently receive letters correcting or amplifying my summaries.

The orthodox method of examination aims at ascertaining the name of the disease and when this is done, the patient is given the so-called " specific " mentioned in the textbooks. Patients have told me that they have been to a considerable number of doctors and consultants for, let us say, epilepsy. Each consultant went more or less perfunctorily through the rite of physical examination and then prescribed the inevitable Bromide and Luminal. Other patients with heart disease had been to numerous doctors, each

of them had tested the heart more or less thoroughly,
and each of them had prescribed the usual Digitalis
with no benefit. Mr. H. S. came to me because of
pernicious anæmia before the liver treatment had
become known. He had visited doctor after doctor,
consultant after consultant. Each of them had prescribed Arsenic and its cumulative action had given
the poor fellow severe Arsenic poisoning.

The method of examination suggested in these pages
is totally different from that employed by doctors.
Novelty attracts, particularly if the novel form of
examination leads to results which were not obtained
by those doctors who employ the mechanical form of
examination with numerous instruments. After all,
the most wonderful instruments of precision are the
human brain and our five senses. The examiner
should employ his five senses and train them by constant use. An experienced doctor is able to diagnose
numerous diseases with his nose. There is a peculiar
smell emanating from consumptives, diabetics, cancer
victims and others. Scarlatina, measles, typhoid,
diphtheria have a specific smell. The clinical thermometer is by no means indispensable. I knew a very
excellent old doctor who carried with him a stethoscope
and thermometer, but he hardly ever used them. He
felt the patient all over in order to ascertain whether
he had a local or a general fever, smelt him, and then
applied his ear to chest and back. Only when the
patient's skin was objectionable he used his stethoscope. He was a magnificent diagnostician.

After an examination, patients often ask anxiously:
" What is the matter with me? " If a patient is told
that there is such-and-such anomaly of his heart which
bears a forbidding scientific name, he becomes
depressed and disheartened. It is much better to tell
him: " It is true your doctor has told you that you
suffer from incompetence of such-and-such valve of the
heart, but I do not agree with the diagnosis. Your
heart has been upset by malfunctioning of the bowel
and the malfunctioning of the bowel has been caused

by your faulty nutrition. By correcting these mistakes your digestion and excretion will improve, your blood will get purer, and the heart will mend itself. The heart is not an ordinary piece of machinery but it is a self-oiling, self-adjusting and self-repairing organ, and you will find that the faulty action of your heart will be miraculously improved before long."

There is a curious unanimity among doctors and consultants. I have handled a number of cases of enlarged prostate. Some of my patients had gone to a number of doctors and specialists and all had told them that there was " no treatment except operation." That information was mistaken, as I have shown in the chapter on enlarged prostates. A number of ladies came to me with fibroid tumours of the womb. Some of them had consulted a number of gynæcologists. Each of them had said that there was no treatment except operation. However, the great majority of them vastly improved under non-surgical treatment. After all, there is a cause for every effect, and the discovery of the cause points to the cure.

Every striking anomaly fault in the patient's life should be considered as a possible cause of his disorder. If a patient takes every day a tablespoonful of salt or a tablespoonful of mustard, or lives on an insufficient diet, or takes large quantities of meat while taking no exercise, or smokes all day long, or lives on salads and raw fruit, these faults should be considered as a probable source of his disease and should be eliminated. Their elimination will certainly result in improvement of his general health and will enable the body to offer a better resistance to the disease, whatever its name.

After the interrogation and examination the patient requires directions and medicine. The directions should regulate his nutrition and whole way of living, as far as necessary, in detail. The often heard advice: "Feed up, take plenty of exercise in the open air, sleep with the window open, be cheerful, pull yourself together, forget about your trouble " is useless. People cannot pull themselves together and be cheerful by order and they do not know how to feed up. It is equally useless to say, " Take 3 pints of milk and 8 ozs. of butter per day." The patient may do violence to himself, upset his digestion and blame, rightly, his adviser.

The suffering individual should be told what to eat and drink at every meal and in between, but there should be no inflexible rules. The patient must be made to co-operate. Hence the last and most important paragraph of my directions usually is worded: *" Act with wise discrimination, but not with mechanical obedience to these directions, for no one understands the working of your body better than you do yourself."* If a patient who has read this italicized warning eats and drinks mechanically, totally disregarding my directions and upsets himself, he has only himself to blame.

Most doctors who give dietetic and other directions either leave it to the patient to come back when he desires to, or they tell him to come back in a month or so. That interval seems to me too long. I have found it best to ask for weekly reports in writing, which enable me to intervene promptly if diet or medicine should prove unsuitable.

It will be objected that an examination of the patient which takes an hour or more, lengthy directions, the dictating of which takes about half an hour, and weekly written reports require so much time that no doctor or specialist can adopt these methods. Underpaid doctors have to do rush work. They see twenty patients in their consulting-room during a time when they ought to see two, and during their visiting hours they race from patient to patient, giving each two or three minutes. Rush work means shoddy work. One can prescribe a cough mixture or a gargle or a laxative in a minute, but one cannot satisfactorily study a difficult chronic case which has proved incurable to numerous doctors and specialists. It is better to treat a limited number of patients with success than to give useless treatments to large numbers.

In cases which prove obscure after the ordinary interrogation and examination, the practitioner must go farther afield. He must study disease tendencies in the two branches of the family. He must enquire into marital relations, social position, business life, etc. I remember the case of a great lady who came to me totally broken down in body and nerves. She had employed more than a hundred doctors and specialists who had treated her with Bromide, Veronal. and other soothing but brain-destroying medicines. I patiently went into her case and discovered only at the second or third interview that her trouble was due to unhappiness in her home. She lived with a young relative whom she had brought up, who sapped her vitality. My discovery was confirmed by members of the household. Therefore the best medicine for the lady was a separation. I obtained it with difficulty. As soon as this was done the old lady improved and she was ever grateful to me.

Fullest details of previous treatments are necessary. Old prescriptions and X-rays should be examined. Very frequently the original disease of the patient is less serious than the treatments which he has received. Many suffer from poisoning with deeply acting dangerous drugs, injections, etc., which have to be antidoted. Last, but not least, the patient should furnish the practitioner with a recent photograph, not touched up by the photographer, which will clearly show his condition at the beginning of the treatment, and which will be invaluable for reference when the patient lives far away. A glance at it will refresh the doctor's memory.

Readers of these pages should bear in mind that a long, searching examination on the lines described is necessary in difficult and obscure cases which have defied treatment by the best physicians and specialists. Without such an examination I could never have obtained successes, such as those mentioned in this volume. On the other hand, the vast majority of cases which come to the ordinary practitioner are obvious and can be efficiently treated after a relatively short interview. If every case needed an hour for the interview and half an hour for dictating the directions, a doctor could see no more than six or eight patients in the course of the day.

In my directions the medicines given are not named. The boxes are marked only with initials. It is dangerous to allow the patient to know what medicine he gets. If a certain medicine to help his digestion has done him good, he may order it and take it month after month although it ought to have been stopped after two or three weeks. There is further the danger that he may object to the medicines chosen. If a box should be marked Phosphorus 6 or Arsenic 30, he may be frightened, but if he is told that the quantity of poison contained in the medicine is infinitely small, he may treat it with contempt. It would be still worse if the patient should know that he was given Tuberculinum in the hope of protecting him against tuberculosis. Initials and figures on the boxes will always tell the prescriber what he has given.

CHAPTER XII

Exophthalmic Goitre

EXOPHTHALMIC goitre, or Graves' disease, is an extremely unpleasant complaint. The goitrous swelling is accompanied by a rapidly beating heart, throbbing of arteries in neck and elsewhere, great nervousness and restlessness, and by protruding staring eyes which occasionally are pressed outward to such an extent that the patient is unable to close the lids in sleep.

Orthodox treatment is very unsatisfactory. The nerves are benumbed with bromides, a cumulative poison, and the heart is quieted with Digitalis, another cumulative poison, injections are used with very questionable results, and frequently the partial excision of the over-active thyroid gland is done. The consequences of this operation are often serious. It is a most disfiguring complaint because of the staring eyes.

In June, 1929, a Mrs. A. J., a young married woman, wrote to me from Tredegar that she suffered from exophthalmic goitre. I saw her on the 28th June. She was strikingly beautiful, 27 years old, and she exhibited the usual great nervousness and restlessness. She had throbbing arteries all over the body, her heart was racing, and her beauty was marred by her protruding eyes.

Homœopaths are not guided by the name of complaints. They have no specifics for this, that and the other disease. Physical examination of organs is a minor matter to them. The individual symptoms are everything. If twelve patients with exophthalmic

goitre go to an orthodox physician, they may be given
the identical advice and medicine. If they go to a
good homœopath, they may be given twelve different
diets and twelve different medicines. After all, one
treats individuals, not scientific abstractions, called
diseases. One must try to deal with the cause of a
disease, not with the disease itself, which is merely an
end-product.

The causation of Mrs. J.'s trouble was clear. I wrote
in my directions:—

"The whites of your eyes are unclear and are slightly
inflamed, you have a good deal of palpitation and one can see
the arteries of the neck throbbing rapidly. Your disease
seems obviously caused by auto-intoxication. You have
always been constipated in the past, going to stool perhaps
once in three days. Urine used to be cloudy, stools were
evil-smelling and apparently are still so, there has been no
perspiration in the past, and the discharge at period time
has been almost nil. All the outlets for the discharge of
body poisons were blocked up. You used to have icy hands
and feet, had terrible pain at period time before marriage,
have heavy vaccination marks, prefer the open air, even
when the weather is cold, cry easily when sympathized with,
are very fidgety, even in bed, developed a lump in the left
groin a year ago, apparently due to accumulations in the
colon. A single diaper used to suffice in the past. There is
no noticeable smell from the arm-pits and from the feet.

"Since the appearance of the goitre, your bowels function
better, your hands and feet are now hot instead of being icy,
and you get occasionally night sweats all over the body, have
developed a huge appetite and tremendous thirst, were sent
to bed by the doctor and were given by him Digitalis, Belladonna, Nux vomica, etc. You pull up your knees almost to
the chin when lying in bed. Your mother is troubled with
rheumatism, your father died of bronchial asthma, and your
mother's brother and sister died of consumption."

Mrs. J.'s doctor had treated her "disease" without
apparently enquiring into her history, general body
condition, bowels, etc., nor did he take any note of
her inheritance. He had given her drugs with no

benefit and had then recommended an operation on the thyroid. The system of poor Mrs. J. was clogged as regards bowels, bladder, skin and menstrual discharges. Things became better when the goitre developed. Consequently the exophthalmic goitre was an attempt of nature to rectify matters, not "a disease" to be combated with medicines, or to be fought by cutting away part of the enlarged thyroid. The thyroid is called upon to detoxicate the system. If too heavy a strain is put upon that gland, it tries to do double and treble work, gets enlarged and its attempts are foiled by incompetent surgeons, who cut out large portions of the thyroid to the injury of the patient.

I told Mrs. J. that the most important thing was to activate bowel, bladder, skin and menstruation. I put her on an eliminating, fleshless diet, gave her liquid paraffin for her bowels, an abundance of bran in puddings, told her to leave off the poisonous dopes which she had been given by the doctor, and gave her Sulphur Iodatum 3X to cleanse the system and to act on the swollen gland, and Thyroid 2X to help the overstrained thyroid. Auto-intoxication was obviously superimposed on a constitution with a distinct tuberculous tendency. There had been much tuberculosis in her family, and she had the beautiful complexion, blue eyes, fair hair and long lashes often seen in the tuberculous. I gave her a few pilules of Tuberculin, each containing a decillionth of a grain, to be taken once a week. She was to gain 2 lbs. per week.

The lady made an excellent beginning. On the 2nd July, after a fortnight's treatment, she told me that she had put on 3 lbs. On the 5th July she wrote:—

"I have been feeling so much better since I commenced your treatment. I do not have any night sweats now and my heart seems much better. I sleep very well. There is less throbbing in my neck, but when I run upstairs or uphill it throbs badly. I empty my bowels twice daily, sometimes more often. I think I am still a bit fidgety. My right eye is somewhat the same but the eyes do not protrude quite as much as they did."

In difficult cases it is always wise to get reports from the patient's family to confirm or refute the patient's statements. I asked the husband to write to me and he told me on the 7th July:—

" The heart does not race quite so badly, although the carotid arteries still throb plainly. The sleeping is more sound and she is not quite so restless. There is evidence of more vitality. The eyes do not show much progress yet. They look more prominent some days than others, although, perhaps, they are not so bulging as they have been. The diet prescribed is certainly doing good in view of her having gained 4 lbs. and, on the whole, there is a general improvement in health. The face certainly is more full and many friends remark on the change seen in a few weeks."

A good homœopath treats his patients according to their symptoms, and with every change of symptoms changes the medicine. After all, the symptoms proclaim the body's needs. Besides, when the symptoms complained of have disappeared one can safely assume that the cause producing these symptoms has disappeared as well. I gave Mrs. J. Calcarea iodata, Iodum in small doses, and, for her throbbing arteries, Belladonna, etc. On the 14th August she wrote:—

" I am feeling very much better. The goitre seems to be a little smaller, my perspiration is much better. I sleep very well these last few nights. My arteries are still throbbing, but not quite so much as they were. I am very, very pleased with myself and I am looking so very much better."

Later on she was given Thuja as a vaccination antidote, Pulsatilla because of her scanty menstruation, and on the 11th August she wrote: " The goitre seems to be much smaller," and on the 16th she reported: " The goitre is much smaller. The arteries in my neck are not throbbing quite so badly." On the 2nd October she wrote: " I think the Iodum and Belladonna pilules together are working wonders. I do not perspire much now and I go to stool regularly. My nerves

seem a little better." On the 16th October she wrote:
" The goitre has gone down a good deal." On the 25th
November: " The goitre is now very small and throb-
bing seems to be getting less."

As she was unable to come up to London again, I
asked her for a photo in January, 1930. I have that
photo before me now. She looked then a completely
different woman, her goitre was gone and the eyes
were no longer protruding. In February she wrote:
" I think you will have a surprise when you see me."
On the 27th February she told me:—

" I saw my doctor yesterday and he thinks that there is a
marvellous change in me, and he wonders what treatment
I am under, but I have not told him as yet. I feel almost
my old self again. My heart never troubles me these days."

In April she told me: " I have no trouble at all
with my heart these days." She was at the time
taking Pulsatilla 30th potency, which suited her particularly well. She came to see me on the 15th May.
After the interview I wrote:—

" I am so glad you have come. You look simply magnificent. There are no throbbing arteries and you need enter-
tain no longer a thought of operation or other violent
treatments. You are no longer the emaciated nervy spectre
who came to me, and are altogether wonderful. You have
worked a veritable miracle in yourself and you will do
still better before long."

The orthodox treatment which Mrs. J. had had with
Digitalis, Belladonna, Nux vomica, etc., in large doses
had been a failure. The poisonous drugs used could,
of course, not overcome the auto-intoxication resulting
from constipation, the effect of a faulty diet, the
absence of perspiration and the totally insufficient
menstrual discharge. Besides, nothing had been
done by her doctor to deal with the pronounced tuberculous tendency. In view of his non-success, the doctor
had urged an operation. Excision of the enlarged
thyroid would not have cured auto-intoxication from
the bowel and elsewhere and the result would have

N

been that the poor grossly disfigured woman would in course of time have succumbed under the mistaken treatments given. She was terribly overwrought when I saw her first, and very possibly an operation would have caused her complete physical and mental collapse.

On the 13th July, 1930, Mr. E. A. A., of Portsmouth, wrote:—

" My wife suffers from exophthalmic goitre, and she has been advised to have an operation, but she feels quite unable to face it. Besides, she is dubious as to the result. Would you kindly help a despairing husband so that my wife may be eased by your treatment? "

I saw her on the 8th August, 1930. She looked ill and worn, extremely nervous and anxious, and it was quite clear that an operation would be the finishing stroke to her. She had been suffering from exophthalmic goitre for 14 years. I summarized her condition in my directions as follows:—

" You are 37 years old, were married in 1919, have no children, and suffer from exophthalmic goitre which began with palpitations in 1916, 3 years before marriage. You were medically advised not to have children. Your worst complaint is the feeling of choking, aggravated when lying down. You sleep badly, tossing about, cannot stand hot sun, hot baths, feel always best in the open air, have very loose bowels, occasionally diarrhœa, swollen ankles, a swelling and great tenderness at the top of the stomach, some tenderness about the uterus region, a very brown, greasy skin, a very rapid and very irregular heart, feel best when eating, memory has terribly suffered, you get train sick, sea sick, tram sick, 'bus sick.

" You are terribly emaciated, look the picture of depression and misery, eyes are getting lustreless, you look despondent and anxious, heart is extremely irregular, palpitations can be felt and seen all over the body. Standing is unbearable to you, you can walk only a few yards, and not at all in the open, are most emotional, dislike fat, had a very unhappy childhood, your mother had two operations on the womb, your father died of bowel cancer."

This was obviously a most unpromising case. The poor woman had had exophthalmic goitre for 14 years, and was a wreck. No doctor would have believed for a moment that treatment could be successful. She had been advised that only an operation might be helpful. An operation would probably have killed her, or driven her into the lunatic asylum. In any case, she had the instinct to refuse it.

I had not much hope of doing her any good, but I consider it a wicked thing for any doctor or non-doctor to refuse a case. Even, if said in the kindliest tones, the pronouncement, " I am afraid I cannot do anything for you" robs the patient of the last spark of hope. Miracles happen every day. One should never refuse help to a patient, even if the patient is dying. I did my best to comfort and encourage the woman, notwithstanding her ghastly inheritance, ghastly condition and ghastly health history.

I prescribed for her Sulphur 6X night and morning, Sulphur being in most obscure cases a useful first remedy. Belladonna produces throbbing of arteries. So I gave her Belladonna 3X, doses to be taken between meals. Cactus grandiflorus produces in large doses a feeling of constriction about the heart, and, as she had complained about constriction, she was to take a dose of Cactus 1X whenever she had that sensation. Furthermore, I gave her a box of Pulsatilla 3, and a bottle of Lycopus virginicus drops, both to be held in reserve. She was given a milky diet with an abundance of vegetables and fruit and was told that she ought to gain between 2 and 3 lbs. per week.

On the 18th August, ten days after I saw her, she sent her first report: " I am pleased to say I am feeling better as I am able to walk better, and am having better nights. I am not nearly so restless. My heart is still irregular, but does not beat so quickly. My weight remains the same."

One of the best medicines for very sick people is encouragement. I wrote to her immediately that I was extremely pleased to hear that she had begun the treatment so well and that she had considerably improved in accordance with my expectations. A week after, on the 25th August, she reported: " I have gained 2 lbs. in weight." Meanwhile she had taken Pulsatilla and it had done her much good. Again I expressed my delight: " You seem likely to become one of my very great successes." The next weekly report told of an increase of 1½lbs. In the following report, on the 15th September, she wrote: " I have gained another 1½ lbs. In fact, now people begin to remark on how much better I look." She also told me that Cactus grandiflorus was a wonderful medicine which had helped her greatly with her choking sensations.

On the 14th January, 1931, after five months' treatment Mrs. A. told me that she had to break off the treatment and I did not hear from her again. I imagined that she had gone back to her doctor and was receiving the usual violent and unsuitable treatments, and I felt very sorry for her. On the 19th November, 1933, nearly three years after her last letter, I took tea in Findon, Sussex, and was talking with a gentleman who bore the same name as my patient. He asked me: " Are you the Mr. Barker who treated years ago Mrs. E. A. A. of Portsmouth?" " Yes." " You have saved her life. Three or four years ago she was in despair. She was terribly ill. The doctors had recommended an operation for exophthalmic goitre. We all thought she was going to die. Now she is perfectly well. We had dinner with her a short while ago. She spoke of you full of gratitude and she is still strictly following the diet you gave her and takes quantities of bran." I wrote to her husband and he replied to me on the 27th November, 1933 : —

" I thank you very much for your kind interest. No one knows better than I, her husband, that she is definitely better in health. Her appetite is always splendid. Of course she still keeps to your diet. She sleeps well and is able to take walks. Everyone remarks upon her rested appearance. We know by experience that diet seems to be the dominating factor, and to have removed part of the thyroid gland, as was suggested by the doctor, would have been disastrous."

Mrs. A. had been given the most incompetent treatment for her goitre during the 14 years before she came to me. She was given in maximum doses dangerous medicines which, according to the textbooks, should be given " for exophthalmic goitre." Not one of the doctors and specialists had ever enquired about her diet, motions, perspiration, and such-like elementary matters of fundamental importance. She was drugged instead of fed, and the disease condition was, of course, immensely aggravated.

CHAPTER XIII

Tuberculosis of the Lungs

ALTHOUGH the mortality from consumption has declined for many years it remains a terrible infliction. The organisms of tuberculosis float in the air and we breathe in millions wherever we are. In 1882 Dr. Robert Koch discovered the tubercle bacillus and it was widely believed that science would rapidly produce a perfect cure. Koch himself felt confident that the discovery of the causative organism would rapidly lead to the finding of a cure. He produced a substance called Tuberculin. It was tried experimentally on many patients who flocked to Berlin. Among them was a relative of mine. The preparation injured patients severely and caused many deaths. Later on Koch produced various other attenuated forms of the hoped-for antidote, but the results were disappointing. The remedy has become discredited. It is dangerous to use.

It should not be believed that Pasteur and Koch are the originators of treatments designed to fight diseases with their modified products. This form of treatment was originated by Dr. Samuel Hahnemann and his successors. Hahnemann himself used Psorinum more than a hundred years ago. His disciple, Dr. Constantin Hering, introduced in 1833 Hydrophobinum, prepared from the saliva of a mad dog, decades before Pasteur, and it has been used ever since by homœopaths. Tuberculinum and Bacillinum were extensively used by Dr. J. Compton Burnett, from 1876 onward, long

before Robert Koch announced his discovery. However, while orthodox medicine, possessed by the mania
of subcutaneous treatments and of large doses, employed huge doses of Tuberculin, giving the unfortunate patients in many cases injections in rapid succession, homœopaths have always employed disease
products, such as Bacillinum and Tuberculinum, in
infinitely small doses, and the medicine is given by the
mouth once a week, once a month or less often. The
largest dose of Tuberculinum currently used is a
billionth of a grain. A billion consists of the figure 1
followed by 12 noughts. As a rule homœopaths give
Bacillinum and Tuberculinum in the 30th potency, by
the decillionth of a grain or higher. A decillion has
60 noughts after the figure 1. Frequently they give
the 100th potency, the 200th potency, etc.

The orthodox treatment of tuberculosis cases by
means of the disease product has been a ghastly failure
—orthodox doctors treating " a disease " are apt to
treat all patients alike—and the other forms of orthodox treatment have not been particularly successful.
It is true that the mortality from tuberculosis has
declined greatly since 1882 when the organism of tuberculosis was discovered. However, a similar decline
had taken place during the years preceding 1882. That
can be seen from the mortality statistics of England
and other countries. Tuberculosis is a poverty disease,
a dirt disease, a bad air disease, a disease which is
spread by infection, lack of ventilation, under-
nutrition, faulty drainage, etc. The improvement of
housing, drainage, the water supply, the food supply,
and the growing knowledge that fresh air is essential
for health have caused the steady decline of the tuberculosis death rate. The medical profession can scarcely
claim any credit for that development.

Before the time of Robert Koch scores of medicines
were prescribed for patients, who were kept in tightly
closed, overheated, stuffy rooms on account of the
fear of draughts. The open-air treatment, which had
been practised by the Greeks and Romans, had fallen

into neglect. Now all medical men recommend nature cure for tuberculosis, and have discarded their drugs.

Nature has a wonderful power over many diseases. The return to nature has saved innumerable tuberculous patients who had been declared incurable by their doctors. The success of the open-air cure led to the rise of sanatoria for the tuberculous, but they have not been an unqualified success. That is known to every doctor. If we wish to cure the tuberculous by nature, it is not sufficient to supply the patients with fresh air. We must also give them fresh, natural food, natural exercise, and keep their bowels in that natural condition of activity which is rarely found among the civilized.

In the sanatoria the patients are only too often fed on devitaminized and demineralized white bread from which the lime is extracted, which the body needs to wall in the tuberculosis germs. In the hope of giving them strength, the sanatoria patients are given a navvy diet, quantities of meat which putrefies in their stagnant bowels and poisons them. They are given little raw fruit and salading, which are indispensable for blood-clearing purposes. In innumerable cases a stay at a sanatorium has done more harm than good. The patient is taught to rest in the open air, but he has not been taught the virtues of internal cleanliness and the elements of wholesome feeding.

A glance at the textbooks shows the resourcelessness of orthodox medicinal treatment of consumption. Orthodox medicine is not aware that the tuberculous can be wonderfully helped by medicine. We read in Osler's and McCrae's *Principles and Practice of Medicine*, 8th edition: "No medicinal agents have any special or peculiar action upon tuberculous processes." Following this depressing statement Kreosote, cod-liver oil, Hypophosphites, and Arsenic are casually and hesitatingly mentioned. In Letheby Tidy's *Synopsis of Medicine*, 3rd edition, we read under "Tuberculosis": "Drugs—none has specific action." As the great textbooks do not recommend any special medicine, "the latest and the most scientific" productions of the great drug houses are readily tried by credulous doctors on their unfortunate patients. Yet, commonsense and homœopathy will supply medical men with the most wonderful weapons with which to fight this insidious disease.

It is easy to learn by rote "for tuberculosis give cod-liver oil" and to declare with assurance that medicines are useless because the orthodox textbooks say so. It is very pleasant for the resourceless orthodox doctor to look with superiority and contempt upon homœopathic doctors and to treat them as cranks and ignoramuses. Homœopathy does not follow fashion. It does not rush from one extreme to the other, first bleeding all patients and then bleeding none, first dosing all patients with alcohol and then banning alcohol, first treating all consumptives with numerous drugs and then treating them without drugs. Homœopathy is guided by a certain law. The medicines which were given by Hahnemann for tuberculosis and other diseases more than a century ago are given by homœopaths to this day and they will continue to be given as long as homœopathy exists. In Boericke's *Pocket Manual of Homœopathic Materia Medica* more than a hundred remedies are enumerated for use in pulmonary tuberculosis. "But what is your specific?" If this question is asked, the homœopath will say: "We have no specific and no specifics. Any one of the hundred and more medicines usable for tuberculosis must be given in accordance with the symptoms of the individual patient." If a conscientious homœopathic prescriber sees a dozen cases of tuberculosis of the left lung, he may give each a different remedy based on his individual symptoms, whereas his orthodox colleague may prescribe cod-liver oil either for all of them or for most of them.

I have handled a large number of desperate tuberculosis cases. I have not examined a single one in the orthodox way. I have found orthodox examination useless in that and in most other diseases. In practically all cases I have been guided exclusively by the symptoms which enable a homœopath to cure people whom he has never seen and who have proved incurable to those doctors and specialists who have carefully but mechanically examined them with all the resources of diagnosis.

On the 23rd July, 1929, I received a letter from Mr. G. E. W., from the Sanatorium, Talgarth Breconshire: —

"I am suffering from pulmonary tuberculosis, and have been at this sanatorium for three and a half months. The diet here consists chiefly of: Breakfast: porridge made from whole wheat, bacon, white bread, tea. Dinner: beef or mutton, preserved peas or beans, mashed potatoes, custard made from custard powder and milk, stewed rhubarb. Tea: white bread, tea. Supper: rice pudding or soup, white bread, cocoa. I think you will agree that the diet is unsuitable. I am inclined to constipation, take liquid paraffin every other day, and eat at least one apple a day. Age 26 years, appetite fairly good."

I replied: "Your diet seems to me as faulty as can be and this is sanatorium treatment! I do not know what you can do as long as you are in the sanatorium." The poor fellow and all the sufferers at the sanatorium were fed on a demineralized and devitaminized diet, instead of being given wholemeal bread, fresh vegetables and fresh fruit in abundance. But then he was treated " scientifically," for his next letter stated: "I have been undergoing treatment here for 18 months and have made little headway. I have had two courses of Sanocrysin treatment (intravenous injections of a double Thiosulphate of gold). I shall be leaving in two weeks' time." I replied: "As far as I can see, the 18 months you have spent at the sanatorium were 18 months wasted, and I imagine that the ultra-artificial treatments given to you have done you no good, and possibly considerable harm." Having received further information and his photo, I sent him on the 10th November my directions, in which I described his condition as follows:—

"You are a plumber, 27 years old, and complain about tuberculosis of the lungs, for which you have been in a sanatorium for some considerable time. You have been treated with injections and have been given a very unsatisfactory diet, and you are no better now than you were previously. You have never been strong, had pleurisy when 15, were always inclined to colds, had a troublesome cough in winter, 1928, and in February, 1929, tuberculosis of the lungs was definitely diagnosed and you went to a sanatorium. There is not much temperature and sputum. You had persistent acne from the age of 17 onward, were constipated and probably vitamin-starved."

I put him on a diet extremely rich in vitamins and essential mineral elements, with an abundance of ordinary bran, coarse wholemeal bread, black treacle, honey, large quantities of vegetables, salads, potatoes boiled in their skins, milk, eggs, and forbade flesh, fish, fowl and everything made of them, strong tea, coffee, alcohol, spices and condiments. In sending him my directions I expressed the hope that within a week he would see considerable progress. For medicine I sent him Sulphur 6X, a dose night and morning, because the persistent acne in his youth pointed to that remedy, and Nux vomica and Carbo vegetabilis combined, a dose before meals, to help his digestion and to counteract the injurious injections he had received at the sanatorium. He was constipated and was to take liquid paraffin and have three evacuations.

The first report was excellent. He wrote on the 18th November, after one week's treatment: "I have gained 2 lbs. in weight and have three evacuations per day." On the 9th December he wrote: "I have gained a further $2\frac{1}{2}$ lbs. and now weigh 10 stone $3\frac{1}{2}$ lbs., which, I think, is more than I have ever weighed." He complained of weakness. I therefore gave him Chininum Arsenicum 3X as a tonic, and he was to take before meals a few pilules of Hydrastis 1X to stimulate his appetite and act on his liver, gall bladder, kidneys, spleen. On the 23rd December he reported: "I have gained 3 lbs." On the 5th January he wrote: "I am now able to take more exercise and feel a general improvement during the past fortnight."

Then he developed a cough and hiccough and he complained about an outbreak of acne, a good sign, nature eliminating disease matter by the skin, which otherwise might have injured the lungs. I sent him Cyclamen 3X for hiccough and acne. On the 27th January he wrote: "Cough and sputum are certainly diminished compared with the period before I consulted you. I am going on satisfactorily."

On the 3rd February he complained that he was seeing spots or rings floating before his eyes. That was a Phosphorous symptom, and, as Phosphorus is also an excellent remedy for consumption, I sent him Phosphorous 12. He told me at the same time: "I gained 3 lbs. during the past week. My weight is now 10 stone 10 lbs. Indigestion is practically non-existent now." I then recommended him to take Garlic as an internal disinfectant.

On the 18th February he wrote: "I have made substantial progress. I have gained approximately 14 lbs. in weight. My cough is less, and sputum is about halved. In outward appearance my chest has improved considerably. Everyone remarks that I look well. I feel that I am on the right road."

On the 4th March he wrote:—

"My weight remains the same and I am going on satisfactorily. I had a rather unpleasant test of my nerves and general constitution last week when I was involved in a motor accident, the car in which I travelled turning over. Apart from a slight chill, I am none the worse for it. I mention this because I feel sure that, had such a misfortune befallen me four months ago, the shock would have laid me up."

On the 18th April he wrote: "My weight remains steady, sputum is slowly but steadily decreasing, and it should cease entirely in a few weeks."

On the 24th April he compared his condition before and after treatment. He told me that his weight had increased by a stone, cough was reduced by half or more, sputum had diminished from one oz. per day to one oz. in six days, that he felt much stronger, that, before I took him in hand, he could only walk two miles, that he could now walk five to six miles. He added: —

" I feel a change in outlook. The future now looks bright, whereas previously, after 20 months of persistent effort to get better, during which I was in the hands of specialists on pulmonary tuberculosis, I was beginning to lose heart. In fact, I was told indirectly, that I had not much of a chance and that my hopes of returning to work were very remote indeed. Thus I was beginning to reconcile myself to prolonged invalidism and a slow fading away."

Later on there came set-backs, cough, pain in the lungs, and in July he had an attack of influenza, a very serious matter in consumptives, for which I treated him with Eupatorium perfoliatum. On the 25th August he wrote: " I am working more now than I have ever done since my illness." On the 22nd September he wrote with indignation: " It is a misfortune that I have not been able to see you, and it is a still greater misfortune that I did not come under your care sooner and let the sanatorium and their fancy treatments go to blazes."

On the 31st October he visited me, after 15 months' treatment during which he had benefited vastly, while the previous 18 months of treatment by tuberculosis specialists had done nothing but harm. I discovered that his skin was a mass of boils, pimples, pustules and acne. Very likely outward applications of ointments had driven in the disease and produced the lung trouble, to which he was predisposed. His mother had died of tuberculosis and his father, also a plumber, had had lead poisoning. It is a well-known fact that lead poisoning of father or mother is apt to injure the child before birth. To clear his skin, I sent him Hepar sulphuris. On the 29th December, 1931, he wrote: —

" I have now been under your care for 13 months and can truthfully say I feel a different person. I have made definite and substantial progress. Previously, I confess, the prospects were poor, and after about two years of sanatorium treatment, I seemed to be slipping back. Further, the doctors did not hold out much hope. I shall always feel grateful to you for putting me on the right road."

Henceforward his letters become infrequent, but they remained satisfactory. On the 3rd May, 1932, he wrote:—

" I am progressing splendidly. I have been rubbing my body with olive oil as a preventative measure against colds, and have not had a cold since I started doing this about three months ago. I am pleased to say that I can do much more work than I could nine months ago and look forward, given ordinary luck, to being completely restored to health in another year."

On the 24th August, 1933, Mr. C. J. N., a business man living at Ilminster, Somerset, wrote:—

" I have been in indifferent health for some years, and would much like to see you. I have a weakness of the right lung. I have not yet found the key to my trouble, but I am convinced that you hold the key. A slight connection of mine had occasion to consult you some time ago for cancer of the breast and, through your advice, she has been cured. Every four months I get a cold with a long crisis of expectoration and have one now which has been running for a fortnight and this is bound to pull me down. I shall not be satisfied until I have seen you. It is all due, I think, to War service in France, gassing, etc."

On the 19th October, Mr. C. J. N. came to my house. He had " a patch on the right lung," high up. Of course one must never admit to a patient that he has tuberculosis, cancer, or anything of the kind. He brought up masses of greenish, jelly-like, saltish-tasting expectoration, had a very dry itchy scaling skin, which a dermatologist might call psoriasis, was losing his hair rapidly, was totally emaciated and did not perspire at all. He had had swollen neck glands, had had treatment for years, looked underfed and anæmic. Although very tall he weighted only 9 stone 10½ lbs., and looked hopeless.

I cheered him up and prescribed for him a diet rich in milk and eggs, an abundance of boiled, unbleached sultanas, vegetables, potatoes, wholemeal bread, 9 heaped tablespoonfuls of bran, intake to be increased gradually and cautiously. I gave him Arsenic 3, a dose before meals, to give him an appetite and help digestion. It was especially indicated as he was very restless. I also gave him Calcarea phosphorica 6X, first and last thing, an excellent strengthening medicine, very helpful to consumptives, and Bacillinum 30, a single dose once a week. He was to gain 2 to 3 lbs. a week. He sent me a dreadful photo, taken immediately after our interview.

On the 5th November he wrote: " In the first ten days of my treatment I put on 4 lbs., the aching in my back has gone, but the stinging feeling in the back persists, I continue to expectorate loads of phlegm, and have bowel movements daily." His next report, dated the 8th November said: " I have put on another lb., my skin is better, scurf on my head is much less, no pains in the kidneys, no backache, am fatter, my clothes feel tighter, I have a better colour, I have made all-round improvement." His next letter, dated 14th said: " Have put on another 3 lbs., bring up loads of dirty coloured mucus, scurf on head is very much diminished." On the 27th November he wrote: " Have a gain of 1¼ lbs." On the 2nd January, 1934, he wrote: " I have put on 3¼ lbs., now weigh 10 stone 9 lbs. 12 ozs., a gain of nearly a stone. I do not get so much stinging pain." In six weeks Mr. C. J. N. had made wonderful progress and had had, according to plan, a gain of 2 to 3 lbs. per week.

On the 1st August, 1928, I was called to the telephone and a lady asked me: " Can you cure threadworms?" " Are you joking? Why do you ask me such a question? Threadworms are a triviality." The lady told me with a shaking voice: " Life is a nightmare. I have been tortured by these worms for years, I have spent more than £100 in Harley Street and I am at the end of my strength. If you cannot help me, I shall do something desperate."

On the 2nd August she came to my house. She told me that she was an actress, that she had been plagued with threadworms for years, that every morning she found a large wriggling mass of worms in her motions, that she had undergone the most searching treatments with poisonous drugs, colon irrigation, etc., which had nearly killed her, that she was in despair.

A good homœopath treats not a single complaint, but the body as a whole. Threadworms and consumption very frequently go together. I discovered that she had lost about 2 stone in weight, felt icy cold, skin did not act, liver and gall bladder were in an unsatisfactory condition, had rheumatism, and the most terribly painful periods. Her dietary was faulty.

I resolved to treat her immediately for tuberculosis, which seemed to me more urgent than threadworms. I explained to her that she was in a very poor condition and that the most urgent thing was to build her up, that I would only then deal with the worms, that I should use no drastic purgatives, enemas, etc. I prescribed a lacto-vegetarian diet, bran porridge to activate excretion and, as a tonic and a vermifuge combined, decoction of Wormwood. I also prescribed Pig bile tabloids to stimulate her sluggish liver. She was to gain about 2 stone. Hot baths were forbidden as weakening. The only Homœopathic medicine was Sulphur in very small doses to stimulate action of the skin.

Threadworms need not appear in the motions. Their presence can be diagnosed by itching at the anus, particularly at night, and itching in the nose. If children rub their nose or dig in the nose with their fingers, one ought to look for threadworms. It appears that these worms emerge at night from the bowel and, when outside the anus, deposit their eggs, causing irritation. The victim scratches or rubs the anus, and, for some reason obscure to me, there is itching in the nose as well. The finger smeared with thread-worm eggs, which may be under the nails, is inserted in the nose, the eggs wander up the nose into the stomach and produce additional masses of worms. I told Miss L. H. to rub Vaseline or Sulphur ointment on her anus when going to bed, protect it with a bandage, wear gloves at night, and never touch the anus at night. Garlic is a wonderful internal disinfectant and very helpful for consumptives. Besides, it is a vermi-fuge. She was to take garlic in milk, and to inject some of it into the bowel. She was to gain 2 lbs. a week.

On the 16th August she wrote: " Two weeks of dieting have certainly made me feel better in health. I begin to feel nice and clean inside and am sure there is an improvement in my skin. Itching of the anus continues, but is less noticeable. Garlic is horrible." As her appetite had improved, I gave her cod-liver oil. On the 5th September she wrote: " I am feeling better and am putting on weight and am getting accustomed to taking garlic." I now sent her Tuber-culinum, 30th potency, to be taken once a week. On the 28th September she wrote: " I am going on splendidly and am gaining flesh. I am certain the worms have not yet departed." On the 30th September she wrote: " I think I have deserved to have a clear skin after taking garlic and wormwood! Everyone is remarking on the difference of my face. I often have a little colour now." On the 2nd October she wrote: " I am quite sure the threadworms are much less."

On the 19th October I thought it time to send her a homœopathic remedy for her worms and sent her Cina 1X. On the 8th December she wrote: " I was 7 stone when I saw you first. I am now 8 stone 7 and am so delighted and everyone remarks upon the clear-ness of my skin. I am in much better spirits and feel I have made good progress." I gave her Pulsatilla to regulate menstruation, China as a tonic, etc., and

o

occasional doses of Tuberculin. On the 15th February, 1929, she wrote: "I have not seen any worms for many weeks."

During the spring she caught bad colds and in view of her poor inheritance, extreme pallor when she came to me, breathlessness, etc., I was much afraid that trouble might develop in the lungs. However, the indicated homœopathic medicines rightened matters rapidly. It was now time to tackle painful menstruation. She had explained to me that during the first day she was in an agony of pain, rolled about on the bed or on the floor, shrieking, pulling her knees up as far as possible and pressing hard on the abdomen, which gave her a little relief. I sent her some Colocynthis to be taken immediately before periods and Pulsatilla in between periods. The former medicine was to deal with the colicky gripes and the latter to regulate menstruation itself which had always been scanty and delayed. On the 8th July, 1932, she wrote: "Once again my period has been quite painless and normal in colour and flow. I am so thankful. Those little sugar pills of yours are wonderful." Ever since Miss L. H. has been in perfect health.

The specialists of Harley Street had tormented the lady for years with the most drastic treatments. They had tried first ordinary enemas and then enemas given by a long tube which is supposed to follow the whole of the big bowel up to the small bowel. They had starved her and then given her the powerful poisonous drugs recommended for worms in the textbooks. In the course of these searching treatments she had declined rapidly in health, strength and weight, and had become a spectre. A few more months of that treatment would have led to tuberculosis and an early death.

Mr. J. C. W., writing from Tawelfan Vale, Denbigh, sent me a letter, dated 14th December, 1932:—

"I am suffering from chronic tuberculosis of the apex of both lungs. The larynx is also affected, and I have completely lost my voice. I have also a chronic cough with about 6 ozs. of sputum daily. I have been suffering for 12 months and am 50 years old."

I asked for full details and a photo, and, on the 5th January, 1933, sent him my directions. This was also a case which I had never seen before treatment. I summarized my findings, based on the patient's letters, as follows:—

" You are 50 years old, a retired draper, are suffering from tuberculosis of the lungs and throat, from which you have been 27 weeks in a sanatorium, where you were given the rest cure without any special diet or treatment, and you gained 8 lbs. in weight, a very inadequate return. You have never been strong, but you come from healthy stock, took formerly much salt, pepper, mustard, etc., do not smoke, do not perspire, are constipated, smell of cooking used to make you sick. You get indigestion, particularly at night time, do not like to get near a fire."

People who do not like to be near a fire frequently need Sulphur. I gave him Sulphur 6X night and morning, Nux vomica and Carbo vegetabilis combined before meals to assist digestion and antidote the medicines which he had previously received and Bacillinum, 30th potency, a dose once a week. I put him on a vegetarian diet rich in milk, eggs, cheese, told him to take 9 heaped tablespoonfuls of bran per day, forbade white flour, white bread, etc. I have found that consumptives do much better without flesh, fish or fowl.

My patients usually go ahead soon after I have started them. On the 16th January he sent me his first report: " I think I am on the right lines. I have gained 2 lbs. I am now 9 stone 11½ lbs., more than I have ever been." As he complained about violent attacks of coughing combined with nausea and vomiting, I sent him helpings of Ipecacuanha 1X, Antimonium tartaricum 3X and Drosera 1X and told him to find out which of the three medicines suited him best.   A week after he told me that his cough was much better. On the 30th January he told me he had gained 2 lbs. " I feel much better." But he complained: "My voice is still a drawback, being unable to speak except in whispers." I told him that I hoped his voice would come back before long. On the 15th February he wrote: "I am feeling very much better and have gained 1 lb. this week. I seem to be filling out a lot these days." I now told him to take raw onions and raw garlic as internal disinfectants, and he was sent Tuberculinum, 100th potency, a dose twice a month. On the 22nd February he told me of further gain in weight, but complained of a cough which " starts when I am washing myself." For this curious cough I sent him Rhus toxicodendron 3X, which has caused this symptom in provers and it was curative. On the 1st March he told me: "I gained another lb. last week. I can now walk a few miles quite comfortably but get short-winded if going up this hill, which, however, tells on most people."

On the 9th March he wrote to my delight: —

" I am pleased to say that I have found a great change since Sunday. My cough and sputum are considerably reduced since then. I wonder if the pills (Tuberculinum 100) did the trick? I took the second dose of that medicine the Sunday on which the great change took place. I have not gained any weight this week, and I have not had that blown-out and bloated feeling.

"I was examined by the T.B. doctor yesterday. It is hard to get anything out of him. There is a decided improvement, he says, but I am still very much affected and must go carefully. I am old enough to know that I am considerably better, and to say that I am 50 per cent. better than when I left the sanatorium is putting it very mildly. I think the doctor must have seen in the report from the sanatorium that I was such an acute case, that it was impossible for me to improve so much in so short a time. I know there is still much trouble to get rid of from my chest, and there is also my absent voice."

I thought it was high time to start on his " absent voice," so I sent him Stannum (tin) 3, a dose of a millionth of a grain to be taken two or three times a day. He went on steadily for a couple of weeks taking

Stannum and reported from week to week gains of
weight.   I then sent him Arsenicum iodatum, an
excellent remedy for consumptives. On the 26th April
he sent me a delightful letter:—

" I have gained 1½ lbs. since last week. Also I had a good
report from the T.B. doctor whom I saw to-day. This time
it was a lady, who was more sympathetic than the usual
doctors. She inspected my chest and she said: ' There is
hardly anything there, and what there is is healing up
nicely.' It is seven weeks since I had the previous inspection
and during that time I have gained 9 lbs. You will say
' wonderful.' Still, my cough is far from cured."

On the 31st May he wrote: "I am still gaining
weight, 15 lbs. since the beginning of January. This
is getting an expensive business, for I am getting so
fat I haven't a suit of clothes to fit me.

So far I had never seen my friend. Feeling so much
stronger he wanted to come to London, partly to see
me and partly to start a new business. I was amazed
and I wrote to him on the 23rd June:—

" From your rather brief letters I had no idea that you
had improved as much as you have done. You looked very
weak and ill on the photo which you sent me at the beginning
of the treatment. Since then you have put on 19 or 20 lbs.
You look sturdy, cough has been reduced to about one-
fourth. Before I took you in hand you were gradually going
downhill. Since then you have improved steadily and very
considerably, and I have every confidence that improvement
will continue and that you will become one of my outstanding
successes, but of course you must help me. You need not
consider yourself an invalid any longer, and I would like you
to return gradually to more normal ways of living. Your
brother-in-law told me that you have never looked so fit
and strong as you do now."

This letter cheered him greatly. The interview had
revealed many new features. I gave him Sulphur,
and then Pulsatilla and Calcarea carbonica. On the
27th July, a month after our interview, he wrote:—

" I had a bad bout of coughing a week ago, but Wednesday
evening the climax came, when I began to spit blood, I

should think 2 ozs. in all. My tubes were very congested, but seem relieved. *I was voiceless for ten months, and I am pleased to say that I am maintaining my power of speech.* The doctor told me not to use it too much."

With regard to the bleeding, which alarmed him greatly, I told him that occasionally a natural blood-letting is advantageous. " If the veins and arteries of the nose get engorged with blood, nature lets off the surplus and no one is alarmed. In your case a similar position arose in the bronchies and you were worried, frightened. You have done splendidly, have put on 20 lbs., have regained your voice, lost for ten months. If matter which has to be got rid of comes away, it is all to the good." One must encourage patients, for cheerfulness and hope are the finest medicines, although they are not mentioned in the pharmacopœia.

On the 30th March, 1932, an anxious-looking lady, living in Tadworth, Surrey, brought me her daughter, Miss B. W. She was 19 years old, a typist in the city of London, and her parents were afraid for her life. She was tall, slender, totally emaciated, weighed only 7 stone, had a most beautiful complexion, blue eyes, long silky eyelashes, blonde hair, perfect teeth, the exact Phosphorus type of the homœopathic textbooks. She was anæmic and strengthless, had a narrow chest with little expansion, bluey whites to her eyes, her breasts were full of hard knots, wrinkled and hanging down like an old woman's, her body skin was extremely harsh and coarse, she did not perspire, could not sleep at night.

Six months previously, in September, 1931, while menstruating, she went for a motor-car ride, got chilled and menstruation had stopped ever since. She had lost 2 stone. The parents had sent her to the panel doctor, but, as she did not cough, he did not trouble to examine her and declared her fit for work. The girl took prodigious quantities of hot tea, large quantities of salt, had indigestion, felt utterly miserable. The danger of consumption was all the greater as two of her aunts had died of that disease. She lived on the usual mixed diet, had no appetite, felt icy cold, went to stool once in four or five days.

I placed her on a lacto-vegetarian diet. Three pints of milk, 3 eggs, 3 ozs. of mild grated cheese, at least 9 heaped tablespoonfuls of bran, 3 tablespoonfuls of black treacle, an abundance of vegetables, wholemeal bread, potatoes, etc. To help her digestive apparatus, she was given Nux vomica and Carbo vegetabilis combined before meals, and Phosphorous 3X night and morning. I told her that I expected her to improve immediately. During the first week she did badly, had diarrhœa, but gained 12 ozs., slept better. Her next report, dated 13th April, was wonderfully good. " I have gained 4 lbs. during the last week, my weight now being 7 stone 5 lbs. My appetite has greatly improved. Also I have much better nights."

The diet, and particularly the bran, began to work. She could reduce paraffin to the vanishing point, and had two good natural motions without medicine every day for the first time in her life. As she had taken enormous quantities of salt and felt always chilly, Natrum muriaticum was indicated, and I gave her that medicine in the 3X potency. On the 28th April she wrote: " I feel much brighter and much more energetic, my appetite has greatly improved, I have gained 1½ lbs. since last week." On the 4th May she reported: " I have made a further gain of 2 lbs. 6 ozs., I have felt much better than I have done for a good many months and it is very gratifying to hear my friends say how much better I am looking."

She visited me on the 11th May, and I found her wonderfully improved. I wrote: —

" I am very pleased with you. You have immensely improved during the six weeks under my care. You have gained 8 lbs. of solid flesh, body skin is vastly better, breasts are less lumpy, bowels act to perfection, sleep is better, appetite has greatly improved, but you are still very, very far from well. You hold yourself badly. You must take deep-breathing exercise, you must try to increase your intake day by day, little by little, and you must gain 20 lbs. Your periods have not yet reappeared."

I ordered her to rub cod-liver oil into chest, back and other parts of the body to be absorbed by the skin. That is preferable to taking it by the mouth which upsets many people. In view of her tuberculous inheritance and appearance, I now gave her Bacillinum 30, a dose every Sunday, and as a tonic Ferrum phosphoricum 3X, first and last thing. Between meals she was to take a dose of Pulsatilla 1X to bring on her period.

Her next letter, dated 19th May, told me: "I have gained 2 lbs. since I came to see you." Her report, dated the 27th May, said: "I am still getting stronger every day and feel a different person from what I did but a few weeks ago. I have not neglected the breathing exercises. My chest measurement is 2 inches more than when I first came to see you. I have gained another 1½ lbs. this week, and feel in excellent health." I told her that she would have to gain 20 lbs. before I could allow her to go to work. On the 5th June she wrote: "I have gained 2½ lbs. this week. I now weigh a stone more than when I first came to you. All my friends are delighted with my progress." On the 14th June she wrote: "I have gained 2 lbs. since writing you last." The next letter, dated 23rd June, said: "I am still making great improvement and have gained 1¼ lbs. this week."

She was to continue Ferrum phosphoricum 3X as a tonic and Pulsatilla, to bring on her menstruation. Her weight increased from week to week. On the 26th July she wrote: "I am wonderfully well, and am sure it is impossible to feel better than I do at present. I feel full of energy." I allowed her to go back to business, and on the 22nd August she wrote: "I have been going up to Town for three weeks now and cannot remember feeling more fit or energetic in spite of the terrific heat of the last two or three weeks which did not fatigue me in the least. I feel perfectly normal."

On the 11th October she wrote: " I have felt marvellously well this last month or two. You will be pleased to hear that my weight is now 8 stone 5 lbs., and I am still steadily increasing. On the 1st of this month my period recommenced for the first time." On the 28th December, 1933, she told me that she had had a motor accident, and added: " My health is excellent. I am now about 9 stone." She had re-gained her health and 28 lbs. of muscle. Had she continued going to business, as advised by her panel doctor, she would not have lived long.

CHAPTER XIV

Fibroid Tumours and other Womb Diseases

MODERN medicine is dominated by the surgeon and the laboratory man. The physician has become a kind of middleman. Many practitioners limit their work to attending to simple ailments, and they hand to their patients laxatives, tonics, sedatives, etc. As soon as they meet a case which presents some difficulty, they either send the patient's excretions and secretions to a laboratory, and a laboratory man, who has never seen the patient, will prescribe a serum or vaccine which may prove utterly unsuitable. Alternatively, the patient is sent to the dentist, a hospital, a specialist or a surgeon.

The domination of the surgeon is particularly striking in the realm of gynæcology. There are numerous textbooks on the diseases of women. I would recommend my readers to glance through some of them. They will find that they are filled with descriptions of surgical operations. Most of them are unnecessary. Dr. Thomas Skinner, the favourite assistant of Sir James Simpson, the greatest gynæcologist of his time, wrote in 1903 : —

" Constitutional treatment alone is all that is necessary for the successful treatment of all mammary, vaginal, uterine, ovarine and pelvic diseases of women, and local treatment is not only unnecessary, but is very frequently hurtful and not devoid of danger, to say nothing of its revolting character. The fearful tide of revolting mechanical and surgical treatments of the disease of women now established is one of the greatest medical scandals of the age."

Professor Bernard Aschner, the eminent gynæcologist and surgeon of Vienna, wrote in his book *Die Krise Der Medizin*, recently published:—

" In going through the hospitals and clinics for women, one is struck by the fact that the female uterus is apparently looked upon as a malignant growth and that it seems to be the principal object of modern gynæcology to extirpate it by the most scientific methods.

" The castration of relatively young women is effected at numerous clinics for women throughout the world on the plea that many women experience no disturbance of their health, or only minor ones. They overlook the fact that the damage done may become apparent only after years and that it may assume very serious forms, such as very high blood pressure, heart disease, severe chronic gout, etc."

Dr. Erwin Liek, the German surgeon, wrote in *The Doctor's Mission*: " I think I am safe in stating that unnecessary operations form more than half of the total." Another eminent surgeon has told me that 90 per cent. of all operations are unnecessary. Some time ago a specialist told me that he had taken out 40,000 tonsils, and that that operation took him only 15 seconds.

It is far more dramatic to say: " I underwent a terrible internal operation and my life was saved by the skill of Mr. or Sir So-and-so, who charged 250 guineas " than to describe a long and dull course of medication which effected the same object at a tithe of the expense. Many women are impatient. A growth in their inside can be cut out in an hour, but it may take two years to get rid of it by medicinal treatment. Lastly, there is the temptation of enormous fees which must not be disregarded. This factor has much to do with the operating mania, especially in women's diseases.

The orthodox textbooks tell us that there is no cure for fibroid tumours, except by surgery. Professor H. S. Crossen's *Diagnosis and Treatment of the*

Diseases of Women says: " The only reliable curative treatment for uterine fibromyomata is removal by operation." Gould and Pyle's *Pocket Cyclopedia of Medicine and Surgery* states: " The treatment of fibroid tumours of the uterus consists in removal." I could quote twenty similar opinions from gynæcological textbooks.

Homœopaths have very different views. Dr. H. M. Guernsey wrote in his textbook *Obstetrics* under the heading " Uterine Fibroid Tumours " :—

" Any remedy in the materia medica may be suitable in these cases. The violent procedures recommended by the gynæcologists of the old school have nothing to recommend them in the way of results, and the old homœopathic practitioner, by carefully choosing a remedy in strict accordance with the principles laid down by Hahnemann, may do much better, and cannot do worse, in these cases, than the dominant school of medicine."

Dr. J. Compton Burnett wrote with justified indignation in *Organ Diseases of Women* :—

" I hold very strongly that it is simply impossible to cure any constitutional disease whatever by any operations. The manifold operations on women are, for the most part, absolutely useless, often harmful, and not seldom fatal. How can anyone cure the quality of a person by cutting a piece off her ? "

Specialists are only too ready to recommend drastic operations. The excision of womb and ovaries is undertaken with the same light-heartedness with which perfectly healthy tonsils and appendices are cut out. I have met scores of women who had been deprived of their womb and ovaries who were ruined for life by that operation, and I must say with great regret that in the vast majority of cases that operation was unnecessary. Some women recover and become more or less normal. Others do not bear the mutilation and become pitiful wrecks. Even for minor troubles surgical proceedings are urged in the textbooks. Women are unnecessarily curetted for a leucorrhœa or some other triviality. Unfortunately the scraping out of the womb very often leads to the grave degeneration of that organ.

The surgeons who specialize in treatment of the male bladder assert that there is no treatment for an enlarged prostate gland except operation. I have shown in another chapter that prostatic enlargement can easily and cheaply be cured in countless cases by diet and homœopathic medicine. Similarly gynæcologists are unanimous in asserting that there is no cure for a fibroid tumour of the womb, except by operation. Yet I have cured a considerable number of such growths by diet and medicine.

There are two kinds of fibroid tumours—bleeding and non-bleeding ones. In the case of bleeding fibroids, the argument in favour of operation is that the woman may bleed to death. That danger exists indeed to the surgically-minded who imagine that uterine hæmorrhage can be stopped only by mechanical means, plugging, etc. However, this is not the case.

On the 25th November, 1928, a Mrs. E. F. wrote to me from Meanwood, Leeds:—

" I have been medically examined and have been informed that I have a fibroid tumour on the womb, and that there is no medicine that is any benefit to me for such a growth, and I am determined not to be operated on. There the matter rests, so far as my doctor is concerned. Now what I want to know is if you can help me in any way. I am just 46 years of age. I have been eating wholemeal bread for the last few months and am certainly not troubled with constipation and never have been. I have always eaten a lot of fresh raw fruit, having lived in the heart of the country until 30 years of age."

On the 1st December I sent her my directions, in which I stated:—

" I shall endeavour to reduce your tumour, or rather cause your system to absorb the tumour, by purifying your blood supply, eliminating morbid material from your system, and reversing the tendency which has caused the growth of the fibroid. Of course this may take some considerable time, and you must have patience and must allow for the fact that the growth, which has been produced in the course of years, cannot be absorbed in a few weeks or months.

" I do not mean to dissuade you from having an operation. The decision whether you are, or are not, to be operated upon lies entirely with you and you must never blame me for having influenced your mind in any way, for nothing is further from me. I put this at the head of my directions so that it should be permanently on record. I take it that the diagnosis of 'fibroid tumour' can be relied upon. I consider your diet very faulty, you lost a great deal of blood at menstruation, you have a hollow cough and do not perspire. We must deal with your various defects one by one."

The lady had been living on fried fish, pork pies, cooked ham, steak and kidney pudding, steamed fish, bacon, plenty of vegetables and fruit and a pint and a half of water taken between meals. As she had been eating white bread until recently, I gave her large quantities of bran and put her on a diet of an eliminating and purifying character. I wrote: " Avoid absolutely flesh, fish, fowl and everything made of them, salt, pepper, mustard, vinegar, sauces, and take the minimum of sugar. Do not eat sweets, pastries, chocolates." As she had cold feet in bed, I gave her a hot footbath every night and for eliminating purposes Thyroid 2X, 2 tablets after meals, and 2 tablets of Aurum muriaticum natronatum 3, to be taken first thing in the morning and last thing at night. Aurum (gold) shares with Iodine the peculiarity of reducing swollen glands and tumours, and Aurum muriaticum natronatum has proved its value in many cases of fibroid tumour in which I have used it.

After a while Mrs. E. F. informed me that she had a sinking feeling at 11 a.m., a well-known Sulphur symptom. Sulphur is a great purifying and blood-clearing medicine. I sent her a box of Sulphur 3X, and then went back to Aurum muriaticum natronatum, which, later on, I alternated with Iodum 3X and Iodum

6X. Orthodox medicine gives Iodine in doses of 5-10 drops of the tincture, and this quantity does fearful injury in innumerable cases which have come to me. I gave Mrs. F. Iodum by the thousandth of a grain and by the millionth of a grain. These small doses are exceedingly effective.

Before long there was considerable improvement. On the 10th March, 1929, the lady wrote to me:—

" My condition is most decidedly one of real improvement. I am always ready for my meals now I have got accustomed to the change of diet. I have gained 4½ lbs. and the tumour is much softer, but I could not say that it is smaller. As to my appearance in general, I get this greeting from nearly all friends: ' My word, you are looking wonderfully better.' My spirits are quite good, I have never let my troubles depress me, and I am determined to carry on and get well with your help, and I am quite optimistic about it."

I went on ringing the changes, giving her Aurum and Iodine. On the 4th April she wrote:—

" The tumour I can scarcely feel at all. It seems about the size of an egg now. I can hardly realize it is not there and I feel an easy, loose movement about my body, which I have not felt for quite a long time. Also I have gone through the winter with only a very slight cold once, which is certainly wonderful for me. I usually have an awful cough for weeks."

When the lady came to me she was taking habitually large bottles of cough mixture sent by her doctor. I stopped these at once.

I had never seen the woman and I had no idea how large the tumour was. When she informed me that it had shrunk to the size of an egg I enquired for its original size. She wrote on the 13th April:—

" The size of the tumour was such that I could just about cover it with my hand, and it felt very hard, and I used to feel a dragging sensation when lying down and the pain at times was so acute that I had no appetite and felt very sick. I do not feel anything of that now and I have had not the least sign of any discharge for two or three weeks."

On the 23rd April she wrote:—

"I am feeling in excellent spirits, and my skin and lips are taking on quite a good colour. My appetite is very good and the tumour is very small indeed. In fact, I can scarcely feel anything whatever. I have also gained another 1 lb. and 4 ozs. in weight, and I feel better in all ways than I have done for years."

On the 2nd May the patient reported:—

"It is a blessing I did not undergo an operation, but my mind was quite made up on that point from the first, although the doctor did not like my decision. I am eating and sleeping well. I can hardly realize the tumour has disappeared so far as I know. I can feel no lump whatever and have not the least discharge."

On the 27th May, Mrs. E. F. wrote:—

"I should like to say how very much better I feel in every way, and I wonder if by a little further treatment I could gain any more benefit. I can sleep better than I have done for years and do not feel at all tired after my day's work, as I used to do. I used to feel weary of being told how ill I looked. Now everyone is greeting me with the remark 'You are looking heaps better.'"

On the 2nd July, 1929, Mrs. E. F. thought that no further treatment was needed and wrote:—

"Since being under your treatment my weight has increased from 8 stone 10 to 9 stone 6. I have had no return or sign of any of the old troubles and I feel perfectly well."

Mrs. E. F. was a poor and very busy woman. I took on her case without having seen her and as she improved from the first, she never thought it necessary to visit me. If a layman can perform such a cure and many similar ones in cases which he has never seen, surely highly trained doctors and surgeons who have seen the patient ought to do at least as well. A cure by diet and medicine is less profitable than a cure by surgery. That fact should be disregarded. A good doctor should find his greatest reward in curing the patient.

On the 2nd September, 1931, I was visited by Mrs. C. L. of Stratford, London, who complained about a huge fibroid tumour, which made it almost impossible for her to stoop, bend and walk up and down stairs. Besides, she suffered from frequent floodings, which were particularly severe at night and they lasted uninterruptedly for three weeks. Then came a remission of a week and then the discharge came again in rushes.

Mrs. C. L. was 50 years old, the trouble had begun at the change of life, and she was as white as chalk. Instead of blood she had a watery serum in her arteries. She had been advised that an immediate operation was necessary, but had refused it. She had been anæmic since childhood. There had been in the past hardly any discharge at menstrual periods. The terrible and almost incessant bleeding drained her. She had loose motions, no footsweat, an evil-smelling perspiration, was never thirsty, and the heart was in a very bad condition, as is usually the case in the very anæmic, for the heart was starved. It fluttered like an insect against a glass pane.

I prescribed a strengthening, blood-making diet. She was to take liver soup every day, made by running 6 ozs. of English liver three times through the mincing machine, dropping it into rampantly boiling water or milk and cooking it only for a minute. In addition, she was to take 2 to 3 pints of milk, 2 to 3 eggs, and any quantity of softly boiled unbleached sultanas and raisins.

She came from poor stock. Her mother had died young of consumption, and one of her sisters also had some unspecified womb-trouble. The doctor had given her a mixture of Gentian, Arsenic and Digitalis, which I stopped. I am not fond of Arsenic and Digitalis in large quantities. They are desperately dangerous. As she looked rather jaundiced and as she had been

P

given these poisonous drugs, I gave her Sulphur 6X night and morning, and Nux vomica and Carbo veg. combined before meals to help her digestion and to antidote Digitalis and Arsenic. I gave her Phosphorus 3, a dose to be taken every hour or so in case of hæmorrhage, her blood being bright red and gushing. I pointed out to her the seriousness of her condition.

On the 9th September her daughter wrote to me: "Mother is feeling a little brighter and has a little more energy. She went to Soho hospital and was examined and they informed her that she had a fibroid tumour." That information was scarcely necessary, for the tumour was as large as a man's head. The question merely was whether it was malignant or not. In view of her inheritance, I was inclined to consider the trouble tuberculous in nature. On the 11th September the mother herself wrote: "I feel brighter and have more energy and my heart feels more steady." I gave her Cinchona rubra, mother tincture, as a blood-making medicine. Then she complained about deadly nausea and was sent Ipecacuanha 3X. A single dose put that trouble right. On the 27th September the lady wrote: "If I could only feel well and strong, it would be a blessing which I have not known for a good many years. Do you think you will be able to disperse the fibroid for me?" I replied: "I certainly hope that your fibroid will leave you, and not with a return ticket." The lady was of the Pulsatilla type, was very affectionate and weepy. So she was given Pulsatilla for constitutional reasons. I had not given her any fibroid medicine as yet. On the 7th October she wrote: "I am still feeling much better, my breathing is much better and I do not have palpitations so much."

On the 24th October, after seven weeks' treatment, Mrs. C. L. called on me for the second time. I wrote to her:—

"I was surprised, amazed and delighted by you appearance, for I had no conception that you had improved as much as you have done. You have less indigestion, eyes are much clearer, skin is no longer jaundiced, you have red lips and gums, pain and throbbing in abdomen are almost gone, heart is much better, catarrh and flushes have improved, and you are in much better spirits and are altogether splendid."

The hæmorrhage had been kept in check. It was clear that her greatly improved body would in due course be able to absorb the fibroid, but building up was still more urgent than dealing with that growth. I sent her Ferrum phosphoricum 3X as a tonic and hæmorrhage preventative. On the 9th December, 1931, after three months' treatment, she wrote:—

"When I first saw you, I was feeling very weak and ill, had no strength, no energy, felt very depressed and irritable, could not walk without puffing and blowing for want of breath, and was suffering from very bad palpitation, and also had bad hæmorrhages. I now am feeling much stronger and brighter, have considerably much more energy, only have a fit of depression now and again, can walk much farther without shortness of breath, do not have palpitations nearly so badly, and have only had two short hæmorrhages. So I think I am progressing very favourably. I am full of gratitude for the restoration of my health so far."

Occasionally constitutional treatment alone will lead to the absorption or expulsion of an internal growth, which has been produced by constitutional factors, the correction of which is apt to reverse the process. The growth or growths of Mrs. C. L. remained practically unchanged for months. Only in February, 1932, I started sending the lady medicines designed to deal with the fibroid or fibroids. I never knew whether she had one or several. I sent her Conium 1X, Thuya 3X, Calcarea iodata 3X, Aurum muriaticum natronatum 6X, and various other remedies for adequate spells, testing each by itself, and alternating these medicines with called-for constitutional remedies, such as Sulphur, Pulsatilla mother tincture, which is very valuable in post-climacteric complaints.

By and by Mrs. C. L. discovered that she could walk and run upstairs and downstairs, could stoop and bend,

which she had not been able to do for years, and then
came letters which told me: " I believe the growth is
smaller." " I am sure it is smaller," " I believe it is
very much smaller." Occasionally there were setbacks
with hæmorrhage, and then I consoled her by suggesting that nature might get rid of the fibroid by
bleeding.

As she was weak, there came intercurrent troubles,
each of which had to be treated by itself, and in the
meantime treatment of the fibroid had to be neglected.
She was given Lachesis for flushes, Ignatia for her
nerves, and so forth. It was a long story. On the
27th June, 1933, she wrote to me: " Of course my
abdomen feels very different from what it did when
I first came to you, and although I can still feel a lump,
it is certainly much smaller. I can draw it in almost
flat now, which I could not do before."

I saw her on the 16th August, 1933. She looked
wonderfully well, and I wrote to her: —

"Everything about you is beautifully normal, but the
pulse is still somewhat weak and slow, and you are still
somewhat anæmic. You looked terribly unwholesome when
I saw you first. Your huge fibroid has shrunk to such small
dimensions that it is really difficult to find it. There are two
fragments now, on the right and on the left side. One may
be as large as a walnut, and the other as large as half a
walnut. You are now thoroughly wholesome."

On that day I sent her a few doses of Tuberculinum,
100th potency, a dose to be taken once a week.

Since then Mrs. C. L. has improved further, but she
has remained a weak and somewhat anæmic woman.
There are certain constitutions in which anæmia cannot be overcome by any means known to me. Occasionally these fibroids disappear completely, ocasionally
they shrivel and leave behind a hard substance.

Possibly the dangerous operation which was proposed might have been carried out by a good and a
lucky surgeon, for luck is as needed as skill, but she
might have been unfortunate. The risk and shock

are great and the risk should not be run if it is avoidable. I have never met an orthodox gynæcologist or doctor who admitted the possibility of dealing with a fiborid tumour of the womb except by operation. Yet homœopaths have cured hundreds of fibroids without operation. Unfortunately orthodox doctors and surgeons take no notice of these cures. From their point of view an unorthodox cure is no cure, and a homœopath need not be listened to, even if he has passed all the orthodox medical examinations with distinction.

On the 13th May, 1929, I was visited by Mrs. E. L., of Swindon. She was 43 years old, had been operated upon for appendicitis, had undergone an operation of the womb, part of which had been taken away, but lately her health had seriously fallen off. Her doctor had discovered a growth on the womb which was pressing on the bowel. He had declared it to be cancerous and had urged another operation. She refused to be operated upon again and came to me.

She was deeply jaundiced, looked desperate, was emaciated, anæmic, terribly flabby, her veins were protruding everywhere through the skin, there were many moles on her body, her hair was dry, and she looked thoroughly unwholesome. She was chronically constipated, had been living on a diet devoid of vitamins and mineral elements, complained of headaches and giddiness.

Although she looked a wreck, I refused to take a pessimistic view, and concluded the introductory part of my directions with the sentence: "Very likely your condition will be vastly improved with the improvement of your intake and excretions." I gave her liquid paraffin three times a day, forbade flesh, fish, fowl and everything made of them, and made her live on 3 pints of milk per day, 3 eggs, 3 ozs. of mild grated cheese, mashed and sieved vegetables, potatoes, black treacle, wholemeal bread, etc. The only medicine which she was given at the beginning was Thyroid 2X to detoxicate her system.

Her first report, dated the 28th May, told me: "I weigh now 6 stone 10 lbs. 12 ozs., I find I have gained nearly 2½ lbs., and I certainly feel much better." The next week she gained 10 ozs., the week after she wrote: "I feel much stronger, my bowels keep in good order, I have had no headaches or giddy attacks, and all this week I have not had any pain at the bottom of my back."

On the 18th June she wrote: "My friends tell me I am looking much better." As her liver was troubling her, I gave her Cholesterin 2X. On the 10th July she told me: "I have been feeling really fine; only yesterday I was saying that headaches and giddiness were getting a thing of the past." On the 23rd July she wrote: "I have gained a good 2¾ lbs." Her next weekly letter informed me: "I have got a little colour which is something new for me." On the 22nd August she said: "I am feeling A.1."

She came to see me on the 20th September, and I found her looking far better than I had expected. As there was pain in the bowel, I gave her Ruta 1X, an excellent remedy in case of cancer of the bowel. Then she got Lilium tigrinum 3, which is valuable for a retroverted womb pressing upon the bowel. On the 22nd October she wrote: "I have gained another 2 lbs., and am now 7 stone 5½, so have put on 11 lbs. since last May. I am feeling very pleased about it." On the 7th November she told me: "I am still feeling all right; it is such a treat to be alive." On the 19th November she said: "I am now 7 stone 9. When I came to you in May I was 6 stone 10¼. It gives me confidence, getting such excellent results."

I now gave her Ferrum phosphoricum as a tonic and Hydrastis for her liver and gall bladder, for Lilium tigrinum had done its duty. On the 15th January she wrote: "That tight uncomfortable feeling at the bottom of my back is a lot better." On the 29th January I was told: "I have gained 2¼ lbs. more in weight. I am now 7 stone 11½. It is splendid."

She was 6 stone 7½ when she came to me first and had therefore gained 18 lbs. and she felt a totally different woman. She considered herself cured and her letters became very rare. On the 5th September she told me: " I am now 8 stone," and she came to see me on the 11th September. After our interview I wrote:—

" You looked five years younger than when I saw you last. You have gained something like 20 lbs. since you came to me, have splendidly firm arms and legs, nice coloured lips, bowels are regular, there seems to be no longer evidence of a growth and there is improvement in every direction. You have lost your jaundiced looks and deep depression, have become comparatively sturdy."

She had been under my care for 16 months, all her pains and discomforts had disappeared, and her doctor could no longer find anything wrong about her womb and an operation was quite out of the question. If she had been operated upon in May, 1929, disaster would have followed. Every doctor and surgeon knows that cancer frequently arises in operation scars, especially in operation scars of people with a very foul blood-stream. If the diagnosis of cancer of the womb was mistaken in 1929 and if part of the womb had been excised and no cancer cells had been found under the microscope, cancer might have developed rapidly after the operation.

CHAPTER XV

Mystery Diseases

THE art and science of diagnosis has progressed with giant strides. The modern doctor can examine the stomach, bowel, heart, lungs and other organs with X-rays and can watch the process of digestion and of elimination. He can introduce tubes, at the tip of which there is a mirror and a small electric bulb, into the bladder, stomach and bowel, and can examine the inside at leisure. He can have a scientific analysis made of all the body fluids, etc.

The doctors have been taught that treatment should be based on an exact diagnosis. Some diseases are easily diagnosable. Others are difficult to diagnose.

An exact diagnosis by means of the numerous scientific tests may take days, and occasionally weeks. In the meantime the patient is kept " under observation," and is frequently not treated at all, although the disease may call for immediate intervention. Occasionally a patient dies before a diagnosis can be made.

The skilled homœopath does not work under this crippling handicap. He may wish for an exact diagnosis, but he need not wait for the findings of the various experts. He can act immediately, guided by the symptoms. Therefore, the homœopath is often able to treat and cure an obscure case while his orthodox colleague is still engaged in its diagnosis. I would describe briefly a few mystery cases which have come my way and which probably would have defied exact diagnosis by the best experts.

On the 11th July, 1928, I received a letter from a Mrs. C. C. J., the wife of an eminent personage residing in an outlying part of the Empire:—

"Last spring I read your book *Good Health and Happiness* and longed for courage to write to you to help me regain my health, but as you mentioned in the book Dr. A., of London, I went to him. He has done me much good, but I cannot get strong, and I am much below weight for my height, 5 feet 5 inches. I am only 6 stone 7½. I always have been liable to tonsillitis, and, when I was 19, I had a tumour on the left lobe of the thyroid which was removed. Of course I have had appendicitis, and had my appendix removed.

"I was most active riding, better at it than most men. My weight was then 8 stone 7, and I was dancing and playing tennis years ago with immense vigour. I am now 37. I got a very bad septic throat with abscesses in my ear. These affected my heart badly and four months later I had diphtheria very badly. The doctors gave me two enormous doses of antitoxin and for weeks I have been critcially ill. Since then I have been struggling to get the poison out of my system. My heart became badly affected and I was a mass of neuritis. Headaches were my daily lot. I was dangerously anæmic. My blood pressure is only 85.

."After all sorts and kinds of orthodox treatment I read your book, but, rather than trouble you, I went to Dr. A. He advised me to eat only twice a day, gave me many exercises, broke down all adhesions due to the neuritis. I was to have two meals, one to consist of green vegetables and farinaceous foods and green salad, and the other of highly cooked roast meat, eggs or cheese and fruit. I have lost the headaches and neuritis, and my heart is strengthened, but I am very thin and have no strength, nor am I able to do a full day like a normal woman. Yet I am so full of the joy of living, and if I get fatigued, I take days to get right.

"Then suddenly, for no reason, I got acute enteritis. I cannot pick up strength again. I have had two nurses and a most enlightened doctor. My face, neck, chest and arms are very thin. I used to have a shocking circulation and religiously do my exercises daily for three-quarters of an hour. Since I had enteritis, I have been troubled with flatulence and indigestion, am not able to take starchy foods, am taking a tonic called Metatone, made by Park Davis. Can you help me? For six months I was under treatment by Mr. E. M., and, as a result, very nearly .died of protein poisoning.

"I am extremely highly strung and live intensely. In 1926 I was in bed for months with a collapsed heart and extreme nervous exhaustion."

I replied:—

"I imagine that I shall be able to rebuild your body, provided you are willing to co-operate with me. I have come to the conclusion that, apart from your being under-fed, over-exercised and over-medicated, there are poisons within you which have to be eliminated."

In view of her weakened condition, I gave her a baby diet, 3 pints of milk, 3 eggs, 2 or 3 ozs. of cheese, she starting with small doses of diluted milk, increasing it gradually to the ideal quantity and taking milk foods as well. I forbade flesh, fish, fowl and their products, and told her to take plenty of bran, if digestible, otherwise Bemax. Medicines and strong disinfectants were forbidden and so were hot baths, which are weakening. Instead of exercise, she was to have massage and was to be strengthened by rubbing into the body olive oil, or, better, cod-liver oil, and to report progress once a week. The medicines were Sulphur 3 night and morning to activate the skin, Hydrastis 1X three times a day before meals to improve functioning of stomach, liver, gall bladder and bowel, and she was to take Thuja to counteract vaccinations and other subcutaneous treatments which she had received in superabundance. I forbade physical exercise. People in her condition cannot get strong by violent exercise.

In her letter, dated 23rd August, she reported to me the effect of the first week's treatment: "I have slept *much* better the last few nights. I am profoundly grateful that you stopped the exercise ordered by the doctor. My weight ten days ago was only 6 stone 7½ lbs., but yesterday, only three days after starting your diet, it had gone up 2 lbs." She informed me that ever since vaccination she had suffered in health. She had been inoculated for typhoid, had had diarrhœa in 1917, and was given " seventeen injections of Emetine which partially paralysed my legs and it took me four months to recover, with hot enemas and electrical treatments." Modern treatments of this character are called " heroic," but the heroism is to be found not on the part of the doctors, but on the part of their victims. Mrs. C. C. J. suffered largely from the violent and unsuitable treatments which she had received.

Soon there was further improvement. On the 6th September she wrote: —

" I am feeling much better and have a much better colour. The ugly yellow-brown round my mouth and down my nose is certainly clearing away rapidly, and my brain is much less clumsy and exhausted. I am feeling radiantly hopeful, especially when I look in the glass. I think the No. 1 pilules are chiefly responsible for the improvement (they contained one millionth of a grain of Sulphur, a very potent medicine with which to begin treatment). There is also very definite improvement in my bowels for the first time for years. For years I had no sensation whatever in my bowels. My stomach also feels very much better. It felt as though the lining were sore and spongy, but that feeling has definitely improved since taking No. 1 pilules. My spirits are soaring high again and I am beginning to feel that you will succeed and make me well, though so many doctors have told me definitely that they will cure me, and all have failed. This time I am almost sure you will succeed, for it is the first time there has been any improvement in the bowels. I used to dread doing my exercises. It was all such a strain and so depressing. My experiences of the last five years have taught me it is so much easier to die than to live. I begin to feel that perhaps, with your help, I may know the joy of living again."

I felt encouraged by her reaction and sent her encouraging letters. She gained weight from week to week. On the 13th September she wrote: " I have again gained about a lb. and a quarter. I am most certainly a far better colour. Everyone notices it. My eyes are clearer." On the 27th September she wrote: " Everyone tells me I am looking tons better. I am getting back my old handwriting. For ages I have not had the strength to form my letters." On the 3rd October she told me:—

" The doctor who tried to help me this summer suffered horribly by his failure. I was wilting under his eyes till the middle of August. I then did not think I was worth saving, but I did dread the long drawn-out death that seemed my fate. I have been weighed and have gained only 2 lbs. in the last three and a half weeks. A man who had not seen me for some time told me he would not have recognized me. I not only looked so much better but so utterly different. I shall send you a snapshot which will show how the shape of my face has altered. It is back to what it was nine years ago. I have improved so much that I feel impatient. I have not had cramps for weeks and used always to be getting them in my feet, legs and back. My ear is better too. What a wonderful work yours is! "

In most cases the personal influence of the practitioner is of supreme importance. Many patients have assured me that my letters were their best medicine. Mrs. C. C. J. wrote on the 18th October: " Your letters are the greatest help to me, and I look eagerly forward to them. My husband last night agreed that I was looking better than I have done since 1915."

It appeared that the treatment I gave without having seen her, suited her better than that of the numerous doctors and specialists in England and abroad who had carefully examined her. On the 26th October she wrote:—

" I wish almost more than anything on earth that you could see me. When I wrote to you first in August of this year my face was yellow with blue and green shadows and not a scrap of flesh on my face and neck. To-day I have a completely pink and white face, with round contours and the cornflower blue eyes of my halcyon days. I think I have made giant strides this last ten days. My skin feels now moister and is certainly better nourished (that was probably the effect of the cod-liver oil and olive oil rubbed into her skin) and I perspire quite freely. I now laugh immoderately at a joke and have not been able to see a joke for at least four and a half years. It amazes me to read that as late as 13th September, 1928, I was still fearing I should never get really well again."

Chronic cases, and particularly chronic cases which have been ill-treated, take long to recover. I had made this clear to the lady. She rewarded me with the most delightful letters. On the 24th January she wrote: " My husband says I look better than for ten years and I feel so well and jolly and, though I am tired at night, I merely want to sleep and not to commit suicide as I used to. I dreaded to be left alone. I dreaded that I would have a collapse or die." She wrote on the 14th February, 1929: " I never feel chilly now. My circulation has improved out of all conscience."

Occasionally I was terrified by set-backs or by threats of dangerous interference on the part of doctors and surgeons. There was hydrophobia about and the grave danger of her being treated subcutaneously if she came near a dog. So I sent her Hydrophobinum 30 as a prophylactic to be taken once a week by the mouth and more often if bitten. Then there was smallpox about. I forbade vaccination, giving vaccination by the mouth with Variolinum and Mallandrinum in the 30th potency.

I had never seen Mrs. C. C. J. but she had fully and faithfully reported to me and had thus enabled me to help her. If there was urgent trouble, she would cable and I cabled back my directions. I had supplied her with a considerable stock of homœopathic medicines and with suitable advice and she knew how to act in all emergencies.

In 1933 she came to England and I saw her for the first time. She was in magnificent condition, felt younger and stronger than ever in her life, had become a champion pedestrian who amazed all her friends by her walking capacity, rode her horse every morning, danced with vigour, took an active part in private theatricals. Her weight had gone up from 6 stone 7½ to 10 stone. She asked me after the name of her disease. I told her that I didn't know and I didn't care. In my opinion the doctor's business consists not in " naming " a disease, but in curing it. Her doctors had diagnosed but had not cured, I had cured but not diagnosed.

On the 11th June, 1930, I received a telephone call from a clergyman in Bath, who was greatly alarmed by the condition of the wife of the manager of a large farm. She was apparently dying from inability to swallow. She had been a magnificently strong woman, had sons who looked like Lifeguardsmen, and she had lost an enormous amount of weight through inability to take food consequent upon the progressive narrowing of the throat, apparently caused by a growth which had been gradually increasing.

I thought of cancer of the throat or of the swallowing tube, and said that the condition seemed to me hopeless. He entreated me to do my best. I reluctantly agreed that I would see her, and she arrived on the 12th June with her son by car. She reached my house about 2 o'clock, had been travelling five hours, and had had no breakfast. She was a shadow of a woman, she dragged herself with difficulty from the gate to my house, and collapsed in a low invalid chair. I told her that she and her son could have any refreshments they liked. The son took an enormous meal, and I hoped that the boy's zest would give an appetite to the mother. However, she took only half a cup of the weakest China tea with the minimum of milk and no sugar and ate part of a single breakfast biscuit. I urged her in vain to take more nutriment. After an interview which lasted nearly two hours she went back by car to Bath. I telephoned my clergyman friend that I took an extremely serious view of her case. I feared that she might collapse and die on the way home from inanition, and suggested various measures in case of emergency

Immediately after having seen the lady, I dictated my directions and a summary of her condition to my secretary:—

"You are 58 years old, married, with magnificent boys, and you have come to me complaining about an absolutely dry mouth, a swelling on the right side of the throat low down which has been in evidence for about two years, very great difficulty in swallowing, bad taste in the mouth, an intense, maddening irritation on the back, especially near the spine, worst in bed, empty retching, bringing up a lot of stomach phlegm, occasional pain in the lower part of the stomach, followed by vomiting of food and relieved by it, the pain being soothed by rubbing the stomach. I cannot make out whether or whether not you have ever vomited stuff like coffee grounds or black stuff, a very important point.

"You are apt to sneeze violently and very frequently, sneezing being followed by vomiting. You drink boiling hot tea, bruise easily, have a very rapid heart with a feeling that you may faint, used to weigh 10 stone, but are now a mere skeleton of bones and skin. After motoring from Bath for hours, you took only half a breakfast biscuit and a cup of weak tea with a little milk and without sugar.

"You are deeply jaundiced, bloodless, and your bloodlessness alone suffices to explain your heart condition and weakness. You are starving to death, and the most essential thing is to feed you up. You have no swollen glands, normal urine, a tendency towards swollen ankles, are constipated, feel occasionally paralytic spasms on the left side. You come from a healthy family, but your father died of tuberculosis, a sister and brother have a tendency towards pneumonia. You have been smashed up seriously in a number of accidents."

The emaciation of the patient, her jaundiced skin, the swelling in her throat, frequent vomiting, etc., strongly suggested cancer. In stomach cancer the vomiting of coagulated blood looking like coffee grounds, or black, is frequent. As there had been tuberculosis and pneumonia in her family, there was further the possibility that the swelling in the throat was tuberculous. The case was a mystery. Exact diagnosis was impossible.

I put her on a milky diet and told her to take per day 3 to 4 pints of milk, 2 to 3 raw eggs, plenty of honey, which is a wonderful heart food, etc., intake to be increased gradually and cautiously. As I thought it possible that one of the numerous violent accidents which she had, she was thrown off her horse as a missionary, might in some way or other be responsible for her troubles, I prescribed for her Arnica 6, a dose to be taken first and last thing, and Spongia, roasted sea sponge, 1X, 3 pilules to be taken three times a day between meals. Spongia is a great medicine for dryness and burning of the throat, anxious and difficult breathing, goitre and goitrous swellings, palpitations with feeling of suffocation, etc.

Mrs. G. reacted favourably almost immediately, possibly because I had raised her hopes, possibly through coincidence. On the 16th June, four days after our interview, she wrote to me with a shaky hand that she was taking 2 or 3 raw eggs per day, more than 2 pints of milk, etc., and she concluded with the words: " Still very weak but think I am distinctly on the mend." I was delighted. But on the 19th June I received a letter which staggered me. Her husband wrote:—

" Mrs. G. is very much weaker and unable to stand, her head going round in a swoon, and she fainted this morning. The heart is desperately weak and we had to resort to champagne, of which I hope you approve. Your diet had a devastating effect and has caused the weakness. No change in the saliva-less state of her mouth. She still continues to retch and has only brought up one glass of milk to-day. Otherwise food has been retained. I carry her about and will not let her walk. I am most anxious about her."

In immediate reply I wrote to the husband that I had told his wife in my directions, as I usually do: " Act with wise discrimination, not with mechanical obedience to these directions, for no one understands the working of your body better than you do yourself," that in view of her desperate condition, she ought to be fed on anything that agreed with her, and that he ought to have communicated with me by telephone every day. As the mouth was still saliva-less, making it practically impossible for her to swallow food, I replaced Spongia, which was to act chiefly on the tumour in the throat, which I thought responsible for the lack of saliva, by two medicines Nux moschata 3X and Cistus canadensis 3X, which cause the greatest dryness of the mouth if taken in large quantities and which, therefore, cure this condition if taken in homœopathic doses. The one box was marked 1 and the other 2 and the patient was to concentrate on the more helpful medicine.

If the symptoms make it not absolutely clear that one particular remedy is called for, if two or three seem to be equally strongly indicated and it is impossible to decide which is the absolutely best, it is wise to give the patient a choice of those competing remedies. Otherwise the patient gets disheartened, gives up, or seeks advice elsewhere.

I telephoned almost daily to Bath, for the position became very threatening. There was nausea with a clean tongue, diarrhœa, vomiting, cold sweat and collapse. For the nausea with a clean tongue I sent Ipecacuanha and for collapse with cold sweat, vomiting and diarrhœa I sent Veratrum album.

I was promptly rewarded by a letter, written in a shaky hand in bed by Mrs. G. herself, dated the 22nd June. Happily it breathed a hopeful and cheerful spirit. Hahnemann taught that the mental symptoms are far more important than the physical ones. If a patient improves physically but is deeply depressed for no obvious reason, I get anxious, but I feel confident that an improvement is at hand if a patient tells me of physical troubles but is more cheerful. Mrs. G. wrote that she was eating regularly and getting down all the food I wanted her to have. She concluded with the words: " I am really quite different."

Q

Apparently Cistus canadensis, which is a wonderful medicine for swollen neck glands, swellings inside the throat and even for malignant disease of the throat, proved more helpful than Nux moschata. I sent further helpings of Cistus and improvement was marked and rapid. She quickly regained weight. She wrote on the 29th June:—

"I have no pain whatever and never retch now, and the phlegm has entirely ceased. I drove to Bath yesterday and was weighed. Another proof of my great improvement is that my stays, which for months, if laced tightly, folded over 2 or 3 inches, would not meet by 2 or 3 inches when I tried to put them on. I now weigh 8 stone and 5 lbs., and must have gained about 6 inches round the waist."

On the 2nd July she wrote:—

"There is nothing fresh to say. The vicar came to see me on Sunday and he said 'Now I see how well you are, I shall not worry any more about you.' The present food makes me very fat."

On the 13th July her husband wrote to me:—

"I think I ought to let you know how Mrs. G. really is from my point of view. She has picked up wonderfully and is really looking better now than I have seen her look for years, but she is chafing under her idleness and it is impossible to keep her from doing a certain amount of work. She says she is feeling perfectly well. The last two nights I have gone for a walk with her. I purposely walked slowly and she was about a yard ahead of me all the way, trying to hurry on. She has been eating very well, but says that she is getting stuffed and is inclined to eat less."

On the 13th July Mrs. G. wrote to me:—

"I am feeling splendid. I am eating terribly well. I have four bowel movements daily. I need exercise. Everyone at the vicar's yesterday exclaimed when they saw me arrive 'How well you look, better than for years, fat and rosy,' etc."

On the 24th September Mrs. G. visited me at my house. I scarcely recognized her. In writing to her I told her:—

"You are an amazing woman. Of course I knew that you were better, but I had no conception that you had improved in the way you have been improving. When you came to me on the 12th June, three months ago, you were a skeleton, and I was wondering whether you would get back to Bath alive. You ought never to have travelled so long in the condition in which you were then, and now you swim, dance, play tennis with the youngest, although you might be a grandmother, and you look strong enough to swim the Channel, or to become a professional athlete. You must have put on 3 or 4 stone, and apparently all your troubles have gone, but there is still the swelling at the right side of the throat and your swollen ankles and feet."

I gave her further helpings of Cistus canadensis for the mysterious swelling in her throat and Arnica for the numerous severe injuries which she had had when she was a missionary. There was further improvement and Mrs. G. considered herself completely cured. The cure held good. She wrote to me on the 30th December, 1933, three and a half years after our first interview: "The swelling in my neck hardly shows at all now. I have been extraordinarily strong and well. You will realize how well I am when I tell you that I have adopted a child." Yet, when she came to my house, she was within an inch of death. Any injudicious treatment, based on a faulty diagnosis, or delay of treatment, would have killed her. And what was her disease? I do not know. Anyway her life was saved and she has been well ever since.

On the 21st January, 1932, I was visited by a Mrs. L. D. of Clapham, London. She was a married woman of 63, complained about a tumour in the left side of the throat which she had noticed for a year and which had steadily got worse, and she was the picture of senile decay and utter hopelessness. She looked cancerous. In my directions I summarized her condition, but I mentioned only incidentally the tumour in the throat, which alarmed me greatly. I was afraid that it might be malignant and I realized that the poor woman would die if she knew what I suspected. Her jaundiced appearance, her way of living, the increasing growth, loss of weight, etc., would strongly suggest malignancy to every medical man. I wrote in my directions: —

" You have come to me complaining about numerous pains. Four years ago you fell, injured both your knees very severely, apparently fracturing them, and since then you have always had pain worse in the left leg, diagnosed as sciatica. You have also pain in the left side of the tongue, and under the tongue, and at the left side of the jaw. During the last 12 months you have been troubled with a feeling of a lump in the throat which is steadily getting worse, which causes pain which radiates from the throat towards the stomach. Swallowing is occasionally difficult. You take tea, boiling hot, cannot take cold water, love heat, cannot stand very hot baths, pain in the tongue is stitching and burning, you have been taking sleeping draughts every night for three months, are thin and look and feel flabby, you never perspire, feel best in the open air in any weather, take insufficient food."

The jaundiced appearance, hopelessness, expressionless eyes, loss of weight, and the habitual taking of boiling hot tea, which often leads to cancer of the swallowing tube and the stomach, made me feel very pessimistic. She had a very stringy throat which suggested over-consumption of salt, and I found that she took salt in huge quantities. Salt-poisoned people are always chilly, have watery eyes, stringy throats and are deeply depressed.

I never allow flesh foods if there is cancer or if I suspect cancer. I put the woman on a diet with an abundance of milk and milky foods, large quantities of ordinary bran, vegetables, potatoes, eggs, mild cheese, and told her to take " the absolute minimum of salt and spices and condiments." She was gradually to increase her intake and was to gain 2 lbs. per week in weight. As her troubles had begun after the change of life at the age of 50, Lachesis was indicated, and the injuries to her knees which crippled her walking power suggested Arnica. I gave her Arnica 3X, a dose to be taken three times a day, and Lachesis 6, 3 pilules to be taken night and morning during three days only.

I cheered Mrs. D. as well as I could, but she looked at me with lack-lustre, expressionless eyes, unable to smile. I took away the doctor's sleeping draught which she had taken every night for three months.

On the 28th January, after a week's treatment, she reported: "Am feeling better in health, and sleeping very well indeed." The second report, written on the 4th February, stated: "My general health is steadily progressing." As she was very restless, I now gave her Arsenic 3X, 3 pilules night and morning, instead of the Lachesis. I was greatly cheered by the immediate and excellent response of this most unpromising case. Improvement continued. On the 18th February she reported "Pains are easier now."

She had not gained any weight, notwithstanding an increasing intake which ought to have caused her to gain. Therefore I gave her Calcarea phosphorica 3X night and morning, combined with Natrum muriaticum 3X three times a day before meals. Natrum muriaticum, ordinary table salt, is a very valuable tonic, especially for chilly people, while Calcarea phosphorica, Phosphate of lime, is a wonderfully strengthening medicine and is particularly indicated in people who are tuberculous or have a tuberculous tendency or inheritance. Improvement became more marked. In her very brief notes sent from time to time there are remarks such as: "I am feeling very much better," "I am feeling very fit and have gained 2 lbs. My people are pleased with the progress I have made," "I am feeling better and am able to take on my work again," etc. As her communications ran as a rule only to three or four lines, I asked her to call. She came on the 27th April, after three months' treatment, and I scarcely recognized the woman. I wrote to her:—

"I was absolutely amazed by your appearance and by the wonderful all-round improvement for which I was not prepared. You are a miracle. Practically all your troubles are gone. You look twenty years younger, an entirely different woman. On the other hand, your varicose veins are unchanged, you cry easily, are always chilly, and take far too little bran."

I ordered her to take milk pudding made with an abundance of bran twice a day, and gave her Natrum muriaticum 30 for her chilliness and frigidity. She rapidly improved. On the 26th May she wrote: "Pleased to say I am feeling very fit and well, eat and sleep well, and can work without feeling any fatigue. I want now to try and do without any further treatment."

Five months later I heard from a friend that he had seen Mrs. D., whom he had known for a long time, and that he had failed to recognize her because she looked like a young woman. I then asked her how she was getting on and she wrote to me on the 21st October, 1932: "I have not felt so well for years. Your treatment did me more good than three years' doctor's medicine. My friends all remark how well I look."

Some months after this she called at my house, a smiling, happy, joyous woman, with a brilliant complexion, apparently free from all her troubles, a joy to herself and to all her friends. She kept well. On the 27th December, 1933, she wrote to me:—

"Am pleased to say I am feeling thoroughly well, and am able to do my work and quite free from pains.

"My friends remark how well and fresh looking I am for my age.

"My weight is now 8 stone 7 lbs., am putting on flesh. My people think I am lucky to be so well for they thought cancer was my trouble."

One must never consider a case hopeless or incurable It has happened to me many a time that a case which came to me with the diagnosis " absolutely incurable " and which I myself thought incurable, got well. There is an unlimited power of repair within us, which can be aroused by right nutrition, right medicine, constant encouragement, and, before all, by the determination of the doctor to cure his patient.

As one of my patients, Mrs. F. E. D., had benefited greatly by my treatment, she urged her son to consult me about his health. I saw him on the 5th December, 1932. He was a tall, powerfully built man, a typical Guards officer. He was 46 years old, had retired from the Army, lived in the south of France, did a great deal of motoring, had served in the War with distinction. He told me that he had never been ill, but for some considerable time he was suffering from an undefinable weakness, and feeling of unwellness, which he could not understand or explain. He was rapidly sliding downhill. There were no positive symptoms, except a dull ache and occasionally excruciating pains in the lowest part of the abdomen, and in the right side of the abdomen high above the appendix region. Besides, there were pains from the right kidney to the bladder, apparently along the line of the right ureter, the tube which connects kidney and bladder.

As there was some gravel in the urine and occasionally blood, I suspected kidney stone. I was not satisfied with this tentative diagnosis on the strength of which I might have suggested an X-ray. However, stones in kidney and gall bladder do not always come out in the X-ray picture. Besides, I did not feel sure that the trouble was purely local.

Major J. D. was tall and well made, but extremely anæmic and jaundiced. He looked nervy and anxious, his skin had a yellow tinge, his hands were fidgety, he had been given numerous injections during the War which might account for his trouble, and he took five or six pieces of sugar in each cup of tea. I looked at his gums, but there was no blue line suggesting lead poisoning. I then looked at his eyes with powerful magnifying glasses and I noticed that on his grey irises there were numerous whitish cloud-like specks, a symptom of Arsenic poisoning. Arsenic might, of course, have upset his kidneys and produced the obscure severe pain. I frankly told him of my suspicion.

He looked horrified and told me: " That is possible.

I have an enemy in France. Perhaps I have been given Arsenic." I replied: "That is very unlikely. These dramatic poisonings happen rarely. Have you any green wall-paper in your house, or have you been given any medicines, washes or ointments likely to contain Arsenic?" "No." "Well, aluminium produces similar symptoms to Arsenic. Do you happen to know whether aluminium is used in your kitchen?" "We use nothing but aluminium."

It was possible that the obscure trouble of my patient was due to aluminium poisoning or to numerous vaccinations and inoculations during the War, or was purely local, arising from the kidneys. In order to be on the safe side, one must treat not only the most likely cause, but also the less likely in order to be sure of prompt success. If a patient has received no benefit during a few weeks' treatment, he goes elsewhere. The modern doctor knows this, and therefore he gives his patient immediately something which will eliminate the symptoms complained of. A little Morphia, Opium, Heroin and such-like things will keep the patient in good humour and ready to come back to the man who has given him relief, although the relief is only temporary and deceptive.

I gave Major J. E. D. Berberis, mother tincture, for his kidneys, to be taken night and morning, Nux vomica and Carbo vegetabilis compound, before meals, partly to improve his digestion and partly because Nux vomica will antidote many drugs dormant in the body. In addition I gave him a little Belladonna to be taken if he should get a violent attack of pain, because Belladonna causes inflammation in substantial doses and relieves inflammation in homœopathic doses. The passage of a stone through a ureter or through one of the gall bladder ducts causes excruciating pain and inflammation, which often can rapidly be relieved by a few doses of Belladonna, particularly in high potency. My favourite strength for this purpose is the 200th potency. As I had to allow for the possibility that his troubles were due to subcutaneous treatments during the War, he was to take a dose of Thuja 30 marked " Injection antidote " every Wednesday, and as I had to allow for the possibility of aluminium poisoning, he was to take a single dose of Alumina 200 every Sunday. I gave him a diet sheet, warned him against overmuch sugar and salt, etc., and sent him away.

His first letter was sent to me on the 18th December, after less than a fortnight's treatment: " Just a few lines to say that I am really much better. I do not think it is fancy when I say that the Aluminium anti-dote made me feel better than the other medicines." On the 4th January, 1933, after four weeks' treatment, Major D. called on me for the second time. He declared himself cured and he was full of gratitude. I summarized the position in a note, in which I wrote : " You looked wonderfully improved, a totally different man, in fact a new man in body, mind and nerves, and I am delighted. I have not given you any further medicine because I do not know whether you need it. In case of need let me know instantaneously so that I can come to the rescue."

I have not seen Major J. D. since then, but from time to time I have heard from his mother and his sisters that he is wonderfully well and very grateful. Naturally he avoids aluminium like the pestilence.

CHAPTER XVI

Diet as an Art

L ORD —— was seriously ill. He was treated by
Dr. S. of Harley Street. He was not very
satisfied with his progress, turned to his doctor and
asked: "What do you want me to eat?" "Anything except roast crocodile." Dr. S. felt very proud
of the smartness of his reply, but the result was that
the patient sent for me and asked me to regulate his
diet and to treat him medicinally as well. Lord ——
bred racehorses. He realized the importance of diet
in health and disease.

Far more people sicken and die of over-nutrition
than of under-nutrition. From year to year our
nutrition has become more artificial and more unwholesome. Most of our diseases are either purely, or
principally, dietetic. We live on food which we would
not give to any animal.

A racehorse worth £10,000 and a cart-horse worth
£10 or less receive the identical food—oats, grass, hay,
bran and so forth and water. No man in his senses
would feed a horse on white bread and butter and other
refined foods, nor would he give it tea to drink. A
woman will say: "Of course I do not add condiments
to my cat's meat," but she will add any quantity to
her own. She will drink poisonously strong, boiling
hot tea with any quantity of sugar, but will say: "*I
am sure it would not be good for 'Fido.' I give him
very weak tea with plenty of milk and one piece of
sugar."

Our cooks endeavour to make our food attractive to our æsthetic sense and our palate. People will eat and drink anything that looks and tastes nice. Whether it is wholesome or not is not considered. A good cook is deeply depressed if most of the food goes' back to the kitchen uneaten and is delighted if she has caused her employers to eat three or four times as much as is good for them. When one glances through a cookery book one finds that most of the dishes recommended require an enormous quantity of butter, eggs, cream. Their existence is disguised in the finished article. A great cook once told me that she was able to make me eat at one meal six eggs and half a pound of butter with plenty of cream added to it, after learning that I never ate more than one egg at a meal and took butter sparingly.

All the dishes mentioned in the cook book are made with refined ingredients, which are deprived of their most valuable food elements, the vitamins and essential minerals. I told a lady who is an excellent cook that she should make all her cakes with wholemeal flour and add plenty of bran to the mixture. She was horrified at the suggestion, told me "that cannot be done," and fetched the cookery book in order to prove her point. "Very well, make me a cake with wholemeal flour and bran and if it is uneatable we will give it to the pigs." She made a cake according to my directions, found it delicious and is now using only wholemeal flour and bran for making cakes, pastries, etc. I then told her to make all her jams with Demerara sugar. Again she told me that it was impossible and quoted the authority of Mrs. Beeton. "Very well, make me a quantity of different jams with Demerara and if it is not to your liking we will give it away." It turned out better than the jam made with refined sugar.

Food manufacturers and cooks have caused us to live on artificialities and their attempts at ruining our health have been ably supported by the chemists and the experts on nutrition. Chemistry, as far as food is concerned, has been a disaster to mankind. It produces unwholesome substitutes for the wholesome natural article. It declared, as Liebig did, that the strength of the meat lies in its extractives. That information was based on abstract notions not on knowledge. Feeding experiments were made on dogs. Meat was cut small and boiled for a long time. The liquid extract was given to one set of dogs and the exhausted fibre to another. The dogs fed on meat extracts died after a few days, while those fed on the exhausted fibre flourished.

For decades chemists and food experts of the Liebig school taught that human beings needed so much protein, carbohydrates, fat. Protein was considered the most valuable element and millions were made chronic invalids and were sent to an untimely grave by endeavouring to get strong in accordance with the teachings of theorists. One fine day it occurred to Sir Gowland Hopkins that the chemical theory of nutrition ought to be put to the test. He discovered that the three food elements would not sustain life. He wrote in 1906:—

" No animal can live upon a mixture of pure protein, fat and carbohydrate, and, even when the necessary inorganic material is carefully supplied, the animal still cannot flourish. The animal body is adjusted to live either on plant tissues or on other animals, and these contain countless substances other than the proteins, carbohydrates and fats." ✓

Students of medicine were taught by professors of nutrition, some of whom suffer from chronic indigestion, that human beings require so many calories, so much protein, etc., to keep them in health. The protein minimum was calculated on the assumption that the average man needed so much meat, so much bread, etc. Elaborate food tables were issued and large laboratories were established in which the new science of nutrition was cultivated. Foods were burned and the residue was included in the scientific analysis under the heading " Ash." No one wants to live on ash.

Ash was considered waste matter. Some scientists analysed the ash and it was discovered that it contains the most valuable mineral elements, which are indispensable to the building up and the maintenance of the body.

When the analytical chemists discovered that their laboratory methods were useless, they re-established the science which had existed before the Early Stone Age. They started making nutritional experiments on animals, as the savages did in the distant past. They threw away their worthless chemical apparatus, and called themselves biological chemists. Biological chemists can produce all the diseases of civilization in laboratory animals by feeding them on those tasty, refined, well-boiled foods on which we live. Sir Robert McCarrison, Professor Plimmer and others produced gastritis, chronic constipation, gastric and duodenal ulcers, appendicitis, colitis, goitre, severe nerve diseases, eye diseases and paralysis by forcing animals to live on the food of the civilized. They produced dental decay and pyorrhœa in animals which, if naturally fed, have magnificent teeth. They produced sterility and insanity by dietetic means. None of the biological chemists thought it worth their while to make experiments on human beings, especially on themselves, except my friend, Dr. M. Hindhede, of Copenhagen, and a few others. It is much easier to torment animals and to draw deductions from their sufferings which may be inapplicable to humans.

The dog is a meat-eater. An English biological chemist fed dogs on oats. Their teeth deteriorated, whereupon she published papers in order to show that oatmeal is bad for the teeth. The Scotch had magnificent teeth as long as they were fed on coarse oatmeal. Their teeth were ruined when they replaced their aboriginal brose, oatmeal cooked only a minute or two, by white bread, deprived of its indispensable mineral elements and vitamins.

Experiments on human beings are far more valuable than experiments made in glass dishes by analytical chemists or on animals by biological chemists. I am a disciple of Dr. Hindhede, and I have learned that the science of nutrition, as generally taught, is worthless. Nutrition is not a science, but an art.

The Liebig school of scientists has probably killed more people than the Great War. Unfortunately, death by faulty nutrition is lingering and far more unpleasant than death on the battlefield. The Germans were high feeders. They had absorbed the Liebig teachings, which encouraged them to eat large quantities of meat, fat, butter, cheese, eggs. Their diabetes death-rate was high. The blockade produced scarcity and the diabetes death-rate was halved. The exact figures may be found in my volume *Good Health and Happiness* (John Murray).

Denmark was blockaded together with Germany. My friend, Hindhede, was made food dictator. The Danes, like the Germans, had lived on large quantities of meat, butter, fat, eggs and bread made from the finest flour, etc. They had imported large quantities of grain for their livestock which also was fed on the bran discarded during the production of white flour. Hindhede placed the nation on pig and cattle fodder. Bread was made from whole wheat to which all the available bran was added. The Danes complained that their bread was dark, required energetic chewing, and was filled with bran, but their health improved miraculously and the death-rate fell to the lowest point ever known. The figures relating to the great Hindhede experiment will also be found in my book *Good Health and Happiness*.

When I was 40 I was a chronic invalid. I suffered from terrible indigestion, accompanied by atrocious pain in the stomach. I looked deeply jaundiced. I had not the strength to walk a mile. It took me two or three weeks to write a little article which I can now dictate in half an hour. Occasionally I could not sign my name or understand the meaning of the simplest newspaper article. I was examined and advised by numerous doctors, went from health resort to health resort. I looked cancerous and felt in the mood which one finds among the cancerous. This was one of the reasons why I started studying cancer.

My doctors had given me medicines and injections and had told me to feed up. I fed up. I ate large quantities of meat, eggs and other concentrated foods, to "keep up my strength," took the strongest tea and coffee, wine, spirits, etc., but got weaker and weaker.

At last it occurred to me that, as the doctors had failed, I ought to try my own hand. I lived for a time on white bread and water in the hope that this was easily digestible. That diet nearly killed me. I then tried other diets and I thought that possibly the strengthening diet which I had tried so far was wrong. I simplified my diet, cut down the quantity of flesh, fish and fowl and at last discarded flesh, fish, fowl and was greatly benefited. I made countless experiments on myself, got well, became enthusiastic for a simple diet consisting, as far as possible, of natural foods in their natural condition, and I induced other people to adopt a similar diet and obtained the most remarkable results.

I am frequently asked "Which is the best diet?" No two people are alike as regards face and figure, and no two people are alike as regards their dietetic requirements. My friend, Dr. John Harvey Kellogg, of the Battle Creek Sanatorium, has made important nutritional experiments on human beings and animals. Pigs are usually given a liquid mixture. Scientifically kept pigs in large piggeries are given a "scientifically balanced diet," evolved by a college professor. Kellogg, instead of feeding pigs on a mixture recommended by a professional theorist, placed in a large piggery a number of troughs, each containing a single food. One trough was filled with potatoes, another with beans, another with grass and so forth. Then he allowed the baby pigs of a litter to make their own selection. It appeared that each piglet had its individual preferences and that the baby pigs knew best what they needed, for they became the finest pigs ever

seen. Describing this experiment, Dr. Kellogg wrote:
" An unlearned pig has a far better knowledge of the
science of nutrition than the most eminent college
professor."

We human beings eat what is put before us, what is
recommended by the nutritional experts, the writers
of cookery books, the food manufacturers and the
cooks. We start with a soup which, according to the
scientists, causes an increase of the secretion of the
gastric juice. Then we eat highly seasoned dishes, and
meat, which have a similar effect. Lastly, we take
food and drink, hot or boiling hot. Heat stimulates
the process of digestion not only by increasing the
supply of the gastric juice, but also by attracting to
the stomach the blood which helps in the process of
digestion. In other words, the dietary of civilization
whips the poor stomach up into an artificial over-
activity which in due course is bound to end in its
exhaustion. The boiling hot food and drink and the
irritating condiments injure the stomach walls and
glands and they injure the liver and kidneys as well.
Hence the ever-increasing number of deaths from
diseases of the stomach, liver and kidneys.

Nutrition must be individual, especially if diet is
used curatively. I have caused thousands of people
to become vegetarians and to live on wholemeal flour
and bran, and I have learned that bran is the finest
health food. Practically every one of my patients is
given bran. If it proves indigestible in the form of
bran porridge, bran puddings, bran cake, bran biscuits,
etc., bran extract is ordered. There are people who
cannot digest roughage, but their percentage is small.
However, I have no standard dietary which cures some
and kills others. Diet depends on individual needs.

Some years ago a retired Local Government official
came to me for advice. He suffered agonies through
indigestion, accompanied by thunderous belching,
which prevented him sleeping in the recumbent
position. He had been treated with medicines by
many doctors without avail, and he lived on a mixed

diet. I gave him a baby diet, and the indicated homœopathic medicines, but his condition did not improve. Then I gave him an exclusive meat diet. It cured his indigestion. The inflammatory condition disappeared and his stomach was gradually taught to digest ordinary foods.

Nature has placed all the food elements which we require into wheat, barley, oats, rice and other grains. Dr. Hindhede has shown by years of experimentation on himself and on a number of his followers that human beings can maintain perfect health and efficiency on a diet consisting almost exclusively of a single entire food, such as whole wheat, whole rye, potatoes, etc. Most people who are ill have been living on what biological chemists call a deficiency diet, on a diet which creates deficiency diseases and they suffer from deficiency diseases. The weakness of their teeth, of the arches of their feet, of the organs of digestion and excretion, etc., shouts out the words " deficiency disease." They have been living on white flour since they were weaned. Consequently it is high time that that age-long deficiency should be made good, and it is made good with bran when they come under my care.

In the parched territories of Africa and Australia, there is often a long-lasting drought. The land is a desert.   Suddenly a rain cloud empties itself and, almost over night, the land is covered with luxuriant vegetation. Sick people respond in the same way to that nutrition which they have lacked for decades. It will be noticed that in most of my cases an amazing improvement takes place within a week. This is largely due to the fact that I place every patient imme- diately on a diet which fulfils his fundamental physical needs.

A Sussex farmer had a very sick horse, a veritable skeleton. The veterinary surgeon had tried his medi- cines to no purpose. At last he had advised the man " Put the poor beast on the grass." I saw the horse in the meadow, hollow-eyed, spectral, haunting.

Three weeks after I passed the same meadow and saw a young horse prancing about in the highest spirits. It had a glossy coat. It was a beautiful animal. The farmer was leaning over the gate. I said to him: "What a lovely horse you have got. What has become of the old spectre horse?" He gave me a broad grin, slowly took his pipe out of his mouth and said: "This is the old spectre horse." One must put sick people on the grass.

Nutrition is not a science. The dietician, like the pig, must be guided by instinct, commonsense, and the effect of the diet chosen. Dieticians who give a standard diet either to all patients or who classify them under headings such as "Stout, thin, diabetic, tuberculous, neurasthenic," etc., giving each class a standard diet, do not know their business.

Emaciated people are usually put to bed and are fed on an intensive milk diet. I have found the tedious rest cure unnecessary. It is best to build slowly but solidly. Many examples of such building up will be found in the pages of this book.

In selecting a diet, one must not be guided by abstract ideas. Hippocrates wrote 2,300 years ago: "An inferior diet liked by the patient is preferable to a superior diet which he dislikes."

Nature curers prescribe diets which do not seem very natural. Patients are given six oranges or 12 glasses of milk a day, or they are fed on salads, raw fruit and nuts. A caterpillar diet is good for caterpillars but not for human beings, and a nut diet suiting maggots may harm humans. Most of the fruit one gets in England is gathered unripe and is deficient in its natural components, in metabolized sunshine, or it is grown under glass, which filters out the most precious rays of the sun. Further, we are given stale nuts which no monkey cares to touch.

The finest food I know is clean, ordinary bran. It should be combined either with coarse oatmeal, which is too heating for some, or with whole wheat. Bran and oatmeal porridge had best be prepared from equal weights of these ingredients and be boiled only a minute or two. Wheat requires about four hours of slow cooking, which will cause the berries to burst. Then bran is added in the proportion most suitable to the individual, and another minute's cooking will make the dish ready for the table. It should be eaten seasoned with milk and black treacle, which is laxative and rich in iron, or with Demerara sugar, honey, stewed fresh fruit, boiled unbleached sultanas, etc. Bran puddings are made like ordinary milk puddings of about equal weights of some cereal, and bran. I prefer semolina because semolina contains the germ of the wheat berry which the millers sift out from our flour. The life essence of the wheat berry is situated in the germ which feeds on the starchy flour, exactly as the budding chicken feeds on the contents of the egg.

White sugar is as objectionable as is white flour. The negroes who chew sugar cane and eat pap made from whole grain have magnificent teeth. White flour and white sugar may be chemically pure, but we were not meant to live on pure chemicals. Our salt is also a pure chemical. The most wholesome salt is pure sea salt, which contains the iodine and other elements which we need in infinitely small quantities. The salt-refiners give us salt lacking iodine which creates various diseases, among them probably goitre. Then they offer us at a high price iodized salt which contains inorganic iodine, the consumption of which is apt to create exophthalmic goitre, the worst form of goitre.

In my directions, I do not consider the question of calories, proteins, vitamins, etc. Theory leaves me cold. The only thing important is success. I endeavour to eliminate the obvious dietetic faults of patients and to supply their dietetic needs. My diet is a curative diet, and if people do not flourish it is changed. Moreover, patients are encouraged to be guided by the spirit of my directions not by their wording.

Nature curers are great advocates of fasting. I occasionally fast myself for one, two or three days if my instinct bids me to, but so far I have never found it necessary to give fasts to patients. Those who habitually order fasts succeed with the plethoric and fail with the emaciated.

A curative diet must be arranged tentatively. One must manipulate dietetic prescriptions like medicine, changing if necessary.

It is a misfortune that most doctors know nothing about diet. A distinguished West End consultant told Lady —— that her anæmic and emaciated daughter was to have a diet which included three-quarters of a lb. of butter. Lady —— placed next morning three-quarters of a lb. of butter on the breakfast table in front of her daughter and told her that she would have to eat it in the course of the day. The girl was just in the middle of her breakfast. She was horrified, vomited and almost had a fit. My diet sheets always contain the sentence: " Increase intake gradually and cautiously towards the ideal." If I wished a delicate and nervous girl to take plenty of butter I should never mention a definite quantity. Besides, I prefer giving butter in the shape of milk which contains butter in the most digestible form, in infinitely small globules, which gives to milk its white colour. In the shape of milk, people can easily take three-quarters of a lb. of butter per day, and more, but it is risky to give milk neat, because it is apt to clot.

I was looking after a very wealthy Society woman who needed feeding up. She was to take 2 to 3 pints of milk a day in every form except neat. She had to rush to a party, gulped down a big tumblerful and got into her car. Presently she suffered the most violent pain because the milk had formed a clot, which refused to enter the bowel. There were violent spasms and cramps. She was in agony and terrified. In the middle of the night she telephoned to a doctor nearby who relieved her sufferings by the injection of Morphia. Milk cannot clot if mixed with plenty of tea, water, etc., or given in the form of bread and milk, milk puddings, custard, junket, and so forth. To digest neat milk, it should be thoroughly insalivated and be taken slowly with a small teaspoon. There are people who find milk indigestible. Toleration can be established either by starting with small doses and increasing gradually, or by giving the patient a few pilules of potentized milk, Calcarea, Sulphur, Aethusa, China.

Intolerance of eggs usually proclaims anæmia. Those who cannot take an egg neat can take two or three embodied in puddings, etc. A few doses of potentized iron will enable people to take eggs who never before had been able to take them.

Every practitioner should carefully observe the instinctive food desires of sick people. Children who wish to eat chalk, coal, lead pencils, need Calcarea; those who crave for meat need Magnesia carbonica, etc. The civilized have lost the instincts possessed by primitive peoples and animals. Curiously enough, the primeval food instincts reassert themselves at times of danger, especially when people are dying. The food desires of child-bearing women and of patients in a critical condition should never be taken lightly.

Twenty years ago a wealthy man in Worthing was dying. His best friend and several doctors and specialists were standing around his bed. The dying man beckoned to his best friend and whispered something into his ear. " What did he say?" asked the doctor. " I—would—like—some—tripe—and—onions." The doctors smiled at one another. One of them said: " The poor fellow is wandering. That happens frequently at the last moment." " If you don't mind, I will get him some tripe and onions," said the friend. " Do, by all means," said the doctor. " He has only about two hours to live. Of course, it may shorten his life." The friend rushed out, looking for a cook shop, and came back with a big dish. Very, very slowly his friend ate the lot, and then whispered: " I

—would—like—a bottle—of—Guinness." He got his
bottle of Guinness—and he lives to this day. I know
another case when a dying man asked for a cold pork
pie and a bottle of ginger beer, a truly horrible combination. However, it saved his life. It is my rule
to allow anything the gravely sick and dying desire
to eat and drink. One can do miracles by diet alone.
Unfortunately that wonderful knowledge cannot be
acquired by scientific tuition, but only by intuition.

CHAPTER XVII

Paralysis and Disseminated Sclerosis

IN the olden days, doctors called the bursting of a blood vessel within the brain "a stroke," and they treated the patients with some success by bleeding them, a reasonable proceeding. The blood of the apoplectic is frequently thick. By withdrawing a considerable amount, the body is compelled to replace it by water from the tissues. The blood is thinned promptly, and it runs more easily through arteries and veins. The patient is relieved. Unfortunately medicine is ruled not by sense but by fashion. Formerly every patient was bled. Now none are bled. On the other hand, every patient is treated subcutaneously until that method of treatment will fall deservedly into the same disrepute into which bleeding fell some decades ago.

Modern medicine claims to be scientific. It is so scientific that the old plain names of diseases which people understand have been abolished. The word paralysis has gone the same way as the word stroke. There has been great scientific progress as regards paralysis from the medico-philological point of view. Learned medical men have divided and sub-divided paralysis into a large number of different diseases which bear most impressive scientific names, to the bewilderment of the public—and of doctors themselves. Among the forms of paralysis to be found in the text-books are Amyotrophic spinal paralysis, Asthenic bulbar paralysis, Atrophic bulbar paralysis, Atrophic muscular paralysis, Amyotrophic lateral sclerosis,

Brachiofacial paralysis, Glossolabiolaryngeal paralysis, Ischemic paralysis, Musculospiral paralysis, Pseudo-hypertrophic muscular paralysis, and scores of others.

Paralysis is supposed to be due to the hardening or degeneration of the spinal cord, brain, etc. According to its presumed causation, it is called Disseminated sclerosis, Diffused sclerosis, Insular sclerosis, Multiple cerebrospinal sclerosis, and there are scores of other names. I do not believe that any specialist could enumerate and describe the bewildering number of forms into which the old-fashioned paralysis has been divided.

While the textbooks have been swelled beyond belief by the description of the numerous forms of paralysis, its treatment is as unsatisfactory as ever. In the standard work, *The Principles and Practice of Medicine,* by Osler and McCrae, there are, under the heading " Sclerosis of the Brain," details regarding Miliary sclerosis, Diffused sclerosis, Tuberous sclerosis, Multiple sclerosis, etc., and after lengthy descriptions of the " morbid anatomy," the appearance of the brain after death, etc., there comes at last a beggarly little paragraph of three and a half lines on treatment: " No known treatment has any influence on the progress of sclerosis of the brain. Neither the Iodides nor Mercury have the slightest effect, but a prolonged course of Nitrate of Silver or Arsenic may be tried."

The advice that some medicines are useless while very poisonous Nitrate of silver and Arsenic " may be tried " is not very encouraging, especially as it follows the sentence: " No known treatment has any influence on the progress of sclerosis of the brain."

Scientific medicine stands under the influence of the pathologist who forgets that disease may be due to faulty living. He searches for the cause of the disease in the bodies of the dead—which show nothing. There have been pathologists who have tried to discover the genius of great men by dissecting their brain. Lenin's brain was cut, according to Hollander, into 30,000 slices which were solemnly examined under the microscope for traces of his genius.

The pathologist looks at the blood clot which follows the stroke, which presses on the brain and causes paralysis, and he may suggest opening the skull and taking out the clot, or he will look at the hardened spinal cord and he will come to the conclusion that nothing can be done. The body is treated by pathologists and surgeons not as a living self-repairing organism, but as a piece of machinery, and if surgery and serums are unavailing, we are told that the disease is incurable and that such-and-such remedies " may be tried."

Practitioners and specialists either frankly tell those who consult them that there is no known cure for paralysis or they prescribe perfunctorily the treatments which, according to the textbooks, " may be tried," and the result is nil. A considerable number of people affected with paralysis in some form or other have come to me. These cases are difficult to handle. I frankly admit that I have never had any full success with paralysis agitans, of which I have had relatively few cases, but I have had gratifying successes with ordinary paralysis. They had been scientifically diagnosed, classified, docketed and labelled when they came to me with the prognosis " incurable." Somehow a number of them got vastly better, or well, but then I disregard the orthodox textbooks in my library because I know their worthlessness.

A Mr. N. L. of Blackpool wrote to me on the 13th September, 1927 : —

" I was a working man, my occupation was model making. I am 58, and suffer from a weakness in the legs which prevents me walking in the street without guidance. I am all right at home where objects are more familiar. I am also restricted in speech, though I can utter a few words in a jerky manner. I call my ailment neurasthenia but that may be wrong. I have a very small belief in doctor's medicine. My ailment dates from 1918."

The poor fellow had been more or less crippled for nine years. He could not travel to London nor could I visit him in Blackpool. I asked him a number of questions regarding his way of living, etc. Mr. N. L. told me that he was normal as regards digestion, excretion, etc. He took daily exercise, massaging himself, did neither smoke nor drink. There were no symptoms to guide me.

His case was a mystery. I gave him a diet rich in vitamins and mineral essentials with an abundance of bran, milk, eggs, fruit, vegetables, told him to take paraffin if necessary to activate his bowel, gave him plenty of water to drink between meals and told him to massage his body vigorously with unrefined cod-liver oil. The patient was surprised at this recommendation. Among his friends were some prominent footballers and they and the chemists had recommended to him a large number of applications for massage. He tried all, but nothing had helped. No one had ever thought of cod-liver oil. I myself had never heard of cod-liver oil for outward application. I said to myself: " As cod-liver oil is full of mysterious power if taken by the mouth, it may be equally valuable if taken by the skin." In puzzling cases I look up all the best books in my library and if I do not find any useful advice in them, I try something of my own invention.

To my great surprise and to that of my patient, my recommendation proved very helpful. After a week, Mr. N. L. wrote: " Being early days, perhaps it is best not to expect much, but so far so good. The muscles of the legs, particularly the calves and guiders behind the knees and at the back of the thighs, are much firmer. These are particularly well massaged and plenty of oil is used." His next letter told me: " Muscles of legs much firmer."

On the 28th September he wrote: " Your diet is entirely satisfactory. I never felt better in my life. I daresay this is to be attributed to the diet. I previously tried massage with olive oil, sweet oil, Elliman's

Embrocation, and with a special liniment used in football training, etc., but none of them gave a quarter of the results of cod-liver oil in the crude state as given to cattle, advised by you." His next report stated: " This massaging, in conjunction with the diet, is effecting wonders. Leg muscles much firmer. As regards speech, I can speak for longer periods." On the 9th October he wrote: " Leg muscles much firmer, speech progressing satisfactorily. I am practising recitations as you advised."

On the 5th September he told me: " I feel that both diet and massage are doing me much good. I have not had the slightest ailment since I started your diet. I had always had the belief that, given the right treatment, which I am sure I now have, I could get well." On the 6th October he wrote: " I thought I would join a family party and see the illuminations by char-à-banc. We had to stand and wait for nearly an hour. I had to walk half a mile to the char-à-banc and back and had to wait for an hour for the vehicle. I had not entered a char-à-banc for over nine years since my weakness began." On the 11th October he wrote: " What gives me every confidence in myself is *your* confidence in me. Your letters are to me like beacons of hope. To-day this is the first time for nine years that I have walked in the street by myself, and I have your treatment to thank for it. My general health was never better."

On the 14th October, after a single month's treatment, he wrote: " Before I came under your treatment I was as careful as you recommend me to be, but with all the care in the world, my exercising, etc., came to nothing, and I made *no progress* until the Ellis Barker treatment was adopted. I shall always regard September 13th as the luckiest day of my life, and I am not regarded as superstitious in the least." (On the 13th September he wrote to me his first letter.) On the 20th October he told me: " I was nine years without hope. At the only time that I was taken before a doctor, he gravely shook his head and assured me that the partial loss of my limbs and of my speech would be *permanent,* and feared it would get *worse.* Under your wise direction it looks as if I should be fully cured."

On the 1st November he wrote: " I am steadily regaining strength as regards walking and speech." In his letter of the 6th November he told me, comparing his then condition with the condition when I took him in hand: " When I wrote to you, I was in very good bodily health, but through neurasthenia or a nervous breakdown I had a peculiar weakness in my legs which prevented me from even walking one yard by myself, even in the quietest streets. At present my general health is even better, and I find no difficulty in walking with my companion. I am practising walking by myself, but the footpath has to be very clear of pedestrians. I am like a child commencing to walk." His next letter told me that he had succeeded in walking 300 yards by himself. On the 13th November, exactly two months after his first letter, my patient wrote: " I feel much better, more sure of myself and can walk by myself for nearly half a mile, and have improved much in my speech also, and am confident that before long I shall be *fully cured.*"

From week to week I guided him along, improving his dietary, devising physical and speech exercises, urging him to walk every day by himself a certain number of additional yards and he pluckily went on. When the cod-liver oil massage seemed to lose its power for good, I made him add Cayenne pepper to the oil. On the 10th January, 1928, he wrote: " I tried and successfully accomplished the measured mile last evening. It was rather stormy and at the commencement it looked rather against its being done. But it *was done* and without the slightest help and I ended up stronger than at the commencement." I was jubilant at the news.

Later on I discovered that before he lost his powers a strong electric current had touched him. I tried to antidote electricity with Phosphorus and gave him in the course of my long treatment whichever homœopathic medicine seemed called for. From week to week and from month to month he improved and at last he wrote to me with joy that he felt a totally different man, could walk miles in the open, etc.

As in so many cases which come to me with the diagnosis "absolutely incurable" or "can only get worse," I felt very sceptical. However, I have learned that there are no hopeless and incurable cases, and I think it the utmost cruelty if a doctor depresses the mind of his patient by an unfavourable forecast which may be wrong. Miracles happen every day. One must have faith in Providence and in the unlimited power of repair of the body if one wishes to cure, and practitioners should remember that hope and faith can remove mountains and can remove many disease conditions which will become truly incurable if the patient is told that nothing can be done.

Disseminated sclerosis is the latest fancy name for creeping paralysis. Doctors become more and more scientific as regards the names of diseases, inventing new ones every day to impress their patients. Bed-wetting is called Enuresis nocturna, rheumatism has been re-christened Fibrositis, and Creeping paralysis has been re-named Disseminated sclerosis. On the 9th March, 1928, Mr. C. de M. wrote to me from near Stockport, Lancashire, that his wife was suffering from Disseminated Sclerosis, for which she had been given Arsenic in large quantities, and exercises, and he enclosed a history of her case and a long opinion of a well-known specialist, dated 3rd February, 1928. The specialist wrote to Mrs. de M.'s doctor.:—

" I think there can be no doubt that the condition is one of disseminated sclerosis. Mrs. C. de M. appears to have varied considerably since I saw her in October, 1925. At that time there were no motor disturbances at all, except that the knee jerk was absent on the left side, and the ankle jerks were absent on both sides. At that time all the trouble appeared to be that of sensation, with special reference to the right hand, and the stereognostic sense was grossly impaired over the right hand . . . When I saw her first I was a little doubtful as to this being disseminated sclerosis, owing to the fact that I had no information as regards the Wassermann determination. As regards treatment, this should consist of intermittent courses of Arsenic with massage, exercise of education, and, in view of the fact that her bladder is occasionally disturbed, I would suggest you letting her have courses of Hexamine from time to time."

Attached to this report there were lengthy notes of findings relating to the central nervous system, motor nerves, sensory, speech, mental state, cranial nerves, teeth, pulse, blood-pressure, heart, lungs, abdomen, urine, etc. Mrs. de M. had consulted a large number of doctors and specialists with the result that she was poorer in pocket and in health. In writing to me and sending me this report, her husband told me: "Her state of chronic constipation was ignored by the specialist, although his attention was drawn to this vital matter. We have read your book on constipation and therefore realize that her illness may be due to constipation."

I studied the bulky enclosures and came to the conclusion that the various nerve specialists had taken no notice whatever of the fact that the patient had been living all her life on a demineralized and devitaminized diet, and had been poisoned by bowel toxins. Specialists who use a bewildering array of scientific instruments frequently overlook the most elementary facts, which would strike an illiterate agricultural labourer. Without having seen her, I sent her on the 20th March provisional directions in which I gave her liquid paraffin three times a day before meals, told her to go to stool three times a day after meals, and gave her a lacto-vegetarian diet, Pig bile tabloids to activate her liver and bowel, and potato water to alkalinize her blood and help her rheumatism. She was to be massaged all over with crude cod-liver oil. She was to stop the use of Arsenic, which had proved absolutely worthless and therefore was probably harmful. I forbade injections which she had received with the usual recklessness and in a great variety. After a short time there was slight improvement. On the 11th April her husband wrote:—

" She continues to improve generally and to have three or four motions a day without any difficulty. Before she commenced your treatment she never felt a motion pass, nor had she control of the bowel, whereas now she has full control. Her bowels functioning in this manner is a constant source of amazement to her. Walking shows continued signs of improvement. She can now walk about 300 yards with the aid of her stick. Her sense of balance has improved, but not as markedly as her walking. Legs feel not nearly so heavy or tight. Our doctor, who does not know she is having your treatment, remarked on her general improvement last week and made special mention of her colour. She has always been pale up to now. He is unable to account for this. On Monday night she perspired profusely generally. This had not happened for months."

She had had no medicine and thought she needed some. So I sent her some unmedicated sugar pills. On the 20th April I received a letter written by Mrs. de M. herself:—

" I find it very difficult to express to you how grateful I am for your treatment. If only I had known of you years ago, the constipation could have been cured and I would not have got this trouble. However, we must go on persevering, and I shall soon be quite normal again, D.V. I have the will to conquer it with the help of your advice. My husband's last report cheered you, but you do not know how your letter cheered me. I want to read it every day.

" You are quite right, my progress is absolutely marvellous. The constipation, I feel sure, is absolutely cured. I am certain I shall never have to take any more medicine, which is a great blessing. I only wish you could have seen me before I started your treatment. I am quite a different creature now, no longer pale and heavy-eyed, and everyone who knows me says I look wonderfully better, and I certainly feel it. My feet are nearly always warm now. Before, they used to be icy cold. I also don't get the burning feeling in them as severely as I used to. My legs still keep cold, and so do my hands, but I am very hopeful for them because of the change in my feet. My hair has now a tendency to be a little greasy. I have never known it to be so before. My hands are not as rough as they used to be. It is all so wonderful to me because the specialist told me I would have to take great care as progress would be very slow, a matter of years. By the way I am progressing it will only be months. I have more control over the bladder."

Three days later Mrs. de M. wrote:—

" My progress is wonderful. I can hardly believe it to be me. It is almost like a dream, only I don't wake up to find everything a myth, but a reality. Walking fairly good and very much easier. I don't walk stiff-legged as I used to before your treatment. I also do not drag my right foot now. I seem to be able to lift both feet clear of the ground. The legs are no longer heavy. My husband remarked this morning how well I walk when I get out of bed."

The lady and her husband visited me on the 3rd May. I examined her carefully without instruments, and summarized my impressions as follows:—

" The extraordinary development of fat on buttocks and upper legs, the fat bags on the insides of the thighs and at the knees, the curious differences between the upper and the lower parts of the body as regards fat, and of the upper and lower arms must be of great significance, and they seem to point either to some glandular anomaly or to the effect of poisoning. The fact that for about 10 years you rubbed in large quantities of Zinc ointment and of precipitate ointment reveals a source of poisoning, which I had suspected. In addition there has been chronic auto-intoxication from the bowel and there is the curious fact that you were given tablets likely to deaden the nerves just before your legs gave way. As you seem a thoroughly sound and exceptionally strong woman, I am full of hope that I shall succeed with you.

" Most important was the discovery that you did not suffer from a vague weakness of the back due to anæmia, but that your spine was seriously affected through a fall."

I gave the lady special spinal massage and asked her to find out what had been injected into her body. I discovered that she had been given Manganese injections. Reference to the textbooks showed that Zinc ointment is a cumulative poison, Zinc attacking particularly the spine and the great nerves springing from it and stopping perspiration, to the great injury of the body, and that Magnanese causes anæmia with destruction of red blood corpuscles, fatty degeneration of the liver, abnormalities of gait, etc. It seemed to me that Mrs. de M. suffered chiefly from medicinal poisoning. Naturally the large doses of Arsenic which the poor woman had lately received were likely to complete the injury. Enquiry from her doctor revealed the fact that she had been given four drops of Fowler's Solution of Arsenic three times a day. She also had been given Heroin and other dangerous drugs. I felt confident that it ought to be possible to recreate the lady's health by antidoting the various poisons, by the old-fashioned but very efficient method of producing profuse sweating, by an eliminating diet, bowel regulations, etc., and I raised her hopes to the utmost. In reply she wrote on the 12th May: —

" You cannot imagine how delighted we are to hear that you have discovered the poison which has been and is responsible for all this trouble, but as you have worked such wonders with me so far, I shall be coming to you with my skipping rope. I am very patiently waiting for your further instructions so that we can work together in a mighty effort to get rid of the fiendish poison which was so wickedly prescribed for me by Dr. C., and by Dr. R., a Manchester skin specialist. If I had not made my doctor show me the specialist's report, I should still be blindly taking Arsenic. What an existence would have been in store for me! "

On the 16th Mrs. de M. wrote, with understandable indignation: —

" I feel furious every time I think of these men we put such faith and trust in. They are not fit to look after animals, and certainly not fit to look after and touch human beings. You could understand these men prescribing these dangerous drugs if they were ignorant of the harm they can do. They take their fees and you are lucky if you survive their treatment. To think that I have more or less been disabled for nearly three years because of these poisonous injections, etc."

Mrs. de M., her husband and myself entertained the highest hopes, but suddenly they were shattered. On the 21st May Mr. de M. wrote to me that his wife had suffered a severe set-back, through influenza.

Practically all the wonderful improvement had disappeared at one blow. Once more Mrs. de M. was unable to use her limbs and crawled about on the floor with the help of her arms. As she had reacted so wonderfully to my previous treatment, I continued treating her on the old lines, but the results were indifferent. I tried one homœopathic medicine after the other and tried to eliminate every new symptom by the indicated remedies, but she always produced new symptoms and on balance there was only little improvement. She and I became disheartened, but I refused to give up. One must never give up a case because occasionally one stumbles on some unsuspected fact or symptom which enables one to effect a cure.

The case was dragging on. In October I was to deliver a lecture at Manchester, and I had arranged that Mr. de M. should bring his wife to my hotel. We met in a drawing-room and I noticed that the poor woman was in a worse state than I had imagined from her cheery letters. In the middle of our conversation, she burst into tears. While talking with me, bladder control had given away. Her husband was not unprepared. She complained about various new symptoms, and told me: " There is a triviality about which I have not written, but which is rather annoying. I have a fearful itching on the lower abdomen." I exclaimed: " The abdomen is red and looks as if you had been badly stung by insects." Mrs. de M. exclaimed: " Oh, this reminds me of something which I have never told you. In July, 1925, before my long illness began, my husband and I were staying at the seaside at a low marshy place, and I got a large number of insect bites. Previously, when bitten by insects, the places showed only small red spots, but at that time every bite raised a huge and very painful lump. Soon after stiffness and loss of control of the limbs began. I thought that these terrible bites were responsible for my condition and I told all my doctors and specialists, but they merely laughed at me. So I never told you about it."

The red patches on the abdomen looked exactly like bee stings. There were numerous lumps and wheals. The pain produced was that of bee stings. There was only a moderate amount of inflammation, and the itching was relieved by the application of cold water. These symptoms pointed to Apis, to bee poison, a frequently used homœopathic remedy. Apis was particularly indicated because it cures burning when urinating, especially at the end of urination, and it produces and cures loss of bladder control. I immediately sent her Apis 3X and very promptly I heard that there was great improvement.

On the 6th January, 1929, Mrs. de M. wrote:—

" I have continued the Apis pilules, three pilules three times a day, and have not taken any other medicine as they were so beneficial. I have gone on improving ever since. I am walking straighter and by myself in the house, but still use two sticks or the pram when I go out. Mr. de M. says I must tell you that this improvement is constant from day to day. I can manage with the help of the sticks or pram for a quarter of a mile without fatigue. I know you will be delighted.

" I feel with you that you have got me to the stage where nature is going all out to effect a cure. Everyone remarks how well I look. I think health and I feel healthy. The urine still continues to be highly coloured and very cloudy, but it causes me no inconvenience and I feel that the organs are throwing off the poisons which are the cause of the disease. I very rarely have backache and my eyes are almost clear of the haziness. I have every confidence and belief that this year will see me a perfectly healthy creature."

On the 21st January her husband wrote to me:—

" My wife has been progressing so wonderfully of late that she says she has no wish to write or think about health. Bowels and bladder are acting normally. Walking has improved to such an extent, that with the aid of two sticks she can walk 500 yards without resting, and yesterday she walked with the pram for a good half-mile. She has not taken any pills or liquid paraffin for more than three weeks, and she gets better so that the neighbours have been remarking on the rapid improvement in her. I am confident that my wife will soon be normal again."

On the 5th March, 1929, a year after the beginning of the treatment, Mr. de M. wrote:—

" My wife can now walk a mile with the aid of two sticks. She can walk without sticks over short distances. She helps in the house, and is hoping to be able to manage without a maid. I do not wish to give you the impression that she is normal in her gait. She is still somewhat wooden in action. Bowels and bladder control are normal. She now goes out for two or three hours at a spell. You remember that she could not hold her water but a few months ago.

" What did her most good? Undoubtedly your spirit of optimism, your disbelief in the term ' incurable.' What pluck you must have to tell a patient that all the specialists are wrong, that there is no such thing as ' incurable.' When my wife used to come from a specialist, although he was most kind to her, when she arrived at my office, she used to weep on account of the feeling of hopelessness that she was given. With you it was quite the reverse. You and your letters inspire confidence.

" If any medicine did her good I think the Apis pilules were the most effective. You see, once the urine became whiteish her walking and everything else improved as if a deposit which prevented nerve action was being removed.

" The correcting of the bowel action in the beginning of your treatment was also highly beneficial to her.

" The fact that you told her some months ago that she could cure herself and that you would help her do so has made her look upon her own powers in a higher way. We avoid all mention of illness in our house, and we do not

encourage anybody to talk ill health; this is the reason I
am writing this letter.

"My wife joins me in thanking you most cordially for
your kindness to us both and for the benefit your treatment
has conferred."

On the 14th February a lady, who acted as almoner
at one of the Liverpool hospitals, wrote: —

"I have been advised to consult you about my mother.
She is 55 years old, and enjoyed good health till four years
ago. About 1926 she became irritable and unreasonable.
We thought this due to the change of life and the doctor
treated her for inflammation of the stomach.

"In January, 1930, she had a very violent fit of coughing,
followed by severe headache and vomiting and temporary
loss of speech. She had similar attacks in July and September. She was then seen by one of our honorary physicians
who told me she had cerebral thrombosis and that nothing
could be done for her. When her speech first became affected
in January of last year, the doctor explained to me that the
coughing had caused the rupture of a blood vessel in the
brain.

"The specialist told me in September that the leakage had
caused cerebral degeneration to commence and that it could
not be improved. She has always eaten heavily and of rich
foods."

From the daughter's account it was quite clear to
me that the lady had had a number of apoplectic
strokes, and as an eminent specialist had explained to
the daughter that the condition could only become
worse, I did not feel very hopeful. Still, I did not
refuse to see the lady because experience has taught
me that those who are officially incurable may be
relieved and may get well.

On the 19th February Mrs. C. E. B. called at my
house. She was deeply depressed, complained of weakness of memory, severe pain in left arm and left leg,
and the left foot dragged distinctly. She was short,
but very stout, weighing about 10 stone, very pale,
extremely flabby, had always been constipated, had a
wet-stocking sensation on feet and lower legs, felt

always chilly, had terrific vaccination marks, felt worse at 11 in the morning, her moods changed easily, she loved eggs, eyes ran with water, she took large quantities of salt, took per day eight cups of tea with sixteen lumps of sugar. I stated in my directions that she suffered largely from over-nutrition.

I gave her a restricted diet with an abundance of bran, to activate her bowels and to supply her with the vitamins and mineral elements which she needed, not only for her general health but also for repairing the weakened walls of veins and arteries. I told her that she was to lose 2 lbs. a week, and gave her Arnica 3X to absorb the clot of blood and to energize her. Further she received Natrum muriaticum 3 for her chilliness, and as an antidote to the masses of salt which she had eaten. She also was given Pulsatilla, because she was affectionate, weepy and chilly, and Hydrastis 1X because she had an enlarged liver and looked jaundiced. She was to take Natrum muriaticum night and morning, Arnica three times a day between meals, but if she felt very weepy she was to take a dose or two of Pulsatilla, and if she felt very liverish she had to take Hydrastis instead of the other medicines. She felt hopeless as doctors and specialists had not given her any hope.

On the 22nd February, three days after our interview, her daughter wrote: " She seems already to be in much better spirits." Six days later, on the 28th February, her daughter wrote: " Her eyes have lost their dullness and her speech has improved. She is losing weight and is certainly more cheerful." On the 5th March, Mrs. C. E. B. herself wrote: " I weigh 9 stone 9½." She had lost 4½ lbs. in the first fortnight. Her letter of the 11th November said: " I weigh now 9 stone 8, and I feel better." On the 19th March she told me: " I weigh 9 stone 7." Her letter of the 25th March said: " I weigh 9 stone 5 lbs. 10 ozs. and I feel fine."

The good lady felt always hungry and wished for

the rich food which she had enjoyed in the past. On the 13th April her daughter wrote:—

"She is now very rarely depressed and to our knowledge has had no weeping fits since her return from London. Her speech is good and her walking is improved, although she still drags the left leg occasionally. She is taking an intelligent interest in most things. My brothers and I are most grateful to you for the remarkable progress she has made. She has been to church regularly since her return, and the improvement in her condition is so obvious that it has given rise to considerable comment among her fellow members."

With pleasant uniformity the lady's weight went down and her spirits went up. On the 13th May she wrote: "My left leg and arm are now well." On the 20th May she told me, "I am 8 stone 11 lbs. 8 ozs." On the 10th June she was 8 stone 8 lbs. 8 ozs. She had now lost 20 lb. of useless fat which of course had terribly hampered her.

On the 29th July, after five months' treatment, she visited me again. She was transformed, and I wrote to her: "You look wonderfully well, years younger, have lost 2 stone, look healthy and happy, have sparkling eyes, a rosy complexion, red lips, action of legs has vastly improved, you are mentally far brighter, are a different woman." As she had terrific vaccination marks I gave her Thuja 30 as a vaccination antidote, twice a week, Calcarea carbonica 3X night and morning because she felt always chilly and had the typical damp-cold feet which point to that remedy, and Veratrum viride 3X for her pain at the back of the head. For emergencies I handed her daughter Aconite 3X and Belladonna 3X to be given if she had throbbing arteries and a red face, indicating the danger of another stroke. On the 6th August her daughter wrote: "Physically my mother is better than I can ever remember her being, but she seems full of self-pity." I then gave her Baryta carbonica in various potencies for her depression.

Her people considered her cured. I received a few satisfactory letters at long intervals. The last letter, written by Mrs. C. E. B. on the 6th May, 1932, told me: " I am pretty well and everybody is saying how well I look." Doctors and specialists had considered the case hopeless and had told the relatives that she " could not be improved, that nothing could be done." She improved marvellously during the fifteen months while she was under my observation and became physically and mentally transformed to her joy and the joy of her family.

The most extraordinary treatments are given for paralysis. Some years ago I saw a charming young woman, a manufacturer's wife from the Midlands, at a West End hotel with her husband. After an injury in childbirth her leg started dragging. She was treated for disseminated sclerosis, and as the local doctors had no success, she was taken to a distinguished nerve specialist in the Harley Street quarter of London and, according to her account, had been injected with 606, had had Mercury ointment rubbed into her body during a month and had been charged a hundred guineas.

I listened to her story with amazement: " Do you know that you have been treated for syphilis? " " Yes, I do." " Was there any reason for treating you for syphilis? Have you had the disease yourself? " " No." " Has your husband had it? " " No." " Has your father or mother had it? " " No. There is not the slightest trace of syphilis either in my family or in my husband's family."

The wretched woman had been poisoned for life with Mercury and Arsenic given subcutaneously. Apparently the distinguished nerve specialist had said to himself: " Syphilis is occasionally followed by paralysis. Consequently one can treat an obscure paralysis exactly in the same way as it was due to syphilis." As a number of paralysis cases, treated in the identical way by that particular specialist, have applied to me for help, I suspect that the man in question uses anti-syphilitic treatment as a routine measure on the paralysed, to their injury, or to their ruin.

CHAPTER XVIII

Enlarged Prostates

THE male bladder contains a small muscular gland, which is about the size and shape of a chestnut, and which is situated about the outlet of the bladder. It corresponds to the womb. After the change of life, the female womb is apt to degenerate and similar degeneration often takes place in the prostate of the elderly male, which may swell to the size of a fist or larger. There are three lobes to this body. The central lobe is near the tube and, if it swells considerably, it interferes with the stream of urine.

Many middle-aged and old men have an enlarged prostate. The holding capacity is much diminished, the urine is dammed back, becomes strong, thick and eventually putrid, causing great irritation and inflammation, which is apt to spread up the ureters to the kidneys producing degeneration in these organs as well. The sufferer from prostatic enlargement can hold his urine only a short time, he must frequently get up during the night, the stream is weak, and often there is great difficulty in starting, anxiety, pain, etc.

Orthodox medicine has practically no treatment for this very frequent condition. Patients are recommended to see a surgeon, and frequently the bladder is opened and the enlarged prostate taken out. This is a grave operation, which gives a great shock to the system. It is a very speculative undertaking. I have known healthy, strong men of fifty or sixty die under the operation. On the other hand, I know men who were operated upon when about eighty with good results. Every avoidable operation should be avoided. It speaks volumes for the low state of modern medicine that the orthodox doctor, but not the homœopath, sends his patients at the first opportunity to the surgeon.

One of my friends, a very eminent surgeon, specializes in prostate operations. He has excised thousands. When I told him that this condition could easily be cured by homœopathy and that I considered it his duty to send to homœopathic doctors, or laymen, all cases in which operation was inadvisable, or was refused, he looked at me with incredulity and said: "There is no treatment for enlarged prostate except operation." He had not the slightest desire to make enquiries. He is a skilled surgical automaton with a tightly closed mind.

In 1932 I was staying at a village in Sussex. There was a smith, a Mr. T., whom I knew slightly, and I was struck by his looking very ill, deeply jaundiced and anxious. I asked: "What is the matter with you?" "I have a terrible difficulty with urination. I have to get up every hour during the night and each time I void only quite a little, perhaps a tablespoonful." He told me his bladder was full to bursting point and therefore he took the minimum of liquid. His urine was extremely thick and dark, acrid and irritating. I felt his abdomen and noticed that his bladder was the size of a football.

It was Sunday, the chemist's shop was closed, I had no homœopathic medicines with me. I went to the garden, collected a large basket of parsley, told his wife to chop it up, fill a teapot almost to the brim, pour boiling water on it, let it draw for ten minutes or so, and that he was to drink it all day long. He was not to touch flesh, fish, fowl or anything made of them, spices, condiments, alcohol, strong tea, and was to abstain from tobacco. I then set out for an all-day walk.

Ten hours after I called on Mr. T., who told me proudly that he had filled a large vessel, that his

urine had become clear and he felt much happier.
Parsley is an old folk remedy for bladder irritation,
gonorrhœa, etc. Returned to London, I sent the smith
Sulphur in a low potency which he needed on constitutional grounds, Pulsatilla 1X for pain in the uretha
and bladder catarrh, and later on Sabal Serrulata,
mother tincture. In the olden days sufferers from
this trouble were given Silica by homœopaths. Sabal
Serrulata is Saw Palmetto, which grows on soil rich
in Silica, and the juice of the plant contains Silica
pre-digested by the plant. I have found it of value
for enlarged prostate. The smith had been terribly
depressed at the time I saw him first. He did not want
to be operated upon. Urination and urine rapidly
became normal.

On June 1st, 1931, Mr. H. C. J. wrote to me from
Cardiff : —

"For some years I have been troubled with my water.
It is too frequent in the day, and, after lying down at
night, I have difficulty in starting. I have had treatment
from my doctor, who told me that my prostate was as large
as an orange and he wanted me to see a specialist. I am
sixty-one years old."

As he did not wish to be operated upon, I put him
on the non-irritating diet, previously mentioned, told
him to take an abundance of fruit, fruit juice, barley
water, and gave him Sulphur for clearing up the case
and Conium 3X to act on the prostate. We read under
the heading "Conium" in Boericke : "Much difficulty
in voiding urine, it flows and stops again, interrupted
discharge, dribbling in old men." Besides Conium is
indicated if there has been an injury. I was under
the impression that there had been an injury in his
case. I alternated Sulphur and Conium, then gave
him Pulsatilla and Arnica, and Chamomilla when
bladder urging became particularly pressing. Then
he received Sulphur in the 30th potency. The man
improved prodigiously. After a few weeks he wrote:
" I weighed myself this morning and am 7 lbs. heavier

than I have ever been. I am feeling well. I keep to your instructions." On June 30th, 1932, he wrote:—

"Last night I had to go to the doctor to have my ear syringed, as the wax had got hard and had made me deaf. When that was over, we had a chat about my old complaint. The doctor passed his finger up my back passage, and told me that the prostatic gland was much larger, and was nearly closing up the bowel and that I had got much thinner during the months when he had not seen me. I told him, as regards my being thinner, I was heavier by a number of pounds. He felt and pommelled me about and admitted that I was in good condition. He asked who had advised me about the prostate and when I mentioned your name he said contemptuously, 'that man is a quack.' I asked him how he accounted for you curing people where doctors had failed. He did not answer, but pressed me to have the operation. Now as regards my own opinion, he told my wife thirteen months ago that I would not be alive in three months' time. Now if he was anyway near right, I could not have improved as I have. Several people whom I told what the doctor had said laughed and told me they had never seen me looking so well as I do now."

Major J. R. brought me on December 21st, 1932, his father, a retired Army surgeon with the rank of lieutenant-colonel. He was seventy-eight years old, had had a very serious attack of influenza, something like a seizure, complained about palpitations, bronchitis, deep depression, and particularly about an enlarged prostate, which made his nights a misery. He explained to me: "Of course, as a surgeon I know that nothing can be done for that trouble except operation, and I am too old for it." Aluminium was used in the kitchen. He was given a dose of Influenzinum 30 every Sunday and a dose of Alumina 200 every Wednesday. In addition he was to take night and morning a dose of Sulphur 6X and a little Nux vomica before meals.

The combination of Sulphur and Nux vomica improved his general condition. On December 30th Sulphur and Nux vomica were exhausted and he was

given Sabal Serrulata mother tincture, ten drops
three times a day, which was alternated with Bryonia,
because of his bronchitis, a sequel of the old influenza
attack. On January 5th Bryonia was exchanged for
Pulsatilla because of pain in the prostatic region.
Later on he was given Ignatia in various potencies
'because of depression and a few doses of Thuja 30 to
antidote numerous vaccinations.

On January 25th the old gentleman wrote: " I am
happy to say I am still sleeping well nearly every night,
so I think the prostatic enlargement must be a good
deal better, because the irritation caused thereby prevented sleep in the past. You have helped me certainly
and I am much obliged to you." In another letter he
wrote: " I am decidedly better and now can sleep for
six or seven hours." On March 12th, 1932, he wrote:
" I am practically well now," and his son, Major R.,
told me: " My father certainly is very much better
in health. My mother tells me that he sleeps quite
well, and I do not think the enlarged prostate is worrying him now." Before he came to me, the patient had
taken strong tea with much sugar, coffee, meat, spirits,
etc. He was given the usual non-irritating diet in
addition to the medicines mentioned.

In June, 1933, I received a letter from a Mr. Laurence
G., Derby, complaining about an enlarged prostate
from which he had suffered for ten years.   " The
doctor says he could take it away by operation, but as
two of my friends did not survive that operation, I do
not feel like taking the risk, especially as the greater
part of my income is derived from a pension which my
wife would lose if I went first."   It is always desirable
to examine an enlarged prostate by way of the bowel
exit where it can be clearly felt, especially as there
may be cancerous enlargement. I sent him Sulphur
6X, to be taken night and morning, told him to take
parsley tea and asked him to come and see me. He
replied that he was an old man, had not been away
from Derby for twenty years and begged me to give
him advice without seeing him.

He was to take the usual non-irritating diet, an abundance of liquid, Sulphur 6X night and morning, and Silica 12X between meals. The success was instantaneous. After a few days he wrote: "I am pleased to say I am already a lot better for following your advice and taking the medicine. On the whole I am decidedly better." On July 23rd he wrote: "I am keeping wonderfully better, I have no urine trouble whatever, and I have a distinct feeling that the gland is reduced. I am sticking to your diet, and like it." On August 1st he wrote: "I am pleased to say I am as well as I have been for years. I have no stoppage of urine at all and very little pain. I am in first-rate health. I think I am cured." This was followed by a letter on August 13th: "I am pleased to say I am keeping better. I have no attacks. I can certainly go much longer without emptying the bladder, and have no, or very little, irritation. I generally wake three times in the night, but mostly without feeling any uneasiness. Still I get out of bed and empty my bladder for fear of trouble."

As the man had been living on a devitaminized and demineralized diet, his diet was greatly improved and he was given an abundance of vegetable water. Notwithstanding a hugely increasing intake of fluid he, like all the other patients, noticed that urging to urinate and bladder control became greatly improved. At first all of them were horrified at the idea of vastly increasing their intake of liquid.

In 1932 I was attending a well-known nobleman. His masseur arrived and told him: "My lord, I am afraid that I cannot treat you to-day. I am too ill." "What is the matter with you?" "I have been bleeding profusely from the bladder for a fortnight and I am at the end of my strength." "See whether Mr. Ellis Barker can help you." Having been told that the blood was bright red, and liquid, I opened my pocket case and gave him a millionth of a grain of Phosphorus, Phosphorus being indicated if there is bright, arterial blood, and Hamamelis when there is

thick, dark blood from the veins. I was in a hurry
and the masseur was anxious. I asked him to get
into my car, and questioned him while driving home.
He had had a very large prostate for ten years, and
on its right side there was a spongy outgrowth which
might have been malignant. I gave him a non-
irritating diet with an abundance of liquid, especially
bran decoction, and Sabal Serrulata, five to ten drops
three times a day, also mother tincture Thlaspi bursae
pastoris, if there should be further hæmorrhage.
Happily the one dose of Phosphorus sufficed to stop
the hæmorrhage for months.

This case was different from the previous ones. Vast
improvement was followed by set-backs. There were
numerous symptoms which made it necessary to use
a large number of remedies. There was the feeling of
a stone rolling in the bladder, which called for
Pulsatilla, burning urine which called for Cantharis,
great pain on movement, which demanded Bryonia,
pain in the perineum when sitting, which was corrected
with Cyclamen 3X, etc. This was the most protracted
case I have ever handled. Happily the soft outgrowth
at the right side of the gland disappeared completely,
urination and bladder capacity greatly improved, but
there were inexplicable set-backs.

One day my patient told me quite casually: " Three
years ago I was examined by a specialist in Harley
Street, who stuck a tube into my bladder and gave me
violent pain." I wondered whether, in addition to the
enlarged prostate, there was an unhealed injury, caused
by the use of the cystoscope.

The most wonderful diagnosis is that which can be
effected without instruments by the reaction of the
patient to homœopathic medicines. There is a herbal
medicine called Staphisagria which is particularly
useful for injuries to the bladder and its sphincter.
I gave a few doses of Staphisagria 3X, which produced
immediate and very great relief. It indicated that
there was a bladder injury, apart from the prostate
enlargement. This shows the danger of orthodox

examination in bladder troubles. I have met a considerable number of people whose bladders were
gravely injured by the unskilful use of catheter or
cystoscope. I then gave him a single dose of
Staphisagria 200th potency and warned him that there
might be an aggravation which probably would be
followed by improvement. During the next day, the
bladder pain became much worse, but then disappeared
completely, and he told me that this had been the most
wonderful medicine he had ever had.

Mr. E. B., a literary man, noticed seven or eight
years ago when he was well over fifty that he had to
pass water more and more frequently, especially at
night. A leading West End physician sent him to
a Harley Street specialist who examined him twice
with a cystoscope, charged thirteen guineas, and told
him that there was an enlarged prostate which would
probably grow larger from year to year and which
could be cured only by operation. No advice as to
diet or medicine was given, for "there is no treatment for that condition except surgery." Mr. E. B.
disregarded his trouble until the end of 1932, when
things became very awkward. He had to get out of
bed every half-hour or so and was afraid to go for
walks, go to the theatre, etc. At last he went to an
eminent homœopath who, like all good homœopaths,
is averse to operations. He examined the prostate
and said: "You have a prostate, the size of a pear,
and I am afraid you have to reconcile yourself to an
operation." The man came to me, I gave him the
usual non-irritating diet, and a number of medicines,
among them Silica, Thuja, Sulphur, Sabal Serrulata,
and Aurum iodatum, and the condition has so much
improved that the patient no longer thinks of an
operation and has practically no discomfort.

It must not be thought that all enlarged prostates
can be cured with Sabal Serrulata and one or two of
the other remedies mentioned. It would only confuse
lay readers if all the medicines given were enumerated.
One must treat in every case the totality of the

symptoms. If the symptoms cry out for Sulphur or
Calcarea or Phosphorus, that remedy must be given,
whatever the disease, but of course a bladder specific
may be interpolated. If a prostate case cannot stand
the heat, must put his feet out of bed because they
burn, feels a sinking at 11 in the morning, and has
other Sulphur symptoms, he must be given Sulphur
in the first place, and Sabal, Aurum, etc., afterwards.
Possibly Sulphur will cure the whole case, including
the prostate. Besides taking note of all the constitutional symptoms, the prescriber must consider the
medical history and inheritance of the patient. If
there is a tubercular tendency or suspicion, he should
receive infrequent doses of Bacillinum or Tuberculinum
in the 30th potency, or higher; if there is a suspicion
of cancer, he should receive infrequent doses of Carcinosinum, or Scirrhinum in the 100th potency or higher;
if there has been vaccineal poisoning or gonorrhœa,
Thuja 30 or Medorrhinum 30 should be given once or
twice a week. The homœopathic prescriber must act
with intelligence, not like an automaton. If Sabal
Serrulata is given to all prostate cases, some will be
cured and others will not be cured, although they might
be cured if the prescriber had used the necessary
industry. Under the heading of enlarged prostate
Boericke enumerates forty-three remedies in his *Pocket
Materia Medica*, while Kent enumerates forty-eight
in his Repertory. Homœopathic prescribing is difficult
if it is done conscientiously.

I have found that cases of prostatic enlargement
respond rapidly and easily to homœopathic treatment,
combined with a judiciously selected diet. Every
physician, homœopathic and orthodox, ought to be
acquainted with this form of treatment which will
give to thousands of unhappy, middle-aged and old
men wonderful comfort. Operation on the part of a
first-class surgeon with nursing homes, etc., means, of
course, a great expenditure, and much anxiety.

On the 27th October, 1933, I was consulted by Mr.
W. H. W. of Orpington, Kent. He was a retired

T

business man, 76 years old, and he informed me that he had a hugely enlarged prostate. He had noticed it first twenty years previously. Periodically he took medical advice, but the doctors had never been able to do him any good. His trouble was caused by faulty nutrition. He liked salted meat and fish, took salt and other condiments irritating to kidneys, bladder and prostate, in large quantities, was constipated.

To my regret he informed me that, six weeks previously, he had consulted an eminent bladder specialist who had told him that, in view of his age and general condition, an operation was out of the question. Nevertheless, with monkey-like curiosity, he forced a large-sized cystoscope into his bladder, causing fearful pain and its withdrawal was followed by terrific bleeding. He had to be taken home in an ambulance. Since then he had been writhing with pain which could be kept at bay only by the use of suppositories which contained a quarter of a grain of Morphia and of Belladonna. They were used when the pain was at its worst, but they did not give permanent relief. Naturally they injured the system as a whole.

I recommended him to reduce the dose by scraping away part of the suppositories, and tried to give him relief with homœopathic remedies and to promote the healing of the bladder injury. Unfortunately all my attempts to relieve him and to cure the prostate were foiled by the cystoscopic injury. I would warn every one of my readers against the use of the cystoscope. It has killed many people, to my personal knowledge, among them Mr. G. D., of Sketty, Swansea, whose story is told in the cancer chapter.

CHAPTER XIX

Drugs and Medicinal Treatments

THE great characteristic of medicine is its confusion. The treatments of yesterday are the
derision of to-day, and the most scientific treatments
of to-day will be laughed at a few years hence.

All who have studied the history of medicine are
aware that what is called medical science is, and always
has been, ruled by fashion. Medicine has rushed from
one extreme to the other. A century ago practically
every patient was bled profusely, guided by the theory
that the morbid blood should be drawn away. Now
no one is bled. A century ago doctors who refused to
bleed were expelled from the medical profession as
quacks. Now doctors who would like to bleed patients
who need bleeding because of their plethoric condition
are afraid to do so because it is no longer fashionable,
and any doctor who bled his patients indiscriminately,
would risk expulsion from the profession. Some
decades ago every patient was heavily dosed with
alcohol owing to the theory of asthenia. Then came
a time when no alcohol was given.

At present medicine is ruled by the bacteriologist.
However, the microbic theory of disease has been
challenged by thoughtful medical men and it will
probably disappear before long. Sir James Mackenzie,
the leading heart specialist of modern times, wrote:
"The detection of a microbe which provokes the ill
health throws no light upon the condition which made
the man ill and which may lead to death." Sir George
Newman, the principal medical officer of the Ministry

of Health, wrote in his *Outline of the Practice of Preventive Medicine*: "If we examine bacteria in a laboratory under conditions wholly unnatural to them, we must expect false returns." Sir Almroth Wright, the leading English bacteriologist, wrote: "Our deterrent in using vaccine therapy may be the possible flaring up of the local infection. The graver kinds of risks, those of a spread of microbes into the blood and a generalization of the infection, should be constantly present to the mind. There is reason to believe that much harm may be done by giving massive doses of vaccine in therapeutic treatment."

Many of the greatest doctors have been the greatest sceptics with regard to the curative power of medicines. Every year hundreds of new medicines and serums appear, are boosted, and disappear, like crops of weeds. Many leading medical men despise drugs. Professor Simon stated in *Infection and Immunity*: "Not one of the hundreds and thousands of pharmaceutical preparations that have been introduced has been shown to be of value." Dr. Oliver Wendell Holmes wrote: "I firmly believe that if the whole materia medica could be sunk to the bottom of the sea, it would be all the better for mankind—and all the worse for the fishes." I could quote scores of similar opinions. Drugs have been terribly abused in the past, exactly as serums and vaccines are abused at present.

Medicine is ruled not by science, but by fashion. Some years ago pepsin, derived from the fresh mucous lining of the stomachs of animals, was proclaimed the most scientific digestive medicine and it was prescribed by every doctor. To-day it is almost forgotten. When Robert Koch discovered the bacillus of tuberculosis, we were promised that in a few years tuberculosis would be a thing of the past. Tuberculin has killed thousands and has become discredited. Then Ehrlich discovered the organism of syphilis and he devised Salvarsan (606), and we were told that it would destroy the organism. It killed numerous patients

Modified forms of Salvarsan were produced by enterprising manufacturers, but all of them, like the Insulin cured diabetes, that that disease had lost its modified forms of Tuberculin, are dangerous. Radium is another disappointment.

The latest craze is Insulin. We were told that terror. The preparation has been well boomed and has been used extensively for years. Consequently the diabetes death-rate should have declined. Unfortunately that is not the case. Insulin was introduced in 1924. The diabetes death-rate per million living has fluctuated in England, as follows:—

Before Insulin.			After Insulin.		
1920	. . .	100	1926	. . .	115
1921	. . .	108	1927	. . .	126
1922	. . .	119	1928	. . .	131
1923	. . .	114	1929	. . .	142
1924	. . .	110	1930	. . .	142
1925	. . .	112	1931	. . .	145

Since the introduction of Insulin, the English death-rate from diabetes has increased enormously. A similar increase has taken place in other countries. Insulin, like Tuberculin, Salvarsan and Radium, is a dangerous drug. I have never seen a cure of diabetes by Insulin, but I have met many diabetics who have been greatly injured by Insulin. It is a habit-creating drug which enslaves the patient. On the other hand, I have seen numerous cases of diabetes cured by diet and homœopathy. I personally refuse to handle cases of diabetes when Insulin has been used because they have become enslaved to the drug. Dr. J. E. R. Macdonagh wrote in *The Nature of Disease Journal*: "Diabetes is a symptom, not a disease, and Insulin, which has nothing directly to do with carbohydrate metabolism, does no more than palliate this symptom. The drug throws no light upon the cause, it does not act in the manner described, and, had the cause been found first and eradicated, as it can be, there would have been no need for its use."

Orthodox medicine is ruled by fashion. The drugs which were used ten or twenty years ago are now derided. Only the latest books on treatment can be used by the up-to-date physician and they will be out of date a few years hence. Homœopathy is ruled by immutable laws. It uses the same medicines now which it used a century ago and these and the new drugs added since then will continue to be used centuries hence.

Orthodox medicine is guided by experiments on animals which prove nothing. Students are told by their professors that such and such a medicine has this or that effect upon the muscles of a frog's legs or on the liver of rats, etc., and that it is used for such-and-such diseases. The experiments made with drugs on animals are crude and useless. It is, of course, foolish to conclude that if a medicine has a certain effect upon guinea-pigs, it will have a similar effect upon human beings. So-called scientists are foolish enough to calculate the tolerance of drugs in human beings by comparing the weight of men and of the animals used experimentally and multiplying the animal dose by the difference between the two weights. That dosage has injured and killed many patients, as was pointed out in the introduction to the *Extra Pharmacopœia*. Scientists tell us that a drug should be given in so many cat units, rat units, etc.

Orthodox medicine is built on shifting sand. Pathologists, forgetting that medicine treats the living, bid doctors to base their treatment on the findings of the mortuary. Hence a vast amount of space in books on treatment is given to what is called " morbid anatomy." Modern medicine is based on morbid anatomy which teaches nothing useful and on unreliable experiments on animals.

Three centuries ago Thomas Sydenham, the English Hippocrates, taught: " Every disease is an attempt of Nature to cure the body." Hippocrates taught the same doctrine 2,300 years ago. Modern medicine, though claiming to be scientific, has not yet grasped this fundamental verity. We frequently read about doctors "fighting" disease. As a rule they do not fight disease, but its curative manifestations, with disastrous results.

Until recently doctors "fought" fever. Fever is not a disease, but a curative effort of Nature. Nature strives to destroy the germs of disease by producing a high temperature, by boiling them to death. That healthful process may be frustrated by bringing down the temperature in some way or other. Formerly patients were immersed in cold water. The temperature went down, but the doctor's triumph was short-lived—and so were his patients. Then the chemical manufacturers of Germany came to the rescue of the fever-fighting doctor and produced a host of "scientific" medicines for bringing down the temperature, Antipyrine, Antifebrin, Phenacetin, Aspirin, etc. In Hare's *Practical Therapeutics* we read: "The objection to the use of all anti-pyretic drugs is that they depress the patient and decrease his power of resisting disease." Unfortunately the great drug houses teach and direct, or misdirect, thousands of doctors by means of their propaganda.

The doctors "fight" skin diseases with poisonous washes and ointments, which drive the disease inward, while Nature tries to drive it outward. A man "cured" of his skin disease is often given asthma or heart disease instead. This treatment is particularly disastrous in syphilis. Syphilis patients are not put on a purifying diet, nor are their bowels regulated, nor is the activity of their skin stimulated, as was done in the past. The body reacts against syphilis by producing the characteristic eruption which proclaims the existence of the disease to all the world. Patients are anxious that their infliction should not thus be proclaimed, and the doctor readily meets their wishes, not by fighting the disease, but by suppressing its natural curative skin manifestations. He thwarts Nature, and the result is deplorable. The skin manifestations are seen no longer. Syphilitics are able to go about and to infect others. Decades ago syphilitic eruptions were common, while syphilis of the nervous system, spinal cord and brain was most uncommon. Treatment by suppression appears to have produced in a large number of patients consequences which formerly were of the utmost rarity.

I have encountered a large number of syphilitics who were pronounced completely cured by all the scientific tests and who had healthy children. However, they died miserably from paralysis or insanity, the most dreaded final manifestations of the disease. Of course it may be that these fearful end-results were not due to syphilis, but to the poisons given in treatment which produce manifestations similar to those of syphilis. I have the uncomfortable feeling that by the suppressive treatments practised at present, syphilis becomes incurable and that it breaks out afresh many years after the nominal cure and notwithstanding negative Wassermann tests which, by the way, are not reliable.

Doctors have abandoned the art of healing to men who know nothing about medicines, diet, treatment, etc. Pathologists, analytical chemists, biological chemists, radiologists and surgeons lay down the law to the doctors, and bacteriologists and other laboratory workers, who have never stood at a sick bed, actually direct doctors how to treat patients whom they have never seen.

Orthodox treatment is dominated by the bacteriologist. However, the connection between the " guilty microbe " and the disease is not always obvious. There is pathological cholera and actual cholera, theoretical tuberculosis and actual tuberculosis, test-tube diphtheria and actual diphtheria, etc. In 1892 there was a terrible outbreak of cholera in Hamburg. The drinking water was swarming with cholera bacilli. Virchow, the greatest pathologist of his time, investigated the position. He went to huge apartment houses, inhabited by scores of families. All of them had been drinking the infected water. The motions of all of them swarmed with cholera bacilli, but only a few of the people had fallen ill or died. From the bacteriological point of view, all the inhabitants suffered from cholera. I understand that there are cholera cases without the cholera bacillus and healthy men who carry millions of cholera bacilli in their bodies. Does the bacillus create the disease, or the disease the bacillus?

The throats of millions of men contain pneumococci. Yet, no one would suggest that every one of the carriers of that germ should be treated for pneumonia.

Formerly a septic throat was called a drain throat and was treated with antiseptic gargles and various medicines which usually produced a cure in a few days. I myself had a " drain throat " two or three times half a century ago. No one thought of taking a swab and sending it to the pathologist. This is done nowadays as a routine measure, and if diphtheria organisms are found, the patient is taken to a fever hospital and is treated subcutaneously for diphtheria. Formerly there were many drain throats but few cases were considered to be diphtheria. Of the few cases of diphtheria, a certain percentage died. Now an enormous number of cases, mostly innocent drain throats, are rushed to the hospitals because the Klebs-Loeffler bacillus has been found. Most of these cases are trivial and need nothing but a gargle. Naturally only a small percentage of these cases die, and then we are told to compare the small percentage of deaths from theoretical diphtheria with the much greater mortality from severe diphtheria years ago and to bless the discoverer of antitoxin.

Some years ago the *Lancet* stated that the Klebs-Loeffler bacillus was absent in 14 per cent. of the cases of clinical diphtheria, while Sir William Osler declared in the *British Medical Journal* in 1926 that the bacillus could not be found in from 28 to 40 per cent. of the cases. The *Lancet* stated a few years ago: " Cases present themselves with all the symptoms and signs of tuberculosis without the presence of tubercle bacilli." Apparently one can have the disease without its "causative germ" and can harbour the causative germ without having the disease. Yet, the majority of medical men and the people in general imagine that the two are always found combined and that it is the most scientific treatment to hunt for the guilty microbe and to destroy it. As a rule the body does the destroying if it is given the necessary stimulus. How it does it, we do not know.

Many of the ablest medical men doubt the wisdom of treating diseases in general in accordance with the microbic theory. Sir Almroth Wright, perhaps the greatest bacteriologist living, stated some time ago that the whole theory of serum therapy rested "upon a foundation of sand." Lord Horder gave some years ago an explanation why, notwithstanding its great risks and doubtful effects, subcutaneous treatments have become universal:—

"At first sight the growing popularity of inoculation treatment among practitioners suggests that its utility is thereby demonstrated. But on a further view we become aware of the fact that to a large extent this accession of practical interest on the part of the doctor is due to the patient forcing his hand. This, and a natural desire not to be left behind, may be responsible for much of the increase in vaccine therapy, as seen to-day, rather than honest conviction, based upon personal experience. Many of us inoculate our patients because it is expected of us, rather than because we feel it is the best way to cure them."

Lord Horder's reference to curing patients reminds me of the saying of Sir J. Goodhart: "The expression 'I cure this or that' heard so often on every side is not a nice one. We *cure* hams! Disease *gets well* while we look on and assist as best we can."

Homœopathy is not guided by fashion, by pathological theories which are praised to-day and gone to-morrow, and by experiments on animals. The materia medica of homœopathy is based on experiments made on human beings, chiefly doctors. The effects of medicines are studied by "provers." The director of a proving gathers around him a number of willing medical men, and gives them day by day a drug unknown to them in increasing quantities. The provers put down every day the symptoms which they observe. If, after a number of days, the majority of the provers report that they experience inflammation in the right side of the throat, congestion of the liver, deep depression, etc., then we know that the medicine used acts on the right side of the throat and on the liver and causes deep depression. Rats and guinea-pigs cannot provide similarly exact information. We can discover in them only the grossest lesions.

The effect obtained by using drugs and injections on animals are published by the experimenters. Soon afterwards we are frequently told that the identical experiments made by others yielded totally different results. Thus knowledge is replaced by confusion. The facts discovered by homœopathic experimentation on human beings in Hahnemann's time have been doubted. New provings were made to check the original ones, and in every case Hahnemann's original findings were brilliantly confirmed.

Homœopaths are not stampeded by drug houses into using unproved and therefore dangerous drugs. The materia medica of homœopathy is enlarged from year to year by the addition of new and reliable medicines. The knowledge obtained of the action of drugs by tests made by medical men on medical men is unchallenged and unchallengeable. The homœopathic materia medica is like a rock, while orthodox medicine is built up on an ever-shifting foundation.

From the popular point of view the most characteristic thing about homœopathy consists in the smallness of the doses given. Orthodox medicine inclines to maximum doses which occasionally produce disastrous results. The orthodox physician, being accustomed to giving medicine in large and very large quantities, laughs at the assertion that a millionth or billionth of a grain of medicine can do any good, and he will say that homœopathy is deception or self-deception. Being the son of a distinguished physician, I had the same idea until I tried homœopathic medicines and I was amazed at the effect of the small doses, but, of course, they must be homœopathically prepared. Otherwise the small dose is ineffective. If homœopathy cured by faith, it would be useless for babies and animals. However, it has produced wonderful results in animals and babies. That is shown in the pages of this work and in my volume *Miracles of Healing and How They are Done*.

Hahnemann discovered the extraordinary fact that every drug has two entirely opposite spheres of action. The effect of the small homœopathically prepared dose is opposite to the effect of the orthodox dose. The most powerful poisons, such as Strychnine and Arsenic, are the most valuable tonics.

Opium in orthodox doses benumbs and is very constipating. Given by the millionth or the billionth or the decillionth of a grain Opium is invaluable for those who are utterly benumbed through apoplexy, coma, etc., and it is a valuable purgative. An old lady came to me with a blood pressure of 300. She was terribly constipated and ordinary laxatives and purgatives had proved useless. I gave her Opium by the decillionth of a grain, homœopathically prepared, and she told me that it was the best purgative she had ever had.

Arsenic in large doses produces bleeding from stomach and bowel. Some time ago my dog developed bloody diarrhœa and he vomited blood. A few doses of Arsenic by the millionth of a grain cured him promptly. Belladonna in large doses causes violent inflammation, throbbing headaches with a flushed head, flaming eyes, throbbing arteries. Such inflammatory conditions are rapidly cured by a few doses of Belladonna in minimum doses. Opium, Arsenic, Belladonna in infinitely small doses have cured the conditions mentioned during 140 years and they will continue to cure them for centuries to come.

Ipecacuanha in large doses produces vomiting. In

small homœopathic doses it stops almost instantaneously violent vomiting, retching and nausea, if accompanied by a clean tongue. "Nausea with a clean tongue" is a key symptom of Ipecacuanha.

Thoughtful doctors recognize the danger of giving drugs in the quantities recommended in the textbooks. One of the most frequently given drugs is Digitalis. It slows the fast and nervous heart and, when it has been given too long, the heart stops or it starts racing and the patient dies. Such a case is described warningly by Sir Lauder Brunton in his book *The Action of Medicines*. Dr. J. T. Kent wrote in his *Materia Medica*: "The time comes when the doctor will be compelled to stop Digitalis and the patient dies of heart failure. Digitalis is never charged with the death and the doctor never seems to learn that Digitalis will kill." Homœopaths also use Digitalis, but they employ it as a rule in infinitely small quantities in which injury is impossible.

Thomas Sydenham, the English Hippocrates, wrote 250 years ago: "The sick man dies of his doctor." Unfortunately this is still true, but doctors do not realize it. According to the death certificates, all die of diseases. The doctors of the present are aware that the copious and indiscriminate bleeding, blistering, purging, vomiting, etc., of the past was deadly. Future generations will look with horror at the aberrations of modern medicine with its insane abuse of the subcutaneous syringe which is more deadly than the lancet was a century ago.

No one can explain why and how the infinitely small doses of homœopathy act, but an explanation is unnecessary. The fact that they act exceedingly well is all-important. We do not know what electricity is. Still, we do not refuse to employ it.

Certain medicines are used for the same purpose by homœopaths and orthodox doctors. Sulphur is used by both schools for treating skin disease. While orthodox medicine gives Sulphur in large quantities, homœopathy gives it in infinitely small quantities.

The usual dose in which I prescribe Sulphur is in the 6X potency, in doses of a millionth of a grain. That will be noticed from the numerous cases in which Sulphur was employed described in this book. One can cure many skin diseases with Sulphur in that potency. If taken at the rate of three doses a day, a single grain of Sulphur would last for a thousand years.

For flatulent indigestion orthodox medicine prescribes vegetable charcoal by the teaspoonful. My favourite potency is the 30th. By the decillionth of a grain it is often far more effective than in large doses. Possibly the higher potencies of homœopathy have so powerful an effect because the medicinal substance is broken up into ultra-fine particles. Hahnemann discovered colloidal chemistry. Homœopathic mecidines are broken up to, and beyond, the atom, are prepared by endless trituration and then by shaking the colloidal drug in a liquid. Therefore the homœopath does not call his ultra small doses dilutions, but potencies or dynamizations. He gives a new and wonderful power to medicinal substances.

The higher the potency is, the more it is triturated and shaken and the more strongly it acts. One can safely give doses of homœopathic medicine by the thousandth of a grain three times a day, every hour, or every few minutes, but it would be dangerous to repeat doses in very high potencies. A dose once a month or so is the most that can be given.

Homœopaths employ hundreds of medicines which are unknown to orthodox doctors. I shall show by a few examples how their value was discovered.

Among the most important remedies employed by homœopaths in treating the diseases peculiar to women is Sepia, the ink of the octopus. Hahnemann had a friend, a painter, who was ill with some obscure disease. One day Hahnemann watched his friend painting with Sepia and he noticed that the artist was moistening the brush in his mouth. It flashed through his mind that the absorption of Sepia from the paint brush might be the cause of his friend's illness. Hahnemann insisted that the brush should be kept out of the artist's mouth and his mysterious illness disappeared.

Having discovered that Sepia was a potent factor in producing disease, Hahnemann wished to discover all the symptoms which Sepia might cause and therefore cure. He did not test Sepia on animals, but started taking daily doses himself and induced some of his medical friends to do likewise.

Dr. Garth Wilkinson went to Iceland on a holiday. He noticed that the animals which fed in the pastures which were covered by the finer ashes of Mount Hecla suffered from hugely overgrown jaws and from similar bony excrescences elsewhere. He collected some of the lava, had it potentized, tested it, and he discovered that in infinitely small doses it cures the very bone disease which it calls forth if consumed in large quantities. Hecla lava is employed with excellent results by homœopaths throughout the world for bony overgrowths.

Some decades ago orthodox doctors became greatly interested in a drug called Condurango, claimed to be a remedy for cancer. It was used in the usual unscientific way for the name of the disease. It benefited some cancer patients and proved ineffective in others, and fell into disuse. Homœopaths use their remedies, guided by the symptoms of their patients. Dr. J. Compton Burnett wished to ascertain what symptoms Condurango would produce and took large and ever-increasing doses of that drug day after day until he had to give up because of his sufferings. The most striking symptom was that it produced a deep crack in the corner of the mouth, which began to ulcerate. It looked cancerous. He stopped taking the drug and the crack healed. Guided by this key symptom, Burnett cured a number of cancer cases, where the patient had a similar unhealing festering crack at the corner of the mouth. Other homœopaths have done likewise.

At first sight it seems absurd to select a remedy by some apparently trivial symptom, such as an unhealing crack in the corner of his mouth. In reality this curious way of choosing remedies acts infinitely better than following the textbooks which tell the doctors that such-and-such remedies " may be tried." Nature calls attention to the needs of the body by certain symptoms. A disease is an abstraction. A patient goes to the doctor not because he has " a disease," but because he cannot sleep after three o'clock in the morning, has gnawing pain, severe itching of the skin, etc. If a patient, complaining of these three symptoms, goes to an orthodox doctor, he will be overhauled. An enlargement of the liver may be found and, on the diagnosis, treatment for the liver may be given which may, or may not, be successful. If it fails to relieve, the patient may be told that his troubles are functional, or purely nervous, etc., with the recommendation that he should take a holiday, or go to Vichy for a cure. If the enlargement of the liver is not the primary cause of his complaints, the liver treatment may injure the patient.

The homœopathic doctor also may discover that the liver is hard and swollen, but he will prescribe for the three symptoms mentioned by the patient and all other symptoms which he can discover, such as ravenous hunger, intolerance for certain foods, desire for heat, etc. He will choose a drug which will produce all the symptoms, and if he has exercised the necessary care, all the vexing manifestations may disappear and the patient will declare himself cured although no liver treatment has been given. If all the symptoms produced by a disease have vanished, the underlying mysterious cause producing the symptoms must have disappeared as well.

It seems to be a law of Nature that likes cure likes. The coughdrops are throat irritants. One of the best remedies for the most irritating cough consists in inhaling Iodine fumes. The orthodox doctor who treats inflammatory conditions by applying a mustard leaf or a Belladonna plaster acts homœopathically and so does the physician who prescribes Mercury for syphilis, for Mercury produces all the symptoms of syphilis. If an innocent girl is employed in a factory where there are quicksilver fumes, she will before long develop a bad throat and an eruption of the skin which will be declared syphilitic by every practitioner who is not aware of the fact that Mercury is the similimum of syphilis.

Diarrhœa may be described as a natural attempt of the body to expel noxious material by way of the bowel. Some orthodox doctors encourage this process by large doses of Castor oil, a dangerous bowel irritant. Others stop the diarrhœa promptly to the danger of the patient by some medicine, usually Opium. The skilled homœopath does not give a specific such as Opium in large doses for diarrhœa. Guided by the law that "likes are cured by likes," he enquires carefully into the character of the diarrhœa. If it is accompanied by severe colicky pain and if there are watery or jelly-like stools with much mucus, he will think of Aloe, which in large doses produces that kind of diarrhœa, and a few doses of Aloe by the thousandth or the millionth of a grain will cure it. If the stools are painless, green, slimy and bloody, he will immediately think of Castor oil, which produces such stools and will give a thousandth or a millionth of a grain and a few doses will cure.

A cough is a commonplace ailment which is treated by the orthodox doctor with his favourite cough mixture, which sometimes cures and sometimes fails to cure. If his prescription has been unavailing, he tries one or two other mixtures and then thinks of inhalations, Morphia, etc. Homœopaths do not give mixtures but single drugs and they have no favourite medicines for coughs. They employ scores of different medicines for coughs and, before prescribing, they enquire carefully whether the cough is dry or moist, difficult or loose, whether the expectoration is stringy, lumpy or thin, what is its colour, taste, smell, whether the cough is hacking, tickling or hard, what conditions make it better and what make it worse, such as lying down, at what hours it is most severe and so forth. After having obtained all this information, a homœopath may cure a cough in a few days or in a few hours which has proved incurable to dozens of orthodox doctors and consultants for years.

Homœopathy has wonderful ways of antidoting poisons. Infinitely small doses antidote large poisonous doses. A man came to me for nicotine poisoning. I gave him a few doses of Tabacum in the 30th potency which cured him promptly. Over-consumption of salt can be cured by a few doses of salt in a high potency. People who have an over-active thyroid and are suffering from exophthalmic goitre, are usually sent to the surgeon, who cuts out part of the thyroid. A far safer course consists in giving thyroid in a high potency in infrequent doses. Patients with enlarged prostates very frequently react well to prostate substance in infinitely small quantities. Those who cannot digest milk can be cured with potentized milk. Many people have an extreme intolerance to the emanations of cats. A young lady who possessed this intolerance was sleeping during a hot summer's night with the window open. She awoke up in a fit of suffocation, and found a cat on her bed. Since then she suffered severely from asthma until she was given by Dr. John H. Clarke a single dose of potentized cat's milk, which cured her.

One of the most striking examples of the power of homœopathy of curing diseases which the practitioner has never seen is afforded by Hahnemann himself. In 1831 a mysterious disease, cholera, advanced from Asia into Europe. Hahnemann had never seen a case of cholera. He read descriptions of the sufferings of those attacked. A modern physician would endeavour to discover the causative organism and to prepare a scientific antidote. As soon as Hahnemann had learned that cholera patients suffered from icy coldness, vomiting, diarrhœa, cramps, etc., he wrote a number of pamphlets in which he recommended for the various phases of the disease Camphor, Cuprum (copper) and

Veratrum album (white Hellebore). Camphor produces icy coldness of the body, with an intolerance of warm, dry clothing, a typical cholera symptom. Cuprum produces terrible colics and cramps, another cholera sequel, while Veratrum album produces icy-cold sweats, vomiting and fearful diarrhœa, combined with intolerance of a warm covering.

The followers of Hahnemann employed these remedies while the great orthodox physicians who had actually seen cholera cases recommended the most unsuitable treatments. In reply to Hahnemann's pamphlets a hundred physicians published their own advice in a document in which copious bleeding was recommended as the principal remedy.

During the last century official treatments for cholera have changed frequently but homœopathy has remained faithful to Camphor, Cuprum and Veratrum album with which it has achieved the most gratifying successes, but it has added to these several other remedies.

In 1854 England was visited by cholera. Of the cholera patients treated in the orthodox hospitals 59.2 per cent. died, while of the patients in homœopathic hospitals only 16.4 per cent. died. These figures were given by Dr. McLaughlin, an orthodox physician, and Government inspector of cholera hospitals.

Orthodox doctors like to demonstrate their progressiveness and scientific knowledge by using " the latest and most scientific " remedies. They will recommend the use of Radium for cancer and of Insulin for diabetes, although, as far as I am aware, Insulin has not cured a single diabetic and Radium has not cured a single cancer patient. On the other hand, Radium and Insulin have killed large numbers. The Ministry of Health found it necessary to broadcast a warning against Radium.

The homœopathic physician, while not disdaining real progress, refuses to be captured by the latest fashion or the latest craze. The latest and the most scientific remedy is usually the most unnatural, the most unproved and therefore the most dangerous. While his orthodox colleague, who knows little or nothing of the curative powers of drugs, tries in sheer despair the latest production of the drug houses, the homœopath will employ with excellent result remedies which have stood the test of centuries. It is quite unnecessary to use serums and vaccines because of the presence of certain disease organisms, such as coli bacilli, etc. The indicated homœopathic remedies given by the mouth will deal with them quickly and safely. The worst cases of septicæmia (blood poisoning) have been cured with Anthracinum, Echinacea, Pyrogen, Lachesis, etc.

Curiously enough the most potent, the most reliable, and the most frequently employed homœopathic drugs are quite unknown to orthodox medicine. Lycopodium, the spores of Club moss, is used every day by every homœopath. It is one of the most potent homœopathic medicines. Orthodox medicine employs Lycopodium only as a dusting powder for pills. Sepia, the ink of the cuttle-fish, one of the most potent remedies in women's diseases, especially in those which are accompanied by prolapse of the womb, is not used at all by orthodox practitioners, as previously mentioned.

Pulsatilla (wind flower), a magnificent remedy for weak girls with delayed and inadequate menstruation, which is used daily by homœopaths, is ignored by orthodox medicine. Chamomilla is a very wonderful herbal remedy which has fallen into disuse. It is not considered sufficiently scientific. Decoction of Chamomile has been used for hundreds of years with excellent results to soothe frayed nerves and to allay severe pain, give sleep, etc. Bromide, Luminal, and Morphia are, of course, more profitable to the great drug houses which have done their best to destroy the use of safe herbs.

Lachesis, the poison of the Surukuku serpent, in infinitely small doses is invaluable for many climacteric troubles of women such as flushes. It is unknown to orthodox medicine. Rhus toxicodendron is invaluable for rheumatism made worse by dampness and relieved by movement. Thuja is of infinite use for the evil effects of vaccination and gonorrhœa. Arnica is used every day for the pain following operations, injury, strain, soreness, fatigue.

For hæmorrhages of every kind orthodox medicine can do little. If Calcium, Adrenalin, and a few other drugs fail, surgical or mechanical methods are used. If the blood is arterial, bright red, spurting, a few doses of Phosphorus, given in homœopathic preparation by the millionth or billionth of a grain, will, in most cases, stop bleeding from stomach, uterus and lungs. A homœopath can frequently with a few doses of medicine stop a hæmorrhage of the womb which would cause his orthodox colleague to rush the patient to the hospital where a terrible major operation would be performed and the woman would be a woman no longer.

CHAPTER XX

Surgical Cases Cured with Medicine

YOUNG surgeons are tremendously keen and enthusiastic. Their first thought when they see a patient is: "How can I use my knife?" They will readily undertake the most risky operations, hoping to acquire fame and to conquer new provinces for surgery. When they advance in years and wisdom they become conservative and will refuse thousands of operations which they would have undertaken in the past. The discovery of anæsthetics and antiseptics has made operations easy and painless to the great advantage of patients and surgeons. Patients are no longer strapped to the operating table, made drunk or held down shrieking and writhing by a number of sturdy hospital attendants until they fainted from pain and loss of blood. The very ease and safety of operations has caused surgery to be abused. The vast majority of operations are unnecessary and harmful.

An eminent homœopathic surgeon, Dr. J. G. Gilchrist, wrote in his book *Surgical Diseases and Their Homœopathic Therapeutics*: "Apart from mechanical injuries, and these are *not* diseases, there can be no such thing as local disease. Tumours, ulcers, and all kinds of abnormal growths are simply *symptoms*, peripheral symptoms of a generally diseased organism." He advocated their medicinal treatment.

Appendices, gall bladders, ovaries, wombs, tonsils, etc., are needlessly excised every year by the hundred thousand, to the harm of the patients. In at least

90 per cent. of the cases, tonsillectomy is not only avoidable, but actually harmful, for the degeneration of tonsils is due to a constitutional fault which should be corrected. If the condition producing the enlarged tonsils remains, swelling will occur elsewhere. The same argument applies to varicose veins and piles. Hæmorrhoids and varicose veins are caused by the weakness of the vessel walls, due to faulty feeding, constipation, pressure from an enlarged liver, etc. If the swollen veins on legs or in anus are cut out or destroyed by injection, the trouble will recur elsewhere unless the causative factor is dealt with. I have seen numerous cases where the destruction of varicose veins of legs and anus has been extremely harmful.

In modern diagnosis the words "Focal Infection" play a large part. If a doctor cannot find the cause of a disease, he is bidden to look for a focal infection, for poisoning from an infected bowel, or gall bladder, from the cavities connected with the nasal passages, etc. Hence patients whose sufferings may be due only to a faulty diet are sent to the dentist to have their teeth taken out, or to specialists to drain antrums, enucleate tonsils, make operations on the abdomen, etc., and they go like sheep to the slaughter.

Some surgeons have advocated the excision of all appendices and of all tonsils as a routine measure, explaining to us that they are useless and dangerous structures. We do not know what the function of the appendix is, but it has probably a useful function, while the tonsils are valuable organs of excretion. If they excrete poisons from the body, doctors, instead of dealing with these poisons, are apt to tell the patient that his tonsils must be cut out. Millions of perfectly healthy tonsils are enucleated, becaue they are slightly enlarged. At the centenary meeting of the British Medical Association in 1932 Drs. Allison Glover and Joyce Wilson, specialists in diseases of the throat, read a weighty paper which concluded with the words: —

"A review of the literature and the epidemiological observations made on a highly tonsillectomized child population suggest, however, that the excellent end-results of tonsillectomy in selected cases have been statistically over-weighted by indifferent end-results in cases in which the operation has been performed without sufficient indications as a more or less routine prophylactic ritual. In our opinion, a large proportion of the tonsillectomies now done in children are unnecessary, entail some risk, and give little or no return."

The ruthless excision of healthy appendices and tonsils by the ten thousand will, of course, be abandoned in time, as was the stitching up of floating kidneys which years ago was done as a routine measure to tens of thousands of women. There is a fashion in operations. Now the straightening out of the septum, the partition between the nasal passages, promises to be a fruitful cause of unnecessary operations. Of a hundred people, about 99 have deflected septums, which means that one of the nasal passages is slightly obstructed. So there is ample scope for normalizing operations which usually injure the patient. A narrow nasal passage can be widened by breathing every day for ten minutes through the malfunctioning nostril, closing the other with the finger.

Some years ago Lord —— was not very well. His doctor recommended him to consult a surgeon. The surgeon strongly advised an operaton. Lord —— was wealthy and shrewd. He thought the matter over, sent for his doctor, and the following conversation ensued: " I have seen your man and he has advised me to undergo an operation. It is rather a big affair and it will cost me hundreds of guineas, but I do not mind the expense. Money exists to be spent and I think I shall have it done." " My lord, your decision is a wise one." Watching the doctor's face closely, Lord —— continued. " There is only one point which we must settle. I mean to be quite certain that your advice is disinterested. There is paper in front of you. Please write me a letter in which you say that you are not financially interested in the operation." The doctor's face grew scarlet. He rose in confusion and protested against a reflection on his honour and that of his profession. Carefully scanning his expression Lord —— enquired: "Are you willing to write that letter here and now or not?" On receiving an evasive reply he rang for the servant and told him: "See this gentleman to his car." He was never operated upon and rejoiced at his escape. I heard the story from Lord —— himself.

Some time ago there was a discussion in the medical journals about the evil of fee-splitting between doctors and surgeons which was imported into England from America and which is particularly prevalent in some parts of the country. Unfortunately the temptation of advising a more or less unnecessary operation is very great when the surgeon's fee amounts to hundreds of pounds.

On the 28th December, 1933, the *Cape Times* published extracts from an address by Dr. T. Wooldridge, President of the Eastern Transvaal Division of the Medical Association, published in the *South African Medical Journal*. He said:—

"Don't you know the case of the child who is quite well in the morning, is a little indiscreet with its appetite, develops an abdominal pain, is rushed into hospital and, according to the doctor who operates, a valuable life is saved. In a large majority of cases a warm soap enema and 12 hours' water diet would have the desired result. But this is not nearly so clever as frightening everybody concerned. Besides, if the doctor carried out this treatment, all chance of an operation and of a 20-guinea fee has gone. I know of certain hostels where a child dare not complain of an abdominal or throat pain, or he will certainly lose his appendix or tonsils."

Good homœopaths can cure without operation 90 or 95 per cent. of all cases of tonsillitis, and most cases of appendicitis. They can deal with most focal infections without destructive surgery. For fistula the only treatment known to orthodox doctors is surgery. It is one of the simplest things to cure homœopathically. I personally have cured a number of them, usually

302 NEW LIVES FOR OLD

with Silica. As a rule a few doses of that drug in a high potency will righten matters.

In most cases of hæmorrhoids and varicose veins surgical treatment is unnecessary and harmful. Medicine and diet will prove curative in 90 per cent. of the cases. The only treatment known to orthodox medicine for fibroid tumours of the womb and enlarged prostates is by operation. The chapters devoted to these two subjects will show that in the great majority of instances operation is unnecessary. These examples could be multipled greatly.

There are purely surgical disorders which may be cured by homœopathy when surgery has failed. It frequently happens that a surgical wound, an amputation stump, an ulcer or an abscess does not heal. The surgical proceeding consists in cutting out the non-healing flesh, or taking off a further piece of the limb in the hope that healing will follow. Unhealing ulcers or abscesses are deeply cut out, and if there is no success, further healthy flesh is cut away. Very frequently non-healing is due to a constitutional factor which responds splendidly to medicinal treatment. A few doses of Silica or of Hepar sulphuris, or some other homœopathic medicine will cause the rapid healing of unhealing wounds, abscesses, ulcers, while broken bones which refuse to unite respond rapidly to small doses of Calcarea phosphorica, Symphytum, etc.

The orthodox treatment of carbuncles consists in vigorous incision, and disinfection, a procedure which is not followed by any good homœopath.

Ruptures are due to the weakness of the abdominal wall. They can frequently be cured by dietetic and homœopathic measures, designed to strengthen this structure.

On the 14th November, 1930, I was visited by Mrs. D. W., of Harringay, London, the wife of a factory manager. Her left hand was hanging loose from her wrist and quite unusable. She was a woman of magnificent physique, very keen at sports, and a passionate motor-cyclist. On the 1st June, four and a half months before she came to me, she was riding a motor-cycle and was flung into the road. She fell on her left arm and had fractured it badly about the wrist. She was taken to the hospital at Bedford, was provisionally treated and then went to Guy's Hospital in London. Her hand and arm were put in plaster. After five weeks, the plaster casing was discarded and it was discovered that she had a useless hand.

X-ray photographs disclosed the fact that an artery and an important nerve had been caught up by the fragments and had been crushed and the arm had badly healed. It was opened up, the broken ends of the bone were joined with plates and screws, a method which was introduced by Sir Arbuthnot Lane, and attempts were made to make the hand usable by daily massage and electrical treatment. It proved a complete failure.

The doctors and surgeons who had treated her had only looked at her fracture. I enquired into every aspect of her life, and I discovered that she had practically no perspiration, very profuse periods, delay in the bowel, a yellow tongue, a slight amount of pyorrhœa and she had been taking Quinine daily in 1924 and 1925 when she lived in Africa. She lived on a diet very poor in vitamins, had vegetables once a week, took boiling hot tea, etc.

I put her on a natural diet with an abundance of vegetables and fruit, told her to leave off massage and electric baths, and gave her Arnica 3X for the shock and injury, and Sulphur 3X to clear up her system.

She came again after ten days and told me that she felt vastly better, her bowels were working to perfection, tongue had cleared up, etc. I resolved now to treat her arm, constitutional preparation having given an adequate chance to the remedies I was going to employ. I sent her Ruta graveolens 1X, which affects particularly the periosteum and tendons, and Hypericum 1X, a great remedy for nerve injuries, to be taken in alternation. After a week's treatment for her injury, Mrs. D. W. wrote: " I think there is just the slightest improvement in my wrist. To-day I appear to have a little wider range of movement. I have great hope of a definite improvement soon now, but of course I realize this must take time."

On the 8th December she came to see me, and I found a vast improvement in the condition of her hand. Lead poisoning produces wrist drop. Arsenic has the same effect. After careful consideration I gave her lead, Plumbum, in the 30th potency, two doses, one at night and the second one next morning. I was not quite satisfied with its action and on the 10th December she was given Plumbum 3, a millionth of a grain of lead to be taken three times a day. Considerable improvement followed. On the 23rd of December she called on me again.

I was delighted with her progress, but as she thought that she had done better while taking in alternation Ruta and Hypericum, I put her once more on Ruta and Hypericum. On the 14th January she wrote: " There is still improvement in my hand, the wrist is fairly strong now and I have the full range of movement. The fingers also are slightly improved. My general health is excellent. I am taking much exercise and am also now doing all my usual housework."

In a few weeks her hand was normal. A few infinitely small doses of homœopathic medicines had succeeded after the resources of one of the greatest hospitals in London had failed.

Some years ago a naval officer bearing a historic name told me over the telephone: " My wife is suffering from an inflamed mastoid and has terrible pain. She would like to avoid an operation. What do you advise?" I replied: " Bring her along in your car as quickly as you can."

The mastoid cells form a most sensitive structure at the back of the ear. Their inflammation is frequently accompanied by fever, swelling and formation of pus, and unless help is promptly rendered, there is the danger of loss of hearing and of inflammation of the brain and death. In slight cases leeches and hot fomentations are applied and sedative drops are instilled to give relief. But if the inflammation does not subside promptly, the mastoid structure is opened and drained. That is the orthodox treatment.

The telephone call came in the afternoon. I asked my secretary to get tea ready and put on the tea table Belladonna 3X, an excellent remedy for inflammation in general, and Capsicum 3X, which is a specific for mastoid inflammation. The pair arrived. The husband was nervy. The wife's face was distorted with pain. I asked them to sit down and take tea and gave the lady a dose of Belladonna. Ten minutes later I gave her a dose of Capsicum. After a further ten minutes she had another dose of Belladonna, followed ten minutes later by a second dose of Capsicum. Meanwhile half an hour had gone by and we had talked with animation about operations, and various other things. I had observed that the expression of Mrs. C. S. had changed, and I asked: "How is the pain?" With wide open eyes the lady exclaimed: "It has gone, completely gone! It is marvellous!" The pair stayed a little longer and went back to their car with two little boxes of pilules, one containing Belladonna and the other Capsicum, with instructions to take doses alternatively at lengthening intervals. There was no further trouble.

On the 27th July, 1933, Mr. O. R. W. and his wife, who live at Lenton, Nottingham, came to me and told me that their little son, the only child, nine years old, was in a terrible condition, that he was getting worse and worse, and that they were afraid that he would become a permanent invalid. They told me that he had been treated at various hospitals, that he suffered from an ever-increasing curvature of the spine combined with increasing paralysis, that numerous treatments had been tried and that apparently the case was quite hopeless.

Instead of having the boy brought to me and making an examination which had been done, probably very well, by a number of doctors and surgeons, I enquired about his history, what started the trouble, or what incident preceded it, such as a fall, injury, fright, illness, etc. It appeared that he was perfectly healthy and normal. Five months before the parents came to me the boy had been in the country and had amused himself jumping over deep ditches. As the trouble began next day, I came to the conclusion that the disorder was either nervous or muscular, or both, that during one of those jumps some muscles might have become badly strained, involving strain of nerves, or that there might have been injury to the spinal cord through concussion. Probably nothing was ascertainable by the usual methods of diagnosis which, though impressive, are often futile. One may discover invisible factors by a little thought, but not by using scientific instruments.

Among the best remedies for injuries and shock is Arnica, and for injury caused by strain of muscles Rhus toxicodrendron. For injuries to nerves and to the spinal cord Hypericum is extremely useful. I resolved upon giving the boy these three medicines, and sent them to the mother with the following letter:

" Dear Mrs. W., your boy is nine years old, and it appears that in March of this year, about five months ago, he jumped over a ditch and next day he started holding himself crookedly. Since then the trouble has steadily got worse. His left side is becoming more and more weak and deformed, he has been treated by doctors and has been kept at hospitals, but apparently treatment has done no good, and you have been told that the boy is suffering from lateral scoliosis, in plain English, curvature of the spine. You have also been told that it might be infantile paralysis. As a baby he had a heavy fall downstairs, but that has probably nothing to do with the present complaint. I hand you herewith three boxes of medicine:

 Arnica 3X (old injury) (1)
 Rhus tox. 3X (old injury) (2)
 Hypericum (nerves) 3 night and morning.

Give the boy 3 Hypericum pilules first and last thing, and

give him three times a day, in between, either 3 Arnica pilules (1) or 3 Rhus tox. (2). Please change every three days from one medicine to the other and observe carefully whether the Rhus tox. or the Arnica medicine suits him best.

"Further, I would like you to get some *unrefined* cod-liver oil, the refined which the chemist has in stock is not much use for the purpose, and rub with it the boy's left side. Rub along the spine downward, and rub arms and legs upward from the hands to the shoulder, and from the toes to the hips. Of course you must study his comfort and must be guided by his sense of wellbeing in massaging him. You should not only rub the oil into his limbs and back, but should try squeezing, pinching, slapping, and other ways to improve circulation, being guided all the time by the boy's feeling of comfort. I hope that in a week's time there will be distinct improvement in him. Of course you must carefully look after his bowels and diet."

This letter was written on July 27th. Treatment was begun a few days later. On August 15th I received the first report from the mother:—

"You will be pleased to hear there is a decided improvement in his condition, and he is much straighter. I think the Hypericum and Arnica pilules have been most effective. Will you please send another supply?"

On September 5th his father reported:—

"Our son Tony has improved wonderfully, and we are delighted with his progress. He is much straighter and at times seems quite normal. He is having his massage as per your instructions and plenty of rest. Will you please send a further supply of Hypericum and Arnica for Tony? He is very lively and active and appears to be perfectly well in himself."

On September 14th the father wrote: "Tony appears to be getting better and better every day, thanks to you." According to the latest reports the boy is perfectly well. The united resources of medicine and surgery which are to be found at the great hospitals had been unavailing in stemming, and still less in curing, the progressive curvature of the spine and paralysis of the youngster, although the specialists consulted had every opportunity of examining the case. A homœopathic layman, who had not seen the boy and who had not received five years or more of medical training, used a little vision and a few homœopathic remedies, and produced a cure.

On the 8th May, 1933, I was consulted by Mr. W. M., a publisher, who had a large carbuncle on the back of his neck, dark-red, raw looking, very painful, and containing a number of depressions which were likely to turn into outlets for the pus. The man looked jaundiced and very ill, had a violent burning pain which was worse at night, he had been poulticing his neck without benefit, and he wished to avoid an operation. He had not been able to sleep during the last four nights.

I explained to him that the inflammation might spread to the spinal marrow and that there was a certain risk, that possibly he would prefer going to a hospital or nursing home. As he wished me to treat him, I gave him immediately a dose of Arsenic in the 30th potency, which relieved the burning there and then, and handed to him two boxes of medicine, one containing Anthracinum 6th potency, and Arsenic 3X, a dose to be taken every hour, the patient changing every hour from one medicine to the other. It was evening, his wife was very anxious, and both looked dubiously at the two little boxes containing a few tasteless sugar pills.

Before leaving he asked me whether he should go on poulticing and he was very surprised to hear that I forbade poulticing and told him to bathe the place occasionally with lukewarm boiled water in which he was to put a few drops of the tincture of Calendula and a few drops of the tincture of Hypericum.

A carbuncle resembles the fearful and frequently deadly boil produced by Anthrax, an acute and infectious bacillary disease of horses. Anthracinum is derived from the discharge of the anthrax boil and it was given to Mr. W. M. in doses of a billionth of a grain. Calendula is a wonderful disinfectant. It is the juice of the Marigold flower which is found in thousands of gardens. It cannot injure the tissues, while all the chemical disinfectants are tissue poisons. Hypericum is the juice of another plant, St. John's Wort, which relieves nerve pain. Both Calendula and Hypericum are not used by orthodox doctors and surgeons, who also do not employ Anthracinum.

The next morning I heard from his wife that Mr. W. M. had had an excellent night, had slept 10 hours without a break, and felt much better. She asked whether he should try to squeeze out matter from the boil. I forbade this.

I then sent him Arsenic and Anthracinum, both in the 30th potency, a dose to be taken in alternation every three hours. Presently a huge core came away without assistance, and in a week's time his neck was practically normal. I then gave him a few doses of Sulphur and Hepar sulphuris to clear up the case. Homœopathy heals quickly and painlessly many surgical cases. The orthodox treatment of carbuncles is excruciatingly painful, it is apt to cripple the patient for weeks, and to leave deep and ugly scars.

Lady P. brought me her Sealyham terrier, who suffered from an ulcer on the eyeball. He was eight or nine years old, the ulcer caused great irritation, the dog wanted to scratch it all the time, and he wore round the neck a huge contraption of solid cardboard, which prevented him touching his eye. The dog was deeply depressed and so was his mistress. She told me that several vets. had treated her little friend without success and that she thought the kindest thing was to put him out of his misery. As orthodox treatment had failed, homœopathy was given a chance.

On enquiring it was discovered that he had suffered from fleshy growths which are produced, and therefore cured, by Thuja. Ulceration of the eye may be induced by Arsenic. Therefore ulceration of the eye may be cured by Arsenic in small quantities. The

v

indication for Arsenic was all the stronger as the dog was very restless and always tried to get near a fire.

I handed the lady boxes of Arsenic 3X and of Thuja 3X. The former were to be given three times a day and the latter only on Wednesdays and Saturdays. The dog immediately improved in general health, became merry and bright, did no longer seek the fire, developed an excellent appetite, but his eye did not improve as much as was hoped. Therefore he was sent Mercurius corrosivus 3X, in the form of pilules and eye drops. Corrosive sublimate in substantial doses produces ulceration of the eyes.

In about a week the eye had become normal, eyelids were no longer inflamed, the desire to scratch the eye had gone, the contraption round the neck could be taken off.

In 1932 I was staying in the country with a clergyman. He introduced me to the postmaster, Mr. P., who suffered agonies from piles. He had been duly examined by a number of doctors, who had informed him that hæmorrhoids were a purely surgical condition to be treated by operation, strangulation, or injection.

The patient was dark haired, dark eyed, nervous, irritable, had a swarthy skin. He seemed a typical Nux vomica case at first sight. A few questions elicited the fact that he was bad tempered, liked highly spiced foods, had a hot skin, felt worse in the morning, was constipated, had frequent ineffectual urgings to stool. The case represented all the symptoms which call for Nux vomica. Some dietetic regulations were given and he was sent a box of Nux vomica 6X. No local examination was made because the conversation took place in the post office.

The postmaster seemed impressed by the consultation and he asked whether he might fetch his daughter. Joan suffered from an exceedingly pronounced and very disfiguring squint of the left eye. Her father explained that some years ago the usual operation had been made, that the squint had disappeared for a time, but had later on re-established itself, and that the doctor had assured him that nothing could be done except another operation, which meant a heavy expense.

No examination could be made as the scene took place in the post office. A glance at the child's head and eyes showed that there was some abnormality of the skull and some abnormality of character and the following conversation took place: —

"Has the child ever had a heavy injury to the side of the skull by the forceps at birth or at any other time?"

"Four years ago she was thrown heavily on the left side of the head and the squint appeared a little later."

"So the whole thing must be due to brain injury, which, of course, cannot be cured by making an operation on a muscle, the action of which is controlled by the injured brain. Has the child's intelligence and character altered since the injury?"

"Very much indeed. Before her accident she was the sweetest-tempered girlie in the world. Since the accident she has become terribly bad-tempered."

I sent Joan a box of Arnica 3X pilules, three to be taken two or three times a day. Both Mr. P. and his daughter seemed incredulous that tasteless sugar pills could do any good for two troubles which had been declared incurable except by operation. However, in a few months a miracle happened, as happens so often in the case of patients treated homœopathically. The father wrote: —

"I must say that I have never felt better, thanks to you. I have had no recurrence of piles and had freedom from that trouble for several months, a freedom which I have not had for years. My daughter, Joan, also seems better, and, strange as it may seem, has become wonderfully sweet-tempered and I think I can safely say her eye is better."

Arnica is a wonderful remedy for strain and injuries of every kind, even for injuries which occurred many years ago and for the after-effects created by these injuries.

CHAPTER XXI

Cancer

FOR decades official medicine has declared: "Cancer is a purely local disease." Guided by this maxim medical men have been urged to send every case suspected of cancer immediately to the surgeon, and the medical organizations have proclaimed: "Cancer is incurable except by surgery." The British Ministry of Health has published a number of monographs from which it would appear that cancer is curable if operated upon in time. Statistics relating to thousands of cases, published by the Ministry of Health, seem to indicate that it is not a very dangerous disease if operation is undertaken promptly, that the proportion of cures after early operation is high.

Tens of thousands of people are rushed every year to the surgeons because of swellings which have aroused the suspicion of doctors. If a perfectly healthy breast has been excised, the surgeon is not very ready to admit that the operation was unnecessary. One cannot help suspecting that the statistics of cures following early cancer operations are swelled by many thousands of cases which were operated upon because of the suspicion of cancer, not because of actual cancer.

Owing to this propaganda, early operation of tumours have increased beyond belief. Hence one might imagine that the cancer mortality had greatly decreased. Unfortunately the statistics published by the English Ministry of Health relating to the apparently easy control of cancer by early operation are contradicted by the statistics of actual deaths published by the Registrar-General. Between 1908 and 1928 the cancer mortality has increased as follows in England and Wales: —

	Total Mortality.	Cancer Mortality.	Proportion of Cancer Deaths to all Deaths.
1908 .	520,456	32,717	1 in 16
1928 .	460,389	56,253	1 in 8
1932 .	484,129	60,716	1 in 8

In my opinion cancer is not a local, but a constitional, disease, and the dreaded tumour is merely its local manifestation, as is the gouty toe. A man with a gouty toe is gouty throughout and a man with a local cancer is cancerous throughout. Many years ago it was assumed that a venereal infection might be treated by the early excision of the primary sore. Nevertheless, early excision, however drastic, has never prevented an outbreak of syphilis. Long before the local sore has appeared, the disease has spread through the body.

If any form of cancer should be purely local, it ought to be the cancer of radiologists. Cancer of the fingers is almost unknown, except in ray workers. Radiologists who have exposed their fingers to the deadly rays are apt to find that cancerous degeneration takes place on the tip of a finger. It is cut off and then the disease appears higher up. Then the whole finger is taken away and it appears in another finger. Then the hand goes the way of the fingers, then an operation is made at the elbow, then at the shoulder, and after years of suffering the victim dies of systemic cancer. That has been the story of numerous radiologists. If operations are useless in the case of X-ray cancers and radium cancers of the fingers, which were purely local at the beginning, why should they be more successful in cases of cancer of the breast, stomach, bowel?

The cancer statistics published by the English Ministry of Health and by Government departments abroad are unreliable. Hospitals and surgeons do not like to admit failure. The way in which operation statistics are manipulated has been revealed by the well-known surgeon, Erwin Liek, and by others. According to Liek, scarcely 10 per cent. of the cancer patients operated upon survive. In many cases an arbitrary and unduly short time limit for survival is set. If the limit is three years, then those who survive the operation for three years are considered as cured, even if it is known that they died of cancer during the fourth year following the operation. Often the officially alive are actually dead.

Official medicine considers surgery the only cure. Doctors do not wish to be censured. They send every case suspected of cancer immediately to the surgeon and wash their hands of all responsibility. The surgeon, if he considers the growth malignant, or suspicious, employs the knife, the cautery, or radium, and then turns to the next case. The result of this division of responsibility is disastrous to cancer patients.

Some years ago Mrs. McF. called on me. She told me that eight months previously she had undergone a very extensive operation on her breast because of a small cancerous growth. Doctor and surgeon had assured her that there was no danger of a recurrence because the operation had been done soon after discovery and the breast, pectoral muscles and glands in the armpit had been cleared out for safety's sake.

The lady looked desperately ill, emaciated, complained of stiffness, pain and swelling throughout the body, and it was clear to me that she suffered from generalized cancer. I immediately visualized the cause of her trouble and asked: "How often do you empty your bowels?" "Sometimes once a week and sometimes once in ten days." "And how long have you been in that condition?" "For I do not know how many years."

The poor woman was poisoned through and through from the bowel. Intensive poisoning had produced general degeneration which had culminated in the growth in the breast. Her doctor had sent her to the surgeon, the surgeon had made an extensive operation, but neither doctor nor surgeon had ever told her of the imperative necessity for keeping her inside clean. One might as well cut off the gouty toe of a man and allow him to drink unlimited quantities of Port.

The woman was not only terribly constipated and toxic, but she lived on the most unsuitable foods, flesh, fish, fowl, white bread, and little else. She was given radium, but, of course, the case was hopeless. If eight months previously she had been told to purify her system, she might possibly be alive and well. The operation shock had probably accentuated the virulence of the cancer and had spread it all over the system, as happens so often after the use of the knife or of radium.

Homœopaths have to their credit a large number of undoubted cures of cancer, declared absolutely incurable by high orthodox authorities. Many of these successes were obtained after microscopic examination of the suspected tissue, or after an exploratory operation. In my book *Miracles of Healing*, I have briefly described twenty or thirty homœopathic cancer cures, effected by physicians of high reputation. I myself have apparently been able to cure cases declared to be cancerous by competent doctors and surgeons.

If orthodox doctors are told of these cures, they are apt to say airily: " Probably the diagnosis was mistaken," and if they are informed " But it was your own diagnosis," they may reply: " I make mistakes like everyone else. I do not claim to be infallible." However, they refuse to investigate the cancer cures of homœopaths. That has been the experience of my friend, the late Dr. John H. Clarke, who had a number of cancer cures to his credit, and of many others.

We do not know what cancer is. Dr. Liek believes that there are two forms of cancer, a malignant and a relatively mild form, and that the latter is curable with, or without, medical intervention. I am not particularly proud of my cancer cures, two of which I shall briefly describe. Possibly the diagnosis was at fault. Still, the argument of a mistaken diagnosis does not arise in cases which died of cancer. Cancer patients come to me, like the late Mrs. McF., when the position is desperate. I have handled a large number of such terrible cases and I am glad to say that in very many instances I have been able to improve the lot of the sufferers very greatly.

A wisely chosen diet, combined with the indicated homœopathic medicines, has produced vast improvement in scores of cases. Many of my patients lost in a few days their jaundiced looks and depression, they got speedily a healthy complexion, their spirits and strength increased and they gained weight and sometimes a considerable amount of weight. Last, but not least, many of them died without pain and without the need of Morphia. I have found that not only the virulence of cancer is often greatly increased by operative or ray treatment, but that pain is terribly intensified. The worst of the orthodox treatments for cancer is probably by lead injection. Some of my patients who were unwise enough to allow themselves to be injected with lead against my advice, suffered the agonies of hell. They seem to add lead poisoning to the original disease.

It is a misfortune that the textbooks and special volumes dedicated to cancer do not consider the obvious common-sense treatment of that disease. Cancer is a disease of civilization. It is practically unknown among primitive races. It is most frequent where civilization is most highly advanced, where life is most artificial. It is highly significant that the cancer mortality is, according to the Registrar-General's statistics, about three times as great among butchers, workers in the drink traffic and merchant sailors as among clergymen and agricultural labourers. Butchers and workers in the drink traffic are unwholesomely fed. The sailors live in the open air and should be healthy, but they are among the unhealthiest men in the community, probably because they live on artificial food, preserved vegetables, white bread, and large quantities of preserved meat.

If we wish to reduce the cancer mortality, we must teach the people to live not like butchers and seamen, but plainly and naturally like agricultural labourers and clergymen. If we wish to relieve cancer sufferers, we must place them on a natural diet, devoid of all heating and irritating foods, condiments, alcohol, strong tea, coffee, spices, etc. Doctors who will try dietetic treatment on these lines may have a revelation. Unfortunately, the textbooks say nothing about diet except that the sufferer should be given an easily digestible diet, fish, fowl, etc. Not one of them forbids flesh foods.

Every doctor who is consulted by a middle-aged man who complains about continuous pains in his stomach should ask some questions about his diet, and if the patient says: "Formerly I was very fond of meat, but now I can scarcely bear the sight and smell of it," the doctor has reason to assume that the patient suffers from cancer of the stomach. Unfortunately people with cancer of the stomach whose instinct bids them to avoid meat are only too often urged to eat meat "to keep up their strength."

If a man suffers from an ordinary abscess, ulcer or skin disease, his doctor will advise him "Do not take anything heating, do not touch meat, alcohol, etc." If he suffers from the worst ulcer, abscess or skin disease, called cancer, the doctor, guided by the textbooks, will tell him "You can eat and drink what you like." That has been the reply which I have received in hundreds of cases.

In the textbooks on cancer, hundreds of pages are dedicated to the microscopic appearance of the growth, to chemical tests, to experiments on animals, and to every other aspect of the problem, while the common-sense question of diet and of treatment for giving relief to the sufferer is not touched at all. The practitioners have been taught that nothing can be done for the cancerous except relieve the last sufferings with injections of Morphia.

I give a small selection from my cases with which I could easily fill a large volume.

On the 1st May, 1929, Miss L. D. W., of Swansea, wrote:— ,

" I am single, 44½ years old, was born in India, have never been robust, had ten years ago an ulcerated stomach, but in October, 1923, I went to the doctor with a pain in my left side, which he said was pleurisy. I was in bed two months, went back to business, had a relapse and then had pleurisy and double pneumonia. Three doctors said I could not live, but oxygen and careful nursing brought me back to a measure of health. Dr. B., the chest specialist, said it would be wise for me to go to a sanatorium. I had little or no cough before I went, but there was a dreadful drawing pain in my left side under the ribs. Dr. B. and Dr. S. thought it was an abscess.

" I went to the Midhurst Sanatorium in June, 1924. After being there two or three weeks, a large swelling, about the size of a duck's egg, came where the pain had been, and then the pain practically ceased, and the doctor thought it was a cold abscess and aspirated it twice, but it quickly filled up again. On the 1st October, 1924, Mr. T. E. operated. It was more serious than he anticipated, the abscess having penetrated the pleura and attached itself to the lungs. I slowly got well, and did not go to the doctor for 18 months previous to March, 1928.

" For several months I had noticed a tiny swelling in my left breast which formed into a tiny lump. Dr. S. and Mr. I., the surgeon, said they did not think it was serious, but it would be wise to have the breast off. This was done in a nursing home on April 10th, 1928. I was cheered to hear from the doctor and surgeon later on that the pathologist's report was that it had been a non-malignant inflamed gland. The breast healed, but three weeks after the operation, as soon as I could stand, I felt pains like nerve pains in my left leg and knee. I found that I could not stoop. It seemed as if 2 or 3 inches of my backbone, lumbar region, had become stiff, and the pain was very bad. Doctor and surgeon examined me on the 7th August, 1928, I was X-rayed, and I was then seen by Dr. L. D., and they agreed that it was a growth in or near the spine which could not be operated upon.

" Dr. S. was anxious to try injections, but I told them that I would not have them until I was forced to. *Dr. S. thereupon told my friends that I could only live six months.* I then went on my own on a diet of raw fruit and salads, used cleansing herbs and lemon juice, my general health greatly improved and the swelling in the back went down and pains nearly ceased, but I was more or less helpless, my back being stiff.

" I seemed to be gradually improving until my periods came on. Then I felt very unwell, and since then I have been conscious of an internal lump in my left side down by the groin. I felt very unwell, and had the pain in my back and leg again. *The doctors have said I have cancer.* I have read your book on cancer and feel sure that, if you will kindly treat me, you will be able to do me good. Please wire when I can see you."

I saw the lady on the 6th May, 1929. After a lengthy interrogation, I sent her my directions, introduced by the usual summary, which concluded with the words: " The diagnosis of malignancy seems to me to lack adequate evidence and appears to me a mere guess. In your past life there is nothing to suggest tendency towards malignancy. Under these circumstances, and in view of your low condition and general flabbiness, you require a diet which purifies you and builds you up at the same time." Notwithstanding this cheerful paragraph, designed to encourage Miss L. D. W., I did not feel at all cheerful about her. At a number of examinations, all the specialists who had examined her had taken a most serious view of her condition. They had told her she had an inoperable cancer. Besides, tuberculous germs had been found when draining the abscess in her chest. Cancer, as is well known, is frequently superimposed upon tuberculosis.

I prescribed for her a milky diet, liquid paraffin to activate her bowel, Kaylene to absorb bowel toxins, Thyroid 2X before meals, to help digestion, and Hydrastis 1X every four hours, a useful remedy in many cancer cases. I cheered her to the utmost because she had been terribly depressed by her previous operations and the pessimistic forecasts. I also asked her to call upon Mr. G. D. of Sketty, Swansea, who had come under my care in the previous year with the prognosis that he had inoperable cancer of bowel and bladder and that he had only a week to live, who had made a marvellous recovery. It is useful to send a new patient condemned to death for some disease to some other patient who had been condemned to death for the same disease and who is alive and flourishing.

She wrote to me on the 20th May, in response to my cheering letters: "I hope to win and am trying to keep a victorious attitude of mind. I have seen Mr. G. D. of Sketty, and gave him your love. He is splendid, so well and happy, and he would like to hug you for all you have done for him. He is a living answer to the maxim 'Cancer is incurable except by operation.'" Miss W. was doing well and was so pleased with her progress that she sent me another lady condemned to die of cancer, Mrs. L. of Swindon, whose story has been told in the chapter on Fibroid Tumours.

On the 20th May she wrote: "I feel a good deal better the last three days, I lost half a lb. last week, but hope to start gaining soon." On the 27th May she wrote: "There seems to be a little improvement. I can sit and walk with greater comfort." On the 4th June she told me: "I think the swelling feels a little less large and it is softer by the groin. My period has been punctual and better than for three or four months. I am half a lb. heavier than when you saw me and weigh now 8 stone."

On the 13th June I was horrified by her telling me of severe cramp-like pain. I sent her Magnesia phosphorica 6X and Cuprum 3. She was to find out which of the two suited her best. I spent anxious days awaiting her next letter which was dated 26th June, and which told me: " I have taken some of the Magnesia phosphorica and Cuprum pilules, and am glad to say the neuralgia sort of pain has ceased. I try to forget that I have a lump." In view of the pain in the left side I sent her Ceanothus 1X which acts magnificently on the spleen and the region around it.

As she was not putting on weight as rapidly as I wished her to, I sent her Nux vomica and Carbo vegetabilis combined. Unfortunately her pain returned and she was given Magnesia phosphorica and Cuprum once more with good results.

On the 12th September, 1929, after four months' treatment, she came again to London. I found that she had made splendid progress and wrote to her: " You look better and there is not much left of your growth." I discovered only then that the milky diet which I had given her was not to her taste. Carrying out my directions with mechanical obedience, she had taken the baby diet with little benefit. I then gave her bran porridge, any kind of fruit, mild cheese, honey, etc. On the 5th October she wrote: " I feel very sure that the cause of my trouble is very much better. I am so much less conscious of my side where the swelling was and the last five or six days I have felt really better, have more vitality, a firmer grip on life."

She had always had a weak chest, had had pleurisy and pneumonia badly and the bacilli of tuberculosis had been found in the chest abscess. I sent her Bacillinum 100th potency, a dose once a week, Spongia 1X, a dose first thing in the morning and last thing at night, and told her to rub cod-liver oil into the whole of the body at night, disregarding the fact that she had to sleep in greasy clothes. I have learned the outward application of cod-liver oil from the Eskimos and am very grateful to them for having taught me its use.

Garlic is an internal disinfectant, excellent in tuberculosis, but, in view of her delicate condition, I did not dare to give it to her by the mouth. So I told her to take footbaths with plenty of garlic in them, which would cause the body to absorb garlic through the feet. Thus taken it cannot upset the stomach Garlic penetrates the body with the most amazing rapidity. If one rubs some garlic on the soles of a man's feet, one can, after a few minutes, smell it in his breath.

On the 29th November, Miss L. W. wrote:—

"I look perfectly well, have not looked so well for many years, everyone is remarking about it, my cheeks are more rounded and a nice colour, my skin very clear and bright eyes, really healthy-looking, and I feel a little stronger and better in every way, except for my leg, for *the swelling* has been steadily getting worse. It was on the thigh when you saw it. It is still there, it *has travelled underneath the buttock*, and has formed into a lump like a duck's egg, very hard, below the groin, which measures 4 to 5 inches thicker than the other leg. I have had very little pain in the leg for the last month.

"I thought it might be a cold abscess which I had five years ago in the pleura that did not yield to aspiration. I can see now that the diet at the Brompton Hospital was anything but helpful to me. They gave me pork, kippers, sausages, fried cabbage and potatoes for supper, and sometimes Shepherd's pie, etc. I think that if my general health can keep as good as it does now, nature will in time get rid of the poison and my leg will be normal again."

I communicated with the late Dr. John H. Clarke, and he and I believed that " something was on the move," that nature was trying to eliminate the trouble in her own way. I told her not to touch the growth and to go on with the garlic footbaths. She steadily improved and her letters became infrequent. The lump became smaller and smaller while it was moving along. On my suggestion, she had seen repeatedly Dr. John H. Clarke, who had encouraged her in his usual kindly, splendid way, and had sent her advice and medicine. On the 24th September, 1931, when I told her of Dr. Clarke's illness, she wrote to me:—

"I feel quite well and look the picture of health, rosy cheeks, rather plump for modern fashion, 8½ stone. I was a little under 8 stone when you saw me. My flesh is firmer and I am full of vitality, and you would laugh if you could hear people say: 'How wonderful you are. You look so well and bright and have such a nice complexion and you do not eat any meat! It's bran you eat, isn't it?' Another will join in and will say: 'No, it's raw carrots,' and a third will exclaim 'It's lemons.'

"Some while ago I met the specialist who was called in in 1928, three years ago, and who gave me six months to live. He was just stepping out of his house to get into his car, and I happened to stand in front of him. So I said: 'Good day. You remember me, Dr. D.?' He replied: 'I know your face quite well, but cannot just recall your name.' I said: 'I am Miss W. You saw me three years ago and you gave me six months to live,' and he exclaimed: 'Good heavens.' I quickly said 'I have been to Mr. Ellis Barker, and I am going to be quite well.' He got into his car as quickly as politeness would allow him.

"I see Dr. S., who used to be my doctor—I haven't any doctor now—sometimes in the street and each Christmas he has paid me a friendly visit and all he can say is: 'You do look well! It's wonderful! Thank God for it!' Poor man, he has heard lots about you and me from some of his other patients who happen to be friends of ours, and, when asked about me, he always replies: "Yes, she does look well, thank God for it."

"I rarely ever think, let alone speak, of my past illness, for I try always to think health and strength, but it would interest you to hear that the hard swelling which I could feel in my side by the hip region gradually dispersed from there and came down just below the groin inside my leg where there was a hard round lump, larger than half a cricket ball, and there was from that a sausage-like swelling below the buttock round to the thigh. At its biggest the left leg measured 5 inches more than the other. I was only

able to sit on the edge of a chair. It took about 9 months
to get to its height and was painful, and it took about
another 9 months to go down. Gradually things improved.

" I have been now normal in every way, no feeling of
swelling inside or out, I can bend over and almost touch
my toes. I lead a busy life and I feel and believe that I am
now *perfectly well* in every way."

I hear from her occasionally that she is keeping
well and is happy. On the 4th January, 1934, for
instance, Miss L. W. wrote to me: " I often remember you with gratitude and you will be pleased to hear
that I am very well, leading a normal life, indeed,
quite a busy one, and that I can get about and bend
over as well as Jeves could. Whatever the trouble
was, *it has entirely disappeared.*" She had been condemned to death on account of cancer six years before
that letter was written. For years, Miss L. W. had
been under treatment by great specialists and one
and all had made the most desperate diagnosis. Her
breast had been amputated, presumably on account of
cancer or incipient cancer, and the depressing forecasts she was given, such as that she had only six
months to live, must have had a powerful effect in
aggravating her obscure disease.

The attitude of the consultant who prophesied three
years before he met her in the street that she would
be dead in six months is not unusual. Doctors and
surgeons are annoyed if unorthodox treatment has
succeeded after they have failed. One would have
imagined that doctors and surgeons would be anxious
to learn how a patient, like Miss L. D. W., regained
her health after having been condemned to death. But
that is not done.

I do not know whether the pathological examination
of excised tissue for cancer is reliable or not. I personally doubt the microscope. I could collect scores
of cases of cancer where an operation was performed,
where only part of the growth could be excised, or
where only a small sample was taken, where the

pathologist had declared the growth undoubtedly cancerous and where homœopathy produced a cure. In
the opinion of the late Dr. John H. Clarke, a very
experienced doctor, the growth of Miss L. D. W. was
cancerous.

On the 22nd February, 1928, I received a letter
from a Mrs. L. D., from Sketty, Swansea: —

" I am a very, very distressed wife. My husband, 57 years
old, has since ten months been very seriously ill. Two
doctors saw him and could not find out what was the matter
with him, and one doctor attended him daily all the time.
I got him as patient into the hopsital here and since Friday
last they have kept him, but on Sunday they chloroformed
him for an examination, and the doctor told me yesterday
it was cancer and too far gone to operate. He is to return
home in five or six days as they can do nothing and they give
me no hope.

" I am just broken-hearted. We have a dear little home
and I can give him anything you may suggest. I am told to
let him eat what he likes and not let him know he has cancer.
It is hard, for my heart is breaking."

Having read this pitiful letter, I turned to my
secretary and said: " Of course nothing can be done
for that poor fellow. Still, I will send him a diet
sheet." I told Mrs. L. D. that her husband should
take liquid paraffin three times a day, half an hour
before meals, live on a milky diet, take an abundance
of wholemeal bread, orange juice, lemon juice, use
honey only for sweetening purposes, and forbade flesh,
fish, fowl and everything made of them.

I learned from the next letter that the husband had
no control over bowels and bladder, that, according to
the diagnosis, there was inoperable cancer of bowel
and bladder, that he had been given only a week to
live. It was apparently a most hopeless case.

On the 28th February, after five days' treatment,
Mrs. L. D. wrote: " Your directions seem already to
be doing good." I thought this a delusion. On the
2nd March after a week's treatment she wrote: " I

w

can see considerable improvement since you came to my aid. I consider your treatment more than wonderful. My dear husband *feels better*."

As I heard that Mr. D. was deeply jaundiced, I ordered Ox Bile Tabloids. I told the wife to rub his weakened legs thoroughly with crude cod-liver oil to strengthen them and to nourish him through the skin. On the 4th March, Mrs. D. wrote: " Your treatment gives me the greatest hope. My dear one seems wonderful to what he was. It is only a week ago that he was so ill and in agony, but it is different now and he has rarely pain." On the 6th March she wrote: " My husband's condition, compared with when he came from the hospital, is considerably improved. He is very cheerful."

Hydrastis canadensis was considered by the late Dr. John H. Clarke almost a specific for cancer. I gave the patient Hydrastis 1X three doses a day. Soon the husband wrote me himself and confirmed the improvement noted by his wife. He wrote on the 11th March: " I have nothing to complain of in any way, and am feeling increasing consciousness of steadfast recovery." On the 15th March he wrote: " I feel sure that the bladder and bowels are yielding under the present treatment." On the 17th March Mrs. D. wrote: " It is absolutely wonderful. My husband feels quite a different man." On the 24th March, after one month of treatment, Mr. D. wrote:—

" Improvement in health has been steadfast. My sleep during the night is unbroken, bowels now act normally. I do not think I have had much colour at any time, but the words of a friend may interest you. He said: ' I have never seen you look so well at any time since you have lived here in Sketty.' I can support this with my own feeling of well-being, and I think my friend is right."

On the 26th March he wrote:—

" My sleep during the last three nights has been of singular restfulness, but not once was I disturbed by a desire or necessity. Such a thing I have not known since June last year. Life, until you took me in hand, was a nightmare. Everything else seems to get to normal functioning.

"It is now one month that I have been under your care and treatment, and I can only say it is a miracle the way I have recovered. I can also affirm that I am increasing in weight, looks and spirits. What seems so remarkable to me is that this result has been obtained in so short a time, through reverting from a solid meat diet to a vegetarian diet."

On the 15th April he wrote:—

"The last two days must be counted as red-letter days in my uphill climb to health, for on either day I was free from any conscious sensation in or about the swelling, although it is still there. I can walk erect and at quite a brisk pace, feeling just fine. All is working well, considering my state of health only a month ago."

His wife wrote on the 17th April:—

"Mr. D. is more wonderful than ever. People who see him remark upon the difference just six weeks ago. I shall never forget how God led me in my absolute hopelessness after the three doctors' verdict at the hospital to Smith's bookshop where in a dazed condition I simply asked for a book on cancer. The man said 'I have only one book on cancer.' I said 'Give it to me,' and before nightfall I had read enough to see that the best thing to do was to write you, which I did. If anyone can cure him, you can."

On the 4th May she wrote:—

"My husband seems wonderfully better. He came to my concert last night. He did splendidly and he is quite hurt now when others look upon him as an invalid."

At the end of February, 1928, three doctors and surgeons, examining him under an anæsthetic at the hospital, had declared that Mr. D. suffered from inoperable cancer of bowel and bladder, and had sent him home to die, telling poor Mrs. D. that he had only a few days to live. Yet I, who had never seen him, was able to produce an extraordinary improvement. I have seen the same thing happen scores of

times in cases of cancer and other diseases which had
been pronounced "absolutely incurable." Unfortunately the textbooks are far too ready to proclaim
that certain diseases are incurable. From my point
of view there are no incurable diseases. Many cancer
cases, apparently in the last stage of the disease, have
recovered under treatment, or spontaneously without
any treatment. I have shown this in my two cancer
books, published by John Murray.

There is a wonderful reserve in most sick people,
which can be mobilized by giving them hope. Unfortunately medicine has become de-humanized. Most
doctors look upon their cases from the scientific point
of view. If more or less careful diagnosis indicates
that the patient has cancer and if operation is impossible, the sufferer is told that nothing can be done for
him. That verdict may kill a patient who is *not*
cancerous.

There is a widespread idea among the people that
cancer is often due to the food. It is based on centuries of observation, and is undoubtedly correct. In
the great majority of cases, cancer occurs in the food
tract. Treatment should be begun by placing the
patient on a fleshless diet, and all artificial foods should
be withdrawn. White bread, white flour, white sugar,
refined salt, are foods which produce deficiency
diseases and should be forbidden. Medicines, such as
Cascara, Aloe, Rhubarb and salts of every kind, are
powerful irritants, and should not be allowed. Bowel
regulation can be effected by giving the patient
adequate quantities of bran and of bran decoction, and
a diet rich in fruit, vegetables, etc. Until the diet
acts adequately, the bowel can be regulated with liquid
paraffin which acts as a lubricant. Homœopathic medication based on the symptoms of the patient should be
added. In scores, if not in hundreds, of cases, I have
been able to effect striking improvement by these
means.

Before all one must give the patient hope. When
a patient comes to me and tells me: "My doctor has

sent me to Mr., Sir or Lord So-and-so of Harley Street, and I have been told that I suffer from an inoperable cancer and that nothing can be done," I look hard at the man and say with quiet confidence: "I cannot accept the diagnosis. Many mistakes occur in these forecasts. There is plenty of good material in you. The body has an unlimited power of recuperation. I have every reason to hope that you will be vastly improved *within a week*." With those words the aspect of the man changes. The despondent creature brightens up, a smile appears on the face. He has been given some hope.

Steady improvement of Mr. D. was checked suddenly and severely by a psychic injury. On the 14th May Mrs. D. wrote:—

"The last few days my husband has complained of all the old pains. He seems to have been told by one of his friends that the hospital doctors had said he had cancer. Ever since he has been worrying."

In my reply I wrote—

"Your husband ought not to be upset if he has been told that his trouble has been diagnosed as cancer. What is in a name? To the incompetent all grave diseases are incurable for they can convert every curable disease into an incurable one. To the competent there is no incurable disease. Every week I receive cases which are 'absolutely incurable,' and the majority of them get better and get well. It is foolish to die of fright if fright is justified, but it is idiotic to be disheartened, or die, of a diagnosis which usually is wrong."

I continued treating Mr. D. with the indicated homœopathic remedies Hydrastis, Arsenicum, Lycopodium, Nux vomica, etc., according to his symptoms, and he continued going ahead. On the 9th July Mrs. D. sent me a very amusing letter:—

"I must tell you of a funny experience which I had the other day. I was in Swansea town with my lady help, and I was passing two gentlemen who were in earnest conversation and one of them said, pointing to me: 'Oh, she is in mourning. Her husband is gone then.' I happened to be dressed in black, and when I heard these words I looked up and I found they were two of the doctors from the hospital. I did not take the slightest notice, but would it not be lovely for me, or for my husband when he is better, to see them. They might think it was his ghost, coming to reproach them."

On the 13th August, 1928, Mr. D. sent a letter to *Truth* signed with his name and address, which was printed on the 22nd of that month:—

"Four months ago I was sent home to die. My wife was told I suffered from inoperable cancer of the bowel and bladder, and that I had not a week to live. I was in agony of pain night and day. I had been for five days at the hospital, and that terrible diagnosis was made after a searching examination under chloroform.

"My wife, when told the terrible news, rushed to the station, asked for a book on cancer, was given that of Mr. Barker, wrote to him, and implored him to help her. He treated me dietetically, and here I am, a man reborn, who is gaining health and strength from day to day, who is almost without pain, who has regained control of bowel and bladder."

On the 24th August, Mrs. D. wrote to me:—

"My husband is simply grand. He looks ten years younger, is quite strong, is putting on flesh daily, and his colour is now a healthy one. I do not think you would know him as the poor invalid he was."

On the 23rd October, Mr. D. had recovered still further and he wrote me a letter from which I learned for the first time the cause of his trouble:—

"In 1916 I had an important post in Philadelphia and caught influenza badly. It was impossible for me to lie up. When I recovered, my kidneys gave me some trouble and it was suggested I ought to have kidneys and bladder examined. The American doctor had to pass a cystoscope into the bladder and found everything normal, but as the instrument was of great size, he forced it in and blood issued freely.

"In 1918 I experienced again pain and burning when passing water. I was then living in Buffalo. Friends suggested my consulting a urinary specialist, Professor Parmenter. He acted in the same way as the doctor in Philadelphia. He forced a cystoscope into the bladder. Upon my returning to England I had another slight attack of the bladder trouble. Then, 10 years after, Dr. M. passed a catheter and later on he forced in a thick instrument, causing an injury. And last of all Dr. J., of Swansea, forced into the bladder the large tube of a cystoscope in February of this year at Swansea Hospital, when I was under chloroform. Reviewing past events, I feel as if I had been through some mediæval tortures."

There is little doubt in my mind that Mr. D.'s disease was started by repeated injuries to the bladder, or to the prostate, or both, by the clumsy use of the cystoscope, a very dangerous instrument, which is unfortunately employed with utter recklessness. Pain is our best friend. It is particularly dangerous to use the cystoscope under a local or general anæsthetic, because then patient and doctor do not realize that an injury is done. As soon as I learned of the bladder injury, I treated Mr. D. with Arnica and Staphysagria. The former is of value for general injuries and their after-effects, and Staphysagria for bladder injuries. The number of patients who have been injured by the abuse of catheter and cystoscope is past counting.

Mr. D., who had been given only a few days to live in February, 1928, did well. He wrote on the 30th July, 1929, after 17 months' treatment:—

"I met the other day one of my late tormentors from the Swansea Hospital, Dr. J. I rated him soundly. He could not look me in the face and walked away like a whipped dog. Wait when I meet Dr. M. He shall have hell for leather. Now in every way my health seems normal. Yet one material and to me very worrying trouble has remained since the almost deliberate injury caused to me by having had those instruments passed into my bladder. I am of opinion that some prostate trouble is the result of all this."

On the 18th July, 1930, two and a half years after the beginning of the treatment, Mr. D. sent me a letter mentioning some trivial complaints, and the correspondence ceased. I was under the impression that he considered himself cured. In January, 1931, I received, to my sorrow, letters from Mr. and Mrs. D., which told me that, after a time of satisfactory health, he had gone downhill. Then he had a violent attack of vomiting. His wife sent for local doctors, who diagnosed his trouble as intestinal catarrh. The bladder trouble also reawakened. He appealed to me once more for help. Unfortunately he had recalled me when it was too late. He reacted no longer to treatment. He died in March, 1931, and the death certificate mentioned convulsions caused by diseased kidneys. I suspect that repeated injuries to the bladder by the misuse of cystoscopes set up the trouble which eventually spread up the ureters towards the kidneys.

This lengthy account shows that so-called incurable patients may be made happy and comfortable for years, or may be saved, by common sense, a carefully chosen diet and homœopathic medicines. Possibly the man might be alive now if he had kept in touch with me.

On the 30th April, 1929, I received a pitiful letter written by a Mrs. E. M. I., from Catford, London:—

"I have a very dear friend living with me who is more than anything on earth to me. She has had a breast off through a growth a year ago last November. She has never been well since and now her doctor says that there is an enlarged gland in the lung, and there is no hope of her recovery, that her death is just a matter of time. She has had a very bad turn of coughing.

"The patient does not know her case is hopeless. Will you kindly word your reply with caution. I would be for ever grateful if you could give some promise of a cure. It is so distressing to watch those we love suffer, especially if one cannot help in any way."

I concluded that, as happens so often, the cancer had spread from the breast into the lungs. On the 10th May, the writer of the letter and her friend, Miss M. E. G., came to my house. I learned that the breast was amputated extensively in December, 1927. At the time she was deeply jaundiced. After the operation there was some improvement, but lately pain had reappeared in breast and back. It became gradually worse, and swellings developed in the operation scar and in the left arm, which became very painful. She coughed up greenish phlegm. It appeared that the pain in the breast was aggravated by delay in the period. Motions and urine had an offensive odour and the urine turned milky on standing. The patient took every morning salts for her bowels, and lived on an ordinary diet with strong tea, bacon, meat, Ovaltine, etc.

I replaced her purgatives by liquid paraffin, told her to take an abundance of bran, vegetables, milk, some eggs, nuts, and boiled raisins or sultanas as a tonic food. Flesh, fish, fowl, coffee, strong tea, spices and condiments, including salt, were forbidden. She was given Hydrastis, a good medicine to begin with in cancer cases, Thuja as an antidote to vaccination, and Thyroid 2X to improve digestion and excretion.

On the 17th May the patient reported that she had great difficulties with the new diet, and that she had lost three-quarters of a lb. in weight. I then added Carcinosin 100, a dose once a week. The next report, dated 24th May, stated: " I am getting along very nicely, I have regained the three-quarters of a lb. lost, my breathing has been rather bad." The next letter, dated 31st May, said, to my delight: " I am certainly very much better than when I saw you three weeks ago. May I eat strawberries and cream? " On the 7th June she wrote: " I am still progressing well. My friend, Mrs. E. M. I., is very pleased with my improvement."

As her letters were very short and obscure, I asked her to call on me. She came on the 19th June, and

I wrote to her after our interview: "I am very pleased with your appearance. You look vastly better, you have gained a lb. in weight, but you complain about breathing difficulty and pain in chest and arm." As she had not sufficiently reacted to the medicines given, I sent her Conium 3, which is indicated in hard cancer. Gradually the strength of the invalid improved. On the 5th July she wrote: " I am walking better now, though not able to exceed five miles per day. I have lost 1 lb. since I came to see you."

The patient's trouble was in the right breast. Below the right breast is the liver. She looked and felt " liverish." I gave her Cholesterin 2X, which is a great medicine for liver cancer, and tried to encourage her notwithstanding her loss of weight. Then I was alarmed by the swelling of glands round about the operation scar. Then came complaints of pain, felt distinctly in the lungs. I refused to be disheartened and gave her Thuja 6X. On the 19th July Miss M. G. wrote: " I am very pleased to report the discharge from the breast abscess has ceased, I am decidedly improving and feel very rejoiced. I have gained 3 lbs. in weight since I mentioned the decrease."

On the 17th September she visited me and told me of terrible itching of the skin, worst at night. Although she had progressed remarkably, her chest condition was as bad as ever, and I came to the conclusion that there was tuberculosis. Cancer is frequently super-imposed upon tuberculosis. I did not have any of the tests made. The diagnosis seemed to me easy and I gave her Bacillinum 30, a dose once every week, and as the skin irritation was improved by heat, I gave her Arsenic 3X, which I followed by Sulphur 6X.

Being an insured city clerk, she required a doctor's certificate to get her weekly allowance. She was determined not to be treated by panel doctors or go to a hospital where she would have been treated by surgery or radium, which she rightly dreaded. I advised her to go to my friend, the late Dr. John H. Clarke, for certificates. Since that time I heard from

her only rarely. On the 9th May, 1930, she wrote:
" I am certain I am progressing, though occasionally
my breath is short and troublesome." Later on there
were fluctuations in her health, and she lost weight.
I dreaded the condition of her chest. However, on
the 2nd January, 1934, she wrote: " I am keeping
very well. I have put on 9½ lbs."

On the 6th August, 1928, a young man, Mr. H. H.,
wrote from Moss Side, Manchester: —

" My father, aged 61, yesterday returned from the Manchester Royal Infirmary, after examination by Dr. R., John
Street, Manchester, whose report was ' Inoperable cancer of
the bowel, and not a fit subject for radium treatment.' I
am writing you in the hope that if your treatment fails
to cure, it will at least alleviate and lighten his burden. I
am sure that there is no need for me to make any effort
to describe my feelings and thoughts."

I told the young man to place his father on a fleshless diet, forbade alcohol, strong tea, coffee, sent some
Hydrastis 1X pilules and asked for further particulars.
On the 10th August, when the new diet and medicine
had been used for only two or three days, the young
man wrote: " My father has remarked on feeling much
easier, except for a kind of toothache pain in the
vicinity of the rectum." I thought the improvement
imaginary. However, as Mr. H. was a butcher and
had been a heavy consumer of meat, I thought that
in due course real improvement would show. On the
15th August, after a week's treatment, the young man
wrote: —

" My father's general condition has improved wonderfully. He is much brighter in himself and is not troubled so
much with his bowels. Yesterday for the first time for
months they were acting normally. So we are only giving
him 1 Hydrastis pilule instead of 3. The toothache pain in
the bowel I wrote of in my last letter is also much easier.
Instead of being continually there it only occurs infrequently. When one considers the fact of the specialist's
verdict: ' It is just a matter of time, nothing can be done,'

there is only one word to describe the improvement in my father and that is ' wonderful.' "

On the 20th August, Mr. H. H. wrote: " We are keeping strictly to the diet prescribed, and he is no doubt receiving great comfort from it. He is now taking a little walking exercise each day." On the 24th August I was told: " I am pleased to say that my father appears to be maintaining the improvement in his condition and he seems to be a little easier from the pain in the rectum. His bowels are now being moved quite easily. He takes exercise just when he feels like it, in the evenings mostly, has quite a colour, and he has now no suspicion of sallowness or greyness."

On the 29th August I was told: " The improvement is still there." Then he felt poorly for a time but he improved once more. On the 30th September the son wrote: " My father is still keeping in about the same condition and at the same time seems to be taking a greater interest in general things, his business and people; his bowels still appear to be acting normally." On the 9th October the son wrote: " My father is still maintaining the improvement, though he is again troubled with flatulence." For this I sent Carbo vegetabilis 3X. The next letter, written on the 2nd November, stated: " My father's condition appears to be unchanged, and at the present I can see a change for the better in his general appearance. On some days, except for being thinner, he looks his old self." On the 15th November I was told: —

" Although my father is still troubled with discomfort in the vicinity of the rectum, in appearance and general looks he does not seem to have lost any ground since the improvement derived from the early period under your treatment. He has quite a good colour, and also I notice an increase in the waist line, which looks more healthy, and this seems to me to be a step forward. The flatulence has not been so troublesome. He is still eating strictly to the diet and takes Hydrastis pilules as he thinks he requires them. When I hear acquaintances talking of cancer cases of which they have knowledge and compare symptoms, it makes all the more obvious the great beneficial effect my father has derived from your advice and treatment."

The son did not write again. He fell ill, his father was taken to the hospital where he was fed on the most unsuitable food and he died in torments.

In scores of cases regulation of the diet, regulation of the bowel with liquid paraffin and the indicated homœopathic medicines have given the most wonderful relief to incurable cancer patients, even in the last stage. They were not only physically relieved, but were cheered up by a new sense of internal cleanliness, health and buoyancy, and their relatives were made happy by the obvious improvement of the patient which occasionally is maintained to the very moment of death. In many of my cases the end was peaceful and painless, and the last days or weeks were not poisoned by the use of the morphia syringe.

On the 5th July, 1929, I was visited by Mrs. M. M., a dressmaker, who complained about a large tumour in her left breast, for which an operation had been urged. She did not want to lose her breast, and was distraught. She was 35 years old, constipated, regulating her bowels with Apenta, did not perspire, had the scantiest discharge at period time. She had been bottling up body poisons for many years and there was a considerable possibility that the tumour might be malignant. The suspicion of malignancy was increased by the fact that her father had died of cancer of the bowel. The lady had a tumour-producing tendency. Her back was a mass of moles. The growth was on the left breast. She had been vaccinated on the left arm, and had many troubles on the left side. There was the further possibility that the swelling stood in some causal connection with the old vaccination.

Mrs. M. M. was in a poor condition, subsisted on unsuitable food, was constipated, did not perspire, had an insufficient menstrual discharge. I told her that no harm would be done if she tried for a few weeks to improve her condition by constitutional means. Possibly a blood-clearing diet and the indicated medicine would lead to the spontaneous shrinkage of the growth. If that should not be the case, she might still be operated upon. A delay of a few weeks would in no way aggravate the existing trouble.

I placed her on a lacto-vegetarian diet with an abundance of fruit and greenstuff, forbade flesh, fish, fowl and everything made of them, strong tea, coffee, alcohol, condiments and spices, all of which she had hitherto enjoyed, and gave her Hydrastis 1X, 3 pilules to be taken three times a day between meals, Scrophularia nodosa 1X, which acts beneficially upon growths on the left breast, a dose night and morning, and Carcinosinum 100th potency, a single dose once a week. She left my house full of hope.

On the 14th July, after a week's treatment, she reported: " I am slightly more energetic, but the lump in the breast is about the same." On the 9th August she wrote: " I am glad to tell you the lump in the breast is very much smaller." I then gave her Thuja, which antidotes vaccinial poisoning. On the 26th August she wrote: " The lump in the breast is considerably smaller and the pain occurs at longer intervals." On the 11th September she wrote: " I am so grateful to you. I am feeling a new woman." She gave no particulars about her breast and then followed a silence of two months, during which she slipped back badly. On the 21st November, 1929, I saw her again, and was horrified by her appearance. I wrote to her:—

" In your last letter of the 11th September you wrote: ' I am so grateful to you. I am feeling a new woman.' To-day you looked an old woman, many years older than when I saw you first, anæmic, weary, pasty-faced, flabby, had lost six lbs., and your left breast was somewhat swollen and tender, causing at times pain and stitches. I must very earnestly urge you to get yourself into order. Otherwise there will be grave trouble."

She promised to change her ways, was given the old medicines with the addition of China 1X as a tonic and for her headaches, and did well. She came to see me again on the 21st May, 1930, nearly a year after her first visit. I wrote to her on that day: "You have magnificently improved since your last visit. There are still lumps in your breasts. Unless you get fundamentally right, you will get all kinds of troubles." She had come to consult me about headaches and depression.

I had urged Mrs. M. M. to keep in touch with me because in my opinion she required continued treatment. She disregarded my advice and I did not hear from her for more than a year and a half. On the 1st December, 1931, she called me to the telephone and told me that she wished to see me immediately. She arrived in the afternoon with her husband and only child, told me that the lumps in her breasts had returned, that they had given pain, that she had gone to a doctor. He had taken the gravest view, had told her that an immediate operation was needed, and had sent her to Mr. D. C. L. Fitz-Williams, the senior surgeon to St. Mary's Hospital, who specializes in treating cancer of the breast, and who is considered the highest authority in England on breast cancer.

He looked at Mrs. M. M.'s breasts and said decisively that there was nothing for her but an operation. The lady demurred, pleading for her breasts. When she asked Mr. Fitz-Williams what was the alternative, he suggested radium. She said in confusion that she wished to think it over. Then she was told quite frankly that, unless the trouble was immediately and drastically dealt with, she would be dead in six months. If a surgeon is convinced that an immediate operation is necessary, he is, of course, justified in putting the strongest pressure on the patient.

Mrs. M. M. was distraught, had not been able to sleep, and her husband and child were worn out by her sufferings. I looked at the breasts, and saw hardnesses more or less identical with those for which she had come to me two and a half years previously. At that time also those growths had been pronounced cancerous and an operation had been urged.

No doctor and no surgeon, however experienced, can say for certain whether a swelling in the breast is cancerous or not. I told her once more, that it would make very little difference whether she was operated upon in two or three days or in two or three weeks, and that the delay would enable her to see whether internal treatment would improve her breasts once more or not. I wrote to her on that day: " As there are no swollen glands in the armpits and no other indications, I do not see any reason for taking at present a serious view of the condition, and I think my view will be shared by sensible specialists whom, of course, you can consult." I gave her Hydrastis, mother ticture, 2 drops to be taken before meals, and Phytolacca, mother tincture, 2 drops to be taken first and last thing. Hydrastis is an excellent medicine for stimulating stomach, liver and bowel, and creating an appetite. Besides, it is a great cancer remedy, while Phytolacca is most valuable for mastitis and other breast conditions, including cancer.

I advised Mrs. M. M. to consult two other surgeons without mentioning that she had seen either Mr. Fitz-Williams or me. She went first to a well-known titled surgeon. He examined Mrs. M. M. and said: " I do not think the growths are cancerous. Very likely they will improve with constitutional treatment, but if you wish to be certain, you ought to consult Mr. Fitz-Williams!" The second authority whom I had recommended was Dr. G. B., a homœopathic surgeon who is also an excellent physician. He never operates if operation can be avoided. He gave a very optimistic view, treated her with homœopathic medicines and the lady did well. From time to time I heard that she was steadily improving. On the 17th January, 1934, she wrote to me: " The breast trouble has cleared up wonderfully. At Dr. G. B.'s request I attended the hospital and two well-known doctors passed the opinion that there was nothing left in my breasts. In fact, they could not be sure that anything had ever been there."

When I saw Mrs. M. M. on the 1st December, 1931, I took the view that the growths in her breasts were not cancer, but that they might become cancerous owing to the condition of her bowel, etc. If she had been operated upon, she would in all probability have been told to her relief that the pathologist had not found any evidence of cancer in the excised breasts. However, I felt certain that cancer was likely to develop in the operation scar because of the foulness of her blood stream.

On the 21st July, 1930, Mr. J. C., a jute merchant of Mincing Lane, asked me to see his wife about an internal swelling for which her doctor had recommended an operation, which the wife had refused. I saw Mrs. J. C. on the 25th July. She was 72 years old, looked bright and I noticed the terrible odour of her breath, which suggested cancer. There was a painful swelling in the abdomen. She was constipated, did not perspire, complained of flatulence, rheumatism, nasal catarrh, frequent attacks of bronchitis, etc. It was clear that her trouble, whether malignant or non-malignant, was due to chronic constipation which her doctor had disregarded.

I prescribed an eliminating fleshless diet, liquid paraffin and gave her Sulphur 6X as a blood-clearing medicine, a dose night and morning, which was indicated because her feet were so hot that she had to stick them out of bed. In addition I gave her Nux vomica and Carbo vegetabilis combined to improve her digestion and Anacardium 3X between meals because she complained of weakness of memory. My suspicion that the obscure growth in the abdomen might be cancerous was strengthened by the fact that she had taken boiling hot tea all her life.

Mrs. J. C. improved promptly. On the 1st August she wrote: "I feel more alert and active, in fact more like myself." Her next letter, dated 8th August, said:

x

"I am feeling much better, quite gay sometimes, my memory is better, my breath, I understand, has improved, there is no internal ache now." On the 13th August I saw the lady and found her much improved and told her so in a letter. On the 20th August she wrote: "I feel better, my breath is still much better." The next week she wrote: "The swelling is less, flatulence much improved, my breath continues the improvement of last week. I am ever so grateful."

There was a discharge from the vagina which she did not like. I told her that very likely the discharge was a blessing, nature trying to rid her of the growth by letting it drain away. It very frequently happens that an internal tumour shrinks by draining away, leaving a hard residue. On the 5th September she reported: "My breath is still getting better, swelling is less, and I feel much more able to do things. The discharge continues. I shall do what you think advisable regarding it. Perhaps it is the natural result of what has been wrong with me. Anyhow, I leave it to you." On the 12th September she wrote: "The swelling has still gone down and I have had my belt made smaller. The discharge still continues and is perhaps freer." Meanwhile I had been giving her Hydrastis 1X. On the 19th September she wrote: "The swelling is still going down and my breath is very much improved."

She visited me on the 26th September and after our interview I wrote to her that she looked ten years' younger than when I saw her first, and that she should not trouble about the discharge which might be of no particular importance. On the 29th September Mrs. J. C. wrote: "There is no appearance of a swelling now." On the 6th October she said: "I am going on all right. The discharge is still there but I don't feel any aching, so I don't worry." On the 30th October she wrote: "The discharge still continues. My general health is much better and all other symptoms have improved."

Mrs. J. C. had improved greatly from week to week during the three months I had looked after her. Her letter of the 31st October closed the correspondence. I wrote to her on the 20th November that I had not heard from her for three weeks, that in my opinion she needed continued treatment, but got no reply. I assumed that she considered further treatment unnecessary.

Four and a half months later, on the 3rd March, 1931, Mr. J. C. called me to the telephone, and told me with a breaking voice: "My wife has just died. It is a terrible tragedy. I must see you at once." He came in his car, and told me a harrowing tale. His wife had told the doctor, who had previously advised an operation, that she had an oozing discharge. Her doctor had told her that the matter was desperately serious, notwithstanding her obvious improvement, and urged her to consult a specialist. She saw a leading gynæcologist and then a surgeon, and all three agreed that immediate action was necessary. People are frequently rushed into precipitate operations. All three men agreed that radium should be used. So a radium specialist was consulted as well. He confirmed the necessity of immediate intervention and the wife was told: "If you go on without having the growth dealt with, you will die in torments before long, but we can guarantee you a healthy, painless life of at least five years if the growth is energetically dealt with."

Mrs. J. C. was taken into a nursing home, was given radium treatment, and in a few weeks the discharge had disappeared. The doctor and the specialists congratulated the lady, and she went home, delighted. Some weeks after, she felt a pain in one of her knees. It became worse and worse, her doctor was sent for and he ordered poulticing. However, the swelling increased still further, the pain became unbearable, a team of specialists was sent for, and X-ray examination disclosed the fact that the knee-cap was eaten up by the foulest pus. An immediate operation was recommended. Mrs. J. C. was rushed to a nursing home, was operated upon, and came home after a few weeks.

Some weeks after this a similar growth appeared in the back. After futile treatment by her doctor, the usual team of specialists appeared, again an operation in a nursing home was effected. After a few weeks the poor woman came back to her home. Then one of her eyeballs started swelling. Her doctor gave her eye drops, then fetched his partner, and then there appeared the usual team of specialists, reinforced by an ophthalmic surgeon. Poor Mrs. J. C. was told that the eye must immediately be taken out because it was filled with the foulest pus.

Then pain developed in new places and became maddening. Further specialists were sent for and they made the obvious discovery that the poor woman suffered from blood poisoning, and she was treated with injections of micro-organisms which drove her almost insane with pain. The injection treatment had to be abandoned abruptly. She could no longer control bowels and bladder. She begged her doctors to ki.l her. They kept her continuously under Morphia and at last she died, tortured to death. After telling me this dreadful story the man broke down and wept: "Why did we abandon you, why did we abandon you? She did so well while she was under your care."

The doctor who first urged her to be operated upon and who had promised her, with the others, "at least five years of a happy, healthy and painless life," wrote out the death certificate. The cause of death was stated to be "streptococcal septicæmia." In plain English this means blood-poisoning by a micro-organism. Of course the woman died of blood-poisoning. She was poisoned by the specialists who sealed up the womb by burning it with radium. They had forced into the blood stream the poisonous discharge which the body tried to eliminate for the poor woman's good.

Unfortunately this is not the only cancer patient of mine who died in torments, a victim of the orthodox treatments which, according to the textbooks, are "the only cure.   I could fill a volume with similar cases.

On the 1st February, 1929, Miss R. L. G., a retired school mistress, wrote to me from Shelton, Stoke-on-Trent:—

"Three weeks ago I casually drew my doctor's attention to my left breast, which has become lumpy lately. There has also come a lump in the left armpit and one in my neck. To my horror the doctor took it seriously and told me I had cancer. Since then I have seen two specialists. One said it was too late, it had got too far, and the other said an operation was possible. The left breast could be taken off and the bone in the neck could be divided. This would leave me a physical wreck and even then he did not guarantee that all would be out. Can you help me? I am 60 years of age, have always been in good health, we are all total abstainers, and I have always been fond of milk foods and fruit, so that I cannot understand this horrifying thing which they call Scirrhus. One specialist said 'Leave it alone!' So I come to you with fresh hope."

I thought it an outrage that the poor lady should have been to'd brutally the dreadful truth. I asked her for the details I needed regarding diet, bowels, etc., and told her: "As no one can tell with absolute certainty whether a growth in the breast or elsewhere is cancerous or comparatively innocuous—yours may merely be a mastitis—I want you not to worry overmuch about the diagnosis you were given. Worry does not help, but hinders, and can make ill the healthiest and strongest." I also asked for her photo.

On receipt of the necessary information I put her on a lacto-vegetarian diet and gave her first Sulphur 3X and then Hydrastis 1X. She had been having meat twice a day, much tea and bread and butter, hardly any vegetables. I told her: "I hope within a week or two you will notice improvement." She gradually improved. On the 18th March she wrote:

" If it were not that I cannot help worrying about my breast, I am feeling well. The paraffin is purifying the bowels and the diet suits me because I now never dream when sleeping and the headaches and acidity of the stomach are gone. I have had only two bad headaches since I have followed your directions and I am very grateful." Sulphur activated her skin. On the 26th March she wrote: " I seem to have perspired more lately and probably that is a good thing."

Unfortunately the poor old lady had been seriously injured by what doctors and surgeons had told her. In every letter she asked questions about her disease and it was difficult for me to cheer her up. On the 16th May she wrote: " I am sure there is an improvement in my breast and arm because they do not hurt so much. What improvement there is, is all due to you. I should have been very hopeless by now if I had only relied on what the doctors have done. They seem to do nothing unless they can use the knife."

Bad days and good days alternated and the poor thing worried and asked me whether artificial sunlight and various patent medicines might not benefit her. I gave her Carcinosinum, Schirrhinum, Scrophularia, Conium, each according to indications. She wrote on the 27th June: " I am sure there is an improvement in my arm and breast, even if the change is only slight. I am very hopeful because I think that if you had not helped me, I should have been much worse now after six months."

Every few weeks she asked me whether I thought she was incurable. On the 3rd February, 1930, after a full year's treatment, she wrote: " I am sure I have made progress. When one looks back over 12 months and thinks what might have been, I am sure your treatment has helped me." So we kept on, I encouraging her all the time although her disease was progressing. Unfortunately I received a letter dated 17th July, 1930, which revealed to me why Miss R. L.

G. had always expressed to me doubts about the future: —

" The doctor who has visited our house for two or three years because of mother, knows all about me. He is the one who knows I have a growth, but when I told him that I had accepted your treatment, he was very gentlemanly about it and left me to you. Now, about a fortnight ago, he informed me very earnestly that he had got in touch with a bacteriologist (I do not know who) who had discovered a germ which by injections will fight the cancer germ in me. I do not know, but I am hoping for great things, and when this growth is galloping, I am ready to grasp at any straw. So I am having two injections a week, and if you will not forsake me over this, I will go on trying and see whether it will stop it. For a while, perhaps, it would be better not to take your pills as well. I shall be glad to know what you think of this and enclose my photo, recently taken at Llandudno."

I replied to her: —

" I am amazed at your photo. You look years younger and ever so much better than on the first photo you sent me. Of course I can understand your trying everything to get better. Did you ask the doctor whether he could tell you of any cases where they had cured the disease and did you ask him what injections they were? At any rate, I would advise you to stop the injections at once if you feel that they do you harm. The worst of all the new treatments are lead injections which give lead poisoning in addition to the original trouble. I earnestly hope that you are not being given lead."

She replied on the 30th July: " I cannot say yet whether the injections are doing any good. I have such funny feelings in all my muscles and in stomach and chest. Doctors are very reticent when you ask pointed questions." Her next letter, dated the 8th August, told me:

" I do not know what is happening to me, but I can hardly move. The doctor says it is not the injections, but I am refusing to have any more, for one leg is so painful that I feel that I should not be able to walk at all if I had any more.

I feel as if all the vitality is going out of me. I have been under you seventeen months with very little pain."

On the 16th August she wrote:—

" The doctor came up and went away rather vexed because I said decidedly I would not have any more injections, but I have had nine and feel as if any more would make me quite helpless. I have never felt like this all the seventeen months. He said it was no use hiding it, I had cancer, it was spreading through the organs of the body, and that the injection was a vaccine for breaking and melting down the growth, but it seems to me to have sent the disease all over the body. I was better before I was given it. You never say whether *you* think it is a cancer or not."

Her next letter, dated 24th August, said: " I have not seen the doctor since I told him I was not having any more injections, and he does not seem to trouble what has happened to me as a result. I daresay he would blame me for not going on with them. If I had done so I should have been laid low. However, I have done with his advice." Her next letter, dated 1st September, told me: " The injections, which I continually regret, seem to upset all my organs. For about five days now I have had piles, which I never had because, ever since I received your diet chart 18 months ago, I was absolutely regular. Now I have gone all wrong." Her last letter, written in pencil, told me: " I can hardly walk, I am going out in a bath chair." Soon after she died, needlessly tortured in body and mind.

On the 16th December, 1933, Nurse E. A. wrote to me from Dublin that she was 63 years old and that eight years ago she began having trouble with her tongue and mouth. The condition got gradually worse and then the throat was affected. She consulted a leading throat specialist who gave her a gargle. Gradually the throat became worse. She could hardly swallow, got very thin, was X-rayed. The doctor took away a specimen from the throat for microscopic examination and she was informed that she suffered from cancer.

I told her not to be depressed by the diagnosis which was apparently based on guesswork, gave her provisionally a diet of the usual kind, sent her Sulphur 6X to be taken night and morning for blood clearing purposes, and Cistus Canadensis 3X to be taken three times a day. Cistus is an excellent remedy for septic throats and for swellings in the throat, both malignant and non-malignant. I also told her to gargle with Hydrastis, mother tincture, a few drops in a tablespoonful of water, and to swallow a little of it at each gargling.

To my great satisfaction she reacted well to the treatment. On the 27th December she wrote: " I do not have the throbbing pain quite so badly in my throat since taking your pills." On the 6th January she wrote: " I can swallow fairly easily and have great hopes that you will be able to cure me. It is such a relief when I am a little better as I have suffered very much and have been in great pain. My tongue is not nearly as stiff as it was."

Miss E. A. was so delighted with her progress that she wished to visit me in London and she had arranged to call on the 17th January, 1934. Unfortunately she was unwise enough to call on her doctor before sailing and the consequences of that visit were terrible. She wrote on the 15th January: —

" I am sorry to say I am unable to cross over to England to-morrow night. I came back from Waterford feeling wonderfully well. I had also put on a lb. Everyone I met said how glad they were as I have been a great source of worry to all my friends. I made an appointment with the doctor and he was delighted and said I could certainly go to London.

" He examined my throat and then put a tube down it. The pain was dreadful. When I got indoors, I just collapsed and have been in bed ever since. My chest, throat and face are dreadfully swollen, and I have such terrible pain in my head and have not been able to swallow until I managed yesterday to get down an egg flip. I cannot write any more because I cannot sit up any longer."

The same man who brutally had told Nurse E. A. that she had cancer and who subsequently noticed that she had vastly improved under my treatment, had the inconceivable stupidity to force an instrument down her throat which injured her. I sent the woman immediately some Arnica 3X to be taken internally and to be used as a gargle, but I very much doubt whether she will recover. Injury to a cancerous growth is apt to spread the disease throughout the system.

Cancer may be created by the misuse of Arsenic, X-rays, radium, etc. On the 19th October, 1932, a lady living in a small town in Gloucestershire wrote:—

" Would you see me about an X-ray rash which I have on my left side? I had my left breast removed for a small lump in 1930, and since then have had X-ray treatment every two weeks, and lately every three weeks. Last Wednesday my side began to be irritable and ever since I have had bad nights and discomfort in the day.

" My doctor frankly says that he does not understand very much about X-rays, but is very sorry. The X-ray treatment was given to me in Gloucester, and this morning I went to the X-ray specialist as usual, but, of course, had no treatment.

" The X-ray doctor was very guarded in what he said and wrote out a prescription and told me that it would only soothe the irritation and not drive the rash in. He now says I have to come for treatment every three months. The rash on my side has spread a lot since it started and it has also come on my right hand where I had X-ray treatment for a little eczema. The X-ray doctor told me quite cheerfully to-day if I didn't look out I should have eczema all over me soon. Can I see you at once? "

Prolonged X-ray treatment is apt to produce X-ray cancer. The fact is known to every medical student. With incredible recklessness Mrs. E. M. S. had been given regular X-ray treatment for two years and the man who gave it was obviously ready to use it for anything and everything, such as a slight rash on the lady's hand.

On the 24th October Mrs. E. M. S. called. I summarized the position in my directions as follows: —

"You were operated upon in May, 1930, for a growth declared cancerous of the left breast which was cut off, and you were told that you were to have X-ray treatment on the place of the scar for eight minutes every fortnight during the next five years. Lately you were also given X-ray treatment of the right hand on account of a slight rash. Recently a terrible itching rash has broken out on the X-ray-treated chest, throat, arm, the left side and on the back of the right hand. The irritation is absolutely intolerable, prevents your sleeping, and you were given by the X-ray specialist a prescription for Lotio Calaminæ, a poisonous Zinc wash."

It seemed to me recklessness bordering on crime for any surgeon to prescribe X-ray treatment following an operation *for five years*. The lady looked the picture of health, had a dairy-maid's complexion and skin, wonderfully clear eyes, magnificent teeth, red lips, looked the picture of physical purity, was mentally well balanced, and was not upset when she was told that cancer had been diagnosed. As she came from exceptionally healthy stock, had healthy children, had had no diseases and lived on a fleshless diet, I felt certain that she had had an innocent lump, which had been operated upon recklessly without any attempt to clear up the case by a few weeks' medicinal treatment. For all I knew, the man at Gloucester had given the woman X-ray cancer.

She had regular bowels, not a single enlarged gland on the body, and the irritation was getting worse from day to day and drove her almost mad. Being determined to help her without delay, I gave her Sulphur 6X night and morning to allay the burning worst at night, a characteristic Sulphur symptom, and I gave her in addition three boxes marked Rhus tox 3X (1), Rhus venenata 2X (2), Petroleum 3X (3). She was to take a small dose of the three other medicines three times a day, trying one after the other during three consecutive days, and she was told to concentrate upon the most helpful medicine. She was to apply outwardly yellow vaseline, olive oil, rich cream, or unmedicated lard, but no disinfectant, which would have irritated the skin still further. Happily she reacted well. She reported on the 4th November:—

"My hand is much better. It is wonderful how much smoother the skin has got the last two days, and it is not so red. I find yellow vaseline suits my skin better than olive oil or cream from the milk. The rash seems gone from my face and went a little from my neck. It seems now to be improving a little and does not irritate so much. My side also seems improving. I had my best night so far since the rash began."

Petroleum is a severe skin irritant. In homœopathic doses it relieves irritation and for outer application in such cases yellow vaseline, acting as a homœopathic counter-irritant, acts far better than the most expensive emollient applications.

On the 15th November she wrote: "I am feeling much better and the irritation is very much less." On the 19th November, exactly a month after the first interview, she called again, and I found that the skin trouble had practically disappeared. Of course I know the extraordinary delay action of X-rays or radium. In many cases radiologists have developed ray cancer only ten or more years after they had had frequent burns. Consequently I wished to keep the lady under observation, but of course I could not give her the reason for wishing to continue giving her treatment.

I feel convinced that, had Mrs. E. M. S. gone on a little longer with the treatment by her so-called X-ray specialist, she would have developed X-ray cancer and then the doctor might have stated in the death certificate that she had died from skin cancer, instead from reckless abuse of X-rays. Unfortunately I have met many similar cases. Many women who were given radium treatment for some relatively minor trouble of womb and ovaries have developed radium or X-ray cancer ten or more years afterwards in the place treated.

GENERAL INDEX